Sarcoidosis: Clinical management

To
Kavita, Keerty, Arion and Tau

Sarcoidosis: Clinical management

Om P. Sharma, BSc, MB BS, FACP, FCCP, DTM & H(Eng.)
Professor of Medicine, University of Southern California School of Medicine, Los Angeles
Physician Specialist at the Los Angeles County-University of Southern California Medical Center
Physician, Barlow Hospital for Respiratory Diseases, Los Angeles, California

Butterworths
London Boston Durban Singapore Sydney Toronto Wellington

All rights reserved. No part of this publication may be reproduced or
transmitted in any form or by any means, including photocopying and
recording, without the written permission of the copyright holder,
application for which should be addressed to the Publishers. Such written
permission must also be obtained before any part of this publication is
stored in a retrieval system of any nature.

This book is sold subject to the Standard Conditions of Sale of Net Books
and may not be re-sold in the UK below the net price given by the
Publishers in their current price list.

First published 1984

© Butterworth & Co (Publishers) Ltd, 1984

British Library Cataloguing in Publication Data

Sharma, Om P.
   Sarcoidosis.
   1. Sarcoidosis
   I. Title
   616.9   RC182.S14

ISBN 0-407-00326-6

Library of Congress Cataloging in Publication Data

Sharma, Om P.
   Sarcoidosis—clinical management.

  Bibliography: p.
  Includes index.
  1. Sarcoidosis.   I. Title.
  [DNLM: 1. Sarcoidosis.
  QZ 140 S531s]
RC182.S14S53 1984   616.9   83-25260
ISBN 0-407-00326-6

Printed and bound in Great Britain by
Butler & Tanner Ltd, Frome and London

Preface

More than a century ago, Jonathan Hutchinson described the first case of sarcoidosis at King's College Hospital, London. The disease now is recognized as a commonplace multisystem disorder which may result in mortality and morbidity due to pulmonary fibrosis, cardiac arrhythmias, renal failure, neurological involvement and blindness.

Almost all physicians, radiologists, pathologists and immunologists face the problem of sarcoidosis at some time, but the disease remains confined to the domain of the chest physician. Although description of the classic features of the disease are relatively clear cut, the diagnosis is often delayed or completely missed because of certain unusual and difficult to recognize manifestations and its close resemblance to tuberculosis, leprosy, berylliosis, coccidioidomycosis, hypersensitivity pneumonias and other granulomas. Also, it has become relatively difficult for a practising physician to keep in touch with changes in this expanding field. This book has been written with such a practitioner in mind.

The book combines the basic science and clinical aspects of the disease with the recent advances in the field of sarcoid immunology. Particular attention has been directed to major areas of importance such as aetiology, epidemiology, pathophysiology, unusual radiological features, immunological alterations, role of T lymphocytes, indications of thallium and gallium nuclear scans and bronchoalveolar lavage. Special problems such as diagnosis, treatment, childhood sarcoidosis, sarcoidosis in the aged, pregnancy and sarcoidosis, cancers, infections, and autoimmunity in sarcoidosis are discussed separately.

The author's aim has been to produce a succinct, easy to read, well-illustrated and comprehensive review providing a plan for the effective management of the patient with sarcoidosis. It is hoped that this book will be of use not only for internists and pulmonary physicians but also for practitioners of other specialties, because sarcoidosis is truly a multisystem disorder that crosses artificial boundaries of modern specialization.

Acknowledgements

It is not possible, of course, to acknowledge individually the help of my friends and colleagues both in the United States and elsewhere who have directly or indirectly contributed to this monograph. I am particularly indebted to Drs D. Geraint James (London), Nathan S. Seriff (New York), John E. Bethune (Los Angeles), Ronald Crystal (NIH, Bethesda), Carol J. Johns (Baltimore) and Kaye H. Kilburn (Los Angeles) for their encouragement and timely advice. My colleagues and the staff of Pulmonary Disease Service, University of Southern California School of Medicine have contributed their ideas and criticisms to this book. I am particularly grateful to the Royal College of Physicians of London for awarding the Prophit Research Scholarship (1967-69) which enabled me to carry out some of my early clinical and immunological studies on sarcoidosis at the Royal Northern Hospital, London, UK.

Permission for reproduction of some of the material which appeared in a previous monograph has been given by Charles C. Thomas, Publishers, Springfield, Illinois, USA. Also, the editors of the following journals have allowed me to reproduce some of the previously published material: *Chest, Archives of Ophthalmology, Journal of the American Medical Association, Journal of Bone and Joint Surgery* and *Journal of the National Medical Association*. Figures 5.3(*a*) and (*b*) were kindly provided by Dr William Jones Williams, National University of Wales, Cardiff, United Kingdom. Dr Russell F. Sherwin and Dr Valda Richters provided *Figures 5.1, 5.2(a), 5.3(c)* and *24.1*. Their kindness is gratefully acknowledged.

I thank Mrs Evelyn Kiyan and Ms Olivia Sheppard for their effort in typing the manuscript. The superb photographic work of Mr Andy Gero speaks for itself.

Finally, the book would never have been completed without the patient and scrupulous assistance of my wife Maggie in proof-reading and improving its organization and language. Needless to say, any inaccuracies and omissions are my own.

Contents

1 **What is sarcoidosis?** 1

2 **History** 2
   The beginning: A dermatological curiosity   2
   Recognition of multisystem involvement   2
   Advent of immunology   3
   The present   3

3 **Epidemiology**   4
   Race   4
   Age   5
   Sex   5
   Familial sarcoidosis   6
   HLA typing in sarcoidosis   7

4 **Aetiology**   8
   Is sarcoidosis caused by tubercle bacillus?   8
   Sarcoidosis and atypical mycobacteria   8
   Viruses and sarcoidosis   9
   Is sarcoidosis an allergy?   9
   Is sarcoidosis an autoimmune disease?   9
   Genetic predisposition   9
   Role of immunological alterations   9

5 **Pathology and pathogenesis**   11
   Pathology   11
   Pathogenesis   16
   Differential diagnosis of sarcoid granuloma   19

6 **Clinical features**   22
   Modes of presentation   22
   Acute (subacute) and chronic sarcoidosis   24

7 Pulmonary sarcoidosis   29
Common presentations   29
Endobronchial sarcoidosis   40
Pulmonary sarcoidosis: Uncommon presentations   42
Lung functions   59

8 Cutaneous involvement   64
Lupus pernio   64
Skin plaques   65
Maculopapular eruptions   67
Subcutaneous nodules   69
Scars   71
Erythema nodosum   71
Other lesions   75

9 Ocular sarcoidosis   76
Uveitis   76
Conjunctivitis and conjunctival follicles   77
Keratoconjunctivitis sicca   78
Miscellaneous lesions   78
Diagnosis of ocular sarcoid   78

10 The reticuloendothelial system in sarcoidosis   80
Peripheral lymphadenopathy   80
Splenic involvement   82
Bone marrow   83

11 Sarcoidosis of the liver   89
Liver granuloma   89
Liver function tests   90
Portal hypertension and hepatic failure   90

12 The kidneys in sarcoidosis   93
Hypercalcaemia   93
Hypercalciuria   93
Granulomatous infiltration of the renal parenchyma   93
Glomerular disease   94
Granulomatous renal arteritis   94

13 Myocardial sarcoidosis   97
Diagnosis   98
Electrocardiographic abnormalities   99
Endomyocardial biopsy   100
Thallium-201 imaging   100
Diagnosis, evaluation and importance   100

14 Neurosarcoidosis   102
Cranial nerve involvement   102
Papilloedema   103
Intracranial involvement   103

Meningitis 104
Seizures 104
Peripheral neuropathy 104
Psychiatric manifestations 104
Spinal-cord involvement 105
Cerebrospinal fluid 105
Miscellaneous studies 105

15 The musculoskeletal system 107
Bones 107
Joints 107
Muscles 111

16 Endocrine involvement 114
Pituitary 114
Diabetes insipidus 114
Hypopituitarism 115
Thyroid 115
Parathyroids 116

17 The parotid glands 118

18 Gastrointestinal tract 122
Oesophagus 122
Stomach 122
Intestines 123
Pancreas 123
Peritoneum 123

19 Upper respiratory tract 125
The nose: Nasal mucosa and the septum 125
Laryngeal sarcoidosis 127
The tonsils 128

20 Reproductive system 129
Male 129
Female 130

21 The immunology of sarcoidosis 132
Cutaneous anergy 132
In vitro: Alterations in delayed hypersensitivity 134
Humoral responses 136
Kveim test 137
Bronchoalveolar lavage 138

22 Laboratory investigations 143
Blood 143
Urine 145
Hypercalcaemia 145
Angiotensin converting enzyme 149

Serum lysozyme 151
Transcobalamin II 151

23 Gallium-67 scanning in sarcoidosis 155
Gallium-67 citrate 155
The technique 155
Gallium-67 uptake in various lung diseases 155
Gallium-67 uptake in sarcoidosis 156
Indications of gallium-67 scans in sarcoidosis 157

24 Diagnosis and biopsy procedures 159
Criteria for diagnosis 159
Biopsy procedures 159
Differential diagnosis 162

25 Treatment 165
Indications 165
Methods 168

26 Sarcoidosis in children 171

27 Sarcoidosis in the aged 172

28 Sarcoidosis and pregnancy 173
Effect of pregnancy on sarcoidosis 173
Effect of sarcoidosis on pregnancy 173

29 Infections in sarcoidosis 174

30 Sarcoidosis and autoimmunity 175
Connective-tissue diseases 175
Sjögren's syndrome 176
Autoimmune thyroiditis 176
Thrombocytopenia 176
Haemolytic anaemia 176
Primary biliary cirrhosis 177
TASS syndrome 177

31 Sarcoidosis, lymphoma and malignancy 179

32 Miscellaneous 180
Sarcoidosis and amyloidosis 180
Sarcoidosis and clubbing 180

Colour plate section between pages 20–21

Index 181

Chapter 1
What is sarcoidosis?

It is hard to provide a concise definition of the disease, whose cause is not known. The following descriptive definition was formulated at the Seventh International Conference on Sarcoidosis, held in New York in 1976:

'Sarcoidosis is a multisystem granulomatous disorder of unknown etiology, most commonly affecting young adults and presenting most frequently with bilateral hilar lymphadenopathy, pulmonary infiltration, and skin or eye lesions. The diagnosis is established most securely when clinicoradiographic findings are supported by histological evidence of widespread non-caseating epithelioid-cell granulomas in more than one organ or a positive Kviem–Slitzbach test. Immunological features are depression of delayed-type hypersensitivity and raised or abnormal immunoglobulins. There may also be hypercalciuria with or without hypercalcemia. The course and prognosis may correlate with the mode of onset. An acute onset with erythema nodosum heralds a self-limiting course and spontaneous resolution, whereas an insidious onset may be followed by relentless, progressive fibrosis. Corticosteroids relieve symptoms and suppress inflammation and granuloma formation.'[1]

Reference

1. SUBCOMMITTEE ON CLASSIFICATION AND DEFINITION (1976) Description of sarcoidosis. *Ann. N.Y. Acad. Sci.*, **278**, 743.

Chapter 2
History

The beginning: A dermatological curiosity

In 1877, Jonathan Hutchinson described a 55-year-old man who presented with large, non-tender purple skin plaques on hands and feet. The patient also had suffered from gout and finally died of kidney failure. It is conceivable that the patient had what we now recognize as sarcoidosis which can produce skin lesions, arthritis, and disorders of calcium metabolism leading to nephrocalcinosis and renal failure.

Hutchinson described another patient, a 60-year-old lady (Mrs Mortimer), who had large symmetrical patches on her face and arms. Hutchinson wrote that the disease:

> '... may not be a tuberculous affection and one of the lupus family, but if so, it differs widely from all other forms of lupus, both in its feature and its course. The disease is characterized by the formation of multiple dusky-red patches which have no tendency to inflame or ulcerate. They are very persistent and extend but slowly. The multiplicity of the patches, their occurrence in groups, their bilateral symmetry and the absence of all tendency to ulcerate or form crusts, are features which separate the malady from lupus vulgaris ...'.

Hutchinson named the disease Mortimer's malady. This lucid description of chronic sarcoid lesions remains a classic to this day.

In 1889, Ernest Besnier, a French dermatologist, described a patient with purple violaceous swellings of the nose associated with ulceration of the nasal mucosa, livid swellings of ear lobules and fingers. He summarized these unusual features and coined a new term, lupus pernio. During the same year, another dermatologist, Cesar Boeck of Norway, described the microscopical feature of the disease and called it 'multiple benign sarcoid of the skin'. Boeck was also the first to point out the multisystem nature of the disease. Tenneson described the detailed microscopic features—'predominance of epithelioid and a variety of giant cells'—in the skin lesions of a patient with lupus pernio. Darier and Roussy described subcutaneous nodules in sarcoidosis.

Recognition of multisystem involvement

Karl Kreibich, of Prague, drew attention to bone lesions and their association with lupus pernio. He examined 60 histological sections of lupus pernio in the search for tubercle bacilli, all of which were negative. He also injected 12 guinea-pigs with the excised sarcoid tissue. In none of the nine surviving animals did any sign of tuberculosis appear. On the basis of these experimental and histological examinations of the sarcoid tissue, Kreibich concluded that lupus pernio did not represent a tuberculous infection. Schumaker in 1909, and Bering in 1910, first noted iritis accompanying cutaneous sarcoidosis. They also observed enlargement of the parotid and submaxillary glands. At the same time, Heerfordt, a Danish opthalmologist, described the clinical association of uveitis, parotid enlargement, and the seventh nerve palsy. He believed that the syndrome was due to mumps. A quarter-century later, Jan Waldestrom convincingly demonstrated the uveoparotid fever of Heerfordt to be a manifestation of sarcoidosis. Jorgen Schaumann's remarkable observations pointed out the uniformity with which the epithelioid granulomas involved lymph nodes, bone marrow, lungs, liver and spleen. He named the disease 'lymphogranuloma benignum' and distinguished it from Hodgkin's malignant granuloma. The syndrome of erythema nodosum and bilateral hilar adenopathy was recognized as an early, acute form of sarcoidosis by Sven Löfgren.

Advent of immunology

The occurrence of hypergammaglobulinaemia was first recognized by Salvesen in 1935; three of his four patients had serum globulin concentrations of over 5 g. $(100 \text{ ml})^{-1}$ $(50 \text{ g.} \ell^{-1})$. Reisner observed that 60% of the patients with sarcoidosis had a negative test. Kveim, an Oslo dermatologist, observed that the intracutaneous inoculation of a heat-killed suspension of a sarcoid lymph node produced a tiny nodule. This simple and non-invasive test was further refined and popularized by Louis Siltzbach of New York. Appropriately, the test is now referred to as the Kveim-Siltzbach test.

The present

Sarcoidosis, as a clinical entity, now had gained a world-wide recognition. Epidemiological, biochemical, immunological, electron-microscopic and radionuclide research began all over the world. There have been nine international conferences during 1958-81. The proceedings of these conferences are the storehouse of available information and knowledge on sarcoidosis. In 1964, spurred by the enthusiasm of Martin Cummings, the National Library of Medicine published a bibliography comprising about 4000 references[1]. Over 100 scientific publications covering clinical and investigative aspects of the disease appear every year. Despite the feverish pitch of extensive research, the aetiology of sarcoidosis remains shrouded in a veil of mystery[2].

References

1. MANDEL, W., THOMAS, J.H., CARMEN, G.T. and MCGOVERN, J.P. (1964) *Bibliography on Sarcoidosis 1878-1963*. Publication No. 1213. (Washington: US Public Health Service)
2. LEVINSKY, L. and MACHOLDA, F. (eds) (1971) In *Fifth International Conference on Sarcoidosis*, pp. 43-68. (Prague: University of Karlova)

Chapter 3
Epidemiology

Sarcoidosis is a common disease with an uneven, world-wide distribution[1]. Most of the epidemiological data collected around the world dealing with the frequency and distribution of sarcoidosis are based on chest radiographic surveys. Autopsy studies indicate that the true prevalence is 4-10 times higher than the number of patients discovered by routine radiographic surveys. Be that as it may, the available data clearly show that the disease has a high prevalence in certain geographic areas; whereas, in other parts of the world, there is little or no sarcoidosis. In Sweden, mass radiography figures show the prevalence rate of 64 cases per 100 000, already the highest in Europe. However, the autopsy studies indicate that actual incidence may be as high as 641 per 100 000 of the population. In Norway, the prevalence rate of sarcoidosis is 26.7 per 100 000, about one-half of that for Sweden. In neighbouring Finland, the disease is much less common (7.5 per 100 000). It is noteworthy that tuberculosis is more prevalent in Finland than in either Sweden or Norway. In Great Britain, a chest radiographic survey of 3 323 910 individuals revealed a prevalence rate of pulmonary sarcoidosis of 20 per 100 000. In North London, the occurrence of sarcoidosis among English born is 27 per 100 000; whereas the figure rises to 155 among Irish immigrants and 183 per 100 000 in West Indians. In Europe, Spain has the lowest prevalence rate of 0.04 per 100 000 for sarcoidosis.

As there have been no nationwide mass radiographic surveys in the United States, the incidence of the disease is being estimated at 11 cases per 100 000 population. In New York City, sarcoidosis occurs at the rate of 31-36 per 100 000, but in certain neighbourhoods an incidence of up to 70 per 100 000 has been reported. The disease is more common in the heavily pine-forested south-eastern region. In Lousiana, an incidence of 71 per 100 000 has been found.

Sarcoidosis is much less frequent in tropical Africa, India and South-east Asia. Surprisingly, in the central mountainous district of Japan the frequency of sarcoidosis is 16 per 100 000. Sporadic case reports have appeared from South American Eskimos, Canadian Indians and New Zealand Maoris, who rarely contract the disease.

Race

In the United States, sarcoidosis shows a definite predilection for Negroes, among whom it is 10-17 times more prevalent than in Caucasians. The disease tends to carry a poorer prognosis in Negroes. It has been suggested that sarcoidosis may be affected by genetic factors and the disease in Negroes might be a different clinical syndrome from that found in non-Negroes. American Indians are rarely affected by sarcoidosis. In the UK, Irish immigrants have a higher prevalence of sarcoidosis than the indigenous population.

Age

Sarcoidosis most frequently occurs in the third and fourth decades of life, but children and elderly persons can also be affected (*see Figure 3.1*). Nauman described a 3-month-old child with sarcoidosis; the first elderly victim of this disease to be described, described by Leitner, was an 80-year-old woman. The first patient of mine to contract the disease in old age was also 80 years old at the time of diagnosis (*see Plate 3.1 a, b*); she is now 92. Another patient, a 92-year-old man, was admitted to the hospital in a coma. He died after a few hours. Autopsy revealed mediastinal and hilar adenopathy which was full of non-caseating granulomas. The cause of death was a massive cerebral haemorrhage. The patient had no previous history of sarcoidosis or any other illness.

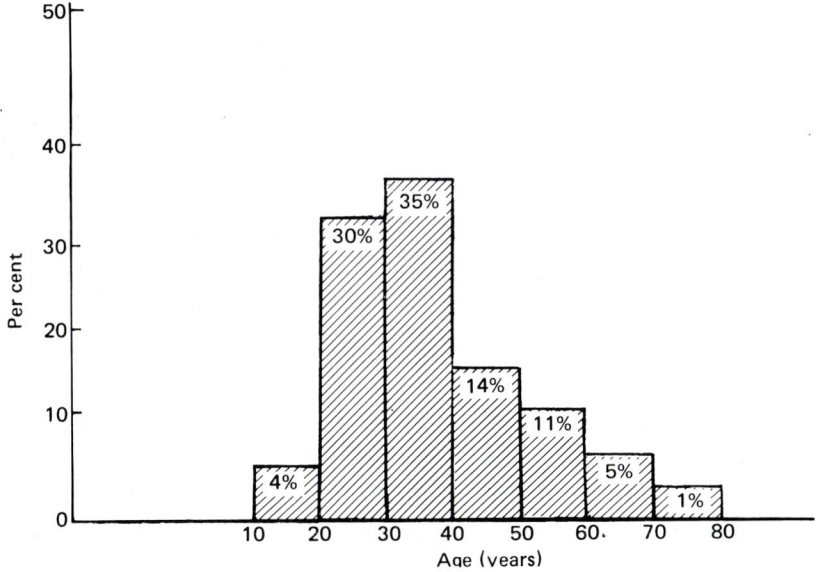

Figure 3.1 Age distribution in sarcoidosis. The disease is more frequent in third and fourth decades of life. (Reproduced from Sharma, O.P. (1975) *Sarcoidosis. A Clinical Approach*, (Springfield, Il.: Charles C. Thomas), by kind permission of publishers.)

Sex

Women usually outnumber men by two to one in a series of predominantly Negro patients. Cowdell's series consisting of all non-Negro patients showed an almost even distribution between the two sexes. In Scadding's series of 275 cases from England, 156 (57%) were men.

6   Epidemiology

In a study of 110 patients attending a private sarcoidosis clinic, Teirstein found that the distribution of sarcoidosis was approximately the same in both sexes. It appears that sarcoidosis affects Negro women twice as often as Negro men; whereas, in non-Negro patients, the distribution between the two sexes tends to be more even.

Familial sarcoidosis

Familial sarcoidosis is recognized with increasing frequency. James reviewed almost 200 patients reported to have familial sarcoidosis during the last 60 years[2]. The most common family relationship is brother–sister, followed in frequency by a mother–child relationship. A father–child relationship is rare and has been reported only once, by Wiman. I also encountered the father–son relationship once (*see Figure 3.2*). The total number of cases involving more than one member of the family is so small that it can be considered to occur no more often than would be expected by chance[3]. Merchant and Utz feel that a complex hereditary trait may be operative in this disease[4]. James believes in a recessive mode of inheritance of sarcoidosis.

The British Thoracic and Tuberculosis Association Research Committee conducted a study of 121 patients in 59 families. The report emphasized the preponderance of

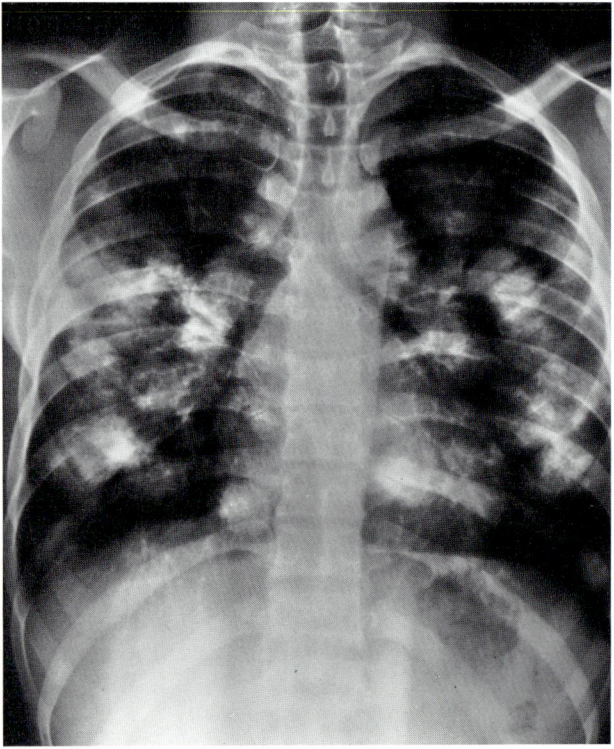

Figure 3.2 The chest radiograph of a 29-year-old Negro man, showing bilateral hilar adenopathy and nodular densities. A transbronchial lung biopsy showed non-caseating granuloma. The patient was asymptomatic. His father had sarcoidosis.

monozygotic over dizygotic twins, females over males, and mother-offspring over father-offspring sets[5].

HLA typing in sarcoidosis

During the last 10 years, conflicting reports concerning the association of HLA phenotypes and sarcoidosis have appeared. Moller et al.[6] and Kueppers et al.[7] have found no relationship between the HLA-B7 phenotypes and sarcoidosis in a German population. Brewerton et al. reported that in sarcoid patients with arthritis, there was an increased incidence of B8 and the haplotype A1-B8[8]. In Turkish sarcoidosis patients, Akokan discovered a significant increase in the frequency of HLA-B5 and A9[9]. Amongst our Negro sarcoid patients there was no increase in HLA antigens in the A and B loci[10]. Newill et al. appreciated an association of the disease with HLA-AW30 and with a group of cell surface antigens which serologically cross-react with AW30[11]. In another interesting study, the sarcoidosis patients who recovered spontaneously had an increased prevalence of B8[12]. It is clear that no significant association exists between sarcoidosis and the occurrence of HLA phenotypes.

References

1. TEIRSTEIN, A.S. and LESSER, M. (1983) World distribution and epidemiology of sarcoidosis. In *Sarcoidosis and other Granulomatous Diseases of the Lung* (ed. B.L. Fanburg), pp. 101-34. (New York: Marcel Decker) (An excellent encyclopaedic review of the epidemiology of sarcoidosis, with 109 references.)
2. JAMES, D.G. (1983) Genetics and familial sarcoidosis. In *Sarcoidosis and Other Granulomatous Diseases of the Lung* (ed. B.L. Fanburg) p. 135. (New York: Marcel Dekker)
3. SHARMA, O.P., JOHNSON, C.S. and BALCHUM, O.J. (1971) Familial sarcoidosis. Report of four siblings with acute sarcoidosis. *Am. Rev. Resp. Dis.*, **104**, 255.
4. MERCHANT, R.K. and UTZ, J.P. (1960) Familial sarcoidosis. *Arch. Intern. Med.*, **106**, 64.
5. BRITISH THORACIC AND TUBERCULOSIS ASSOCIATION (1973) Familial association in sarcoidosis. *Tubercle*, **54**, 87.
6. MOLLER, E., HEDFORS, E. and WIMAN, L.G. (1974) HL-A genotypes and MLR in familial sarcoidosis. *Tiss. Antigens*, **4**, 299.
7. KUEPPERS, F., MUELLER-ECKHARDT, HEINRICH, D., et al. (1974) HL-A antigens of patients with sarcoidosis. *Tiss. Antigens*, **4**, 56.
8. BREWERTON, D., COCKBURN, G., JAMES, D.C.O., et al. (1977) HL-A antigens in sarcoidosis. *Clin. Exp. Immunol.*, **27**, 227.
9. AKOKAN, G., CELIKOGLU, S., GOKSEL, F., et al. (1977) Antigens in Turkish patients with sarcoidosis. *N. Engl. J. Med.*, **296**, 759.
10. EISENBERG, H., TERASAKI, P., SHARMA, O.P., et al. (1978) HLA association studies in Black sarcoidosis patients. *Tiss. Antigens*, **11**, 484.
11. NEWILL, C.A., JOHNS, C.J., COHEN, B.H., et al. (1981) Sarcoidosis, HLA and immunoglobulin markers in Baltimore Blacks. In *Sarcoidosis and Other Granulomatous Disorders* (eds Chretien, J., Marsac, J. and Saltiel, J.C.), pp. 253-6. (Paris: Pergamon Press)
12. SMITH, J.J., TURTON, C.W.G., MITCHELL, D.N., et al. (1981) Association of HLA-B8 with spontaneous resolution in sarcoidosis. *Thorax*, **36**, 296.

Chapter 4
Aetiology

The cause of sarcoidosis remains unknown. Some authorities believe that sarcoidosis is a syndrome, like bronchial asthma, with many causative agents (tuberculous sarcoid, beryllium sarcoid, fungal sarcoid, etc.); whereas others believe that sarcoidosis is a single disease the cause of which is not known.

Is sarcoidosis caused by tubercle bacillus?

Originally, the disease was thought to be an unusual type of tuberculous infection. Schaumann thought that sarcoidosis represented an infection either by a non-acid-fast variant of human tubercle bacillus or an attenuated form of bovine bacillus[1]. Pinner believed that sarcoidosis was a non-caseating type of tuberculosis[2]. However, in an exhaustive study, Bowman et al. were not able to isolate any form of bacteria—acid fast or non-acid-fast—from sarcoid granulomas[3]. Furthermore, because of obvious epidemiological, clinical, radiological and immunological differences between sarcoidosis and tuberculosis, the idea of these two diseases sharing a common aetiology seems extremely unlikely.

Sarcoidosis and atypical mycobacteria

The possibility that sarcoidosis may represent a hypersensitive response to atypical mycobacteria has been considered. Chapman and Speight reported that 90% of their patients with sarcoidosis had significant titres of serum antibodies to atypical mycobacteria[4]. Reid and Wolinsky, on the other hand, found no evidence of precipitating antibodies to atypical mycobacteria in 29 patients with sarcoidosis[5]. Mankiewicz suggested that sarcoidosis results from invasion of the tissues by phage-infected lysogenic mycobacteria which produce a granulomatous response in individuals who lack the capacity to form phage-neutralizing antibodies[6]. There are two objections to this hypothesis: first, in sarcoidosis the humoral or circulating antisystem is intact; and secondly the animal experimental studies show that inoculation of mycobacterium tuberculosis alone, mycobacteriophage alone, or a mixture of both given subcutaneously do not produce granulomas similar to that of sarcoidosis.

Viruses and sarcoidosis

A viral aetiology of sarcoidosis has been considered by Lofgren, who isolated mumps–influenza–Newcastle group virus from six cases with cutaneous sarcoidosis[7]. Reagan demonstrated virus-like particles attached to the red cells of a patient with sarcoidosis[8]. Hirshaut et al. noted high serum titres of antibody to herpes-like virus (HLV or Epstein-Barr virus) in 131 patients with sarcoidosis. They, however, regard HLV as a 'passenger' virus which possibly multiplies in individuals with depressed delayed-type hypersensitivity[9]. Mitchell and Rees have demonstrated a transmissible agent from human sarcoid tissue[10].

Is sarcoidosis an allergy?

Allergy to pine pollens has been postulated as an aetiological factor. Baer proposed that the habit of chewing pine needles might be a cause[11]. Cummings and Hudgins found that intradermal injection of pine pollen extract in tuberculin-sensitive guinea-pigs produced epithelioid-cell granulomas, both at the site of injection and in the neighbouring glands[12]. However, epidemiological studies from countries other than the United States have not confirmed the relation between the distribution of sarcoidosis and pine forests. Likewise, the role of inhalation of peanut dust and hair sprays, and clay eating have never been clearly defined as a causative agent of sarcoidosis. Beryllium and zirconium are known to produce a localized granulomatous reaction. Drugs that are known to be associated with the production of pulmonary granulomas include mineral oil, talc, cromolyn sodium, BCG and methotrexate. Goldstein described a patient who developed fever, rash, lymphadenopathy and hepatosplenomegaly after 6 weeks' treatment with phenylbutazone; liver and scalene node biopsies showed non-caseating granulomas[13].

Is sarcoidosis an autoimmune disease?

Investigators who believe that sarcoidosis should be regarded as an autoimmune disorder do so largely on the basis of hypergammaglobulinaemia, a therapeutic response to corticosteroids, the coexistence of Sjögren's syndrome, scleroderma, systemic lupus erythematosus, and primary biliary cirrhosis; and the occasional occurrence of non-specific circulating antibodies. But, there are so many clinical, radiological and immunological differences between sarcoidosis and other autoimmune diseases that any casual relationship between the two seems unlikely (*see* Chapter 30).

Genetic predisposition

The high prevalence of sarcoidosis amongst Negroes in the United States, Irish and West Indians in London, and Puerto Ricans in New York indicates the possibility of some yet unrecognized genetic and constitutional factors in the aetiology of sarcoidosis (*see* Chapter 3).

Role of immunological alterations

Although we have not made much progress as far as the search for the causative agent of sarcoidosis is concerned, we have made tremendous strides in solving the immunological mysteries of the disease. We know now that cell-mediated immunity function is depressed in the peripheral tissues and the blood, but it is carried out with vigour in the lung by activated T lymphocytes. In addition, B-cell activity is stimulated in the disease. It is unclear whether the patient inhales, ingests or even absorbs from the skin an antigen that causes these immunological abnormalities. Are there more than one causative agents? Hedfors suggests that a viral and a mycobacterial agent might interact and disturb the balance between T and B lymphocytes[14].

The initial alveolar injury results in the influx of inflammatory and immune effector cells. The alveolitis may resolve or become chronic, resulting in the formation of granulomas or fibrosis. While the cause of the initiation of the alveolitis remains obscure, the formation and perpetuation of the granulomatous process is carried out by activated T lymphocytes which secrete chemotactic factors that recruit circulating monocytes and macrophages which, in their turn, continue the alveolitis and granuloma formation[15].

This brings us back to the mysterious granuloma—Cunningham raised interesting questions regarding the aetiology of sarcoidosis. Why is the granuloma oval or round? Why are epithelioid cells arranged radially? It has been suggested that perimeter defence occurs when the inciting agent is small or circular as in tuberculosis, histoplasmosis, coccidioidomycosis and in the case of talc and beryllium granulomatosis. The granuloma of sarcoidosis may be an immune response to the focal deposition of the antigen. But why does the granuloma guard the secret so zealously?

References

1. SCHAUMANN, J. (1936) Lymphogranulomatosis benign in the light of prolonged clinical observations and autopsy findings. *Br. J. Dermatol.*, **48**, 399.
2. PINNER, M. (1937) Noncaseating tuberculosis. *Am. Rev. Tuberc.*, **36**, 706.
3. BOWMAN, B.V., KOEHLER, R.M. and KUBINA, G. (1973) On the isolation of infectious agents from granulomas of patients with sarcoid. *Am. Rev. Resp. Dis.*, **107**, 467.
4. CHAPMAN, J. and SPEIGHT, M. (1964) Further studies of mycobacterial antibodies in the sera of sarcoid patients. *Acta Med. Scand.*, **176**, (Suppl. 425), 61.
5. REID, J.D. and WOLINSKY, E. (1971) The relationship of atypical mycobacterial infection to sarcoidosis. In *Proceedings of the Fifth International Conference on Sarcoidosis* (eds Lavinsky, L. and Macholda, F.), p. 85. (Prague: Charles University)
6. MANKIEWICZ, E. and VAN WALBECK, M. (1962) Mycobacteriophages: their role in tuberculosis and sarcoidosis. *Arch. Environ. Hlth.*, **5**, 122.
7. LOFGREN, S. and LUNDBACK, H. (1950) Isolation of a virus from six cases of sarcoidosis. *Acta Med. Scand.*, **138**, 71.
8. REAGAN, R.L., PALMER, E.D., DELAHA, E.C. and BRUECKNER, A.L. (1955) Study by electronmicroscopy of erythrocytes from a patient affected with sarcoidosis. *Texas Resp. Bio. Med.*, **13**, 350.
9. HIRSHAUT, Y., GLADE, P., VIERRA, L.O.B.D., *et al.* (1970) Sarcoidosis, another disease associated with serologic evidence of herpes-like virus infection. *N. Engl. J. Med.*, **283**, 502.
10. MITCHELL, D. and REES, R.J.W. (1976) The nature and physical characteristics of a transmissible agent from human sarcoid tissue. *Ann. N.Y. Acad. Sci.*, **277**, 88.
11. BAER, R.B. (1960) Familial sarcoidosis: Epidemiological aspects with notes on a possible relationship to the chewing of pine pitch. *Arch. Intern. Med.*, **105**, 60.
12. CUMMINGS, M.D. and HUDGINS, P.C. (1958) Chemical constituents of pine pollens and their possible relationship to sarcoidosis. *Am. J. Med. Sci.*, **236**, 311.
13. GOLDSTEIN, G. (1963) Sarcoid reaction associated with phenylbutazone hypersensitivity. *Ann. Intern. Med.*, **84**, 35.
14. HEDFORS, E. (1974) *Immunological Studies in Sarcoidosis.* Thesis, Department of Thoracic Medicine. Karolinska, Stockholm.
15. JAMES, D.G. and WILLIAMS JONES, W. (1982) Immunology of sarcoidosis. *Am. J. Med.*, **72**, 5.

Chapter 5
Pathology and pathogenesis

Pathology

Basic lesion

The basic lesion in sarcoidosis is a well-defined round or oval granuloma made up of compact radially arranged epithelioid cells with pale staining nuclei, a few multinucleate giant cells and a scanty rim of lymphocytes (*see Figure 5.1a and b*). Because of the absence of a well-developed lymphocyte cuff, the sarcoid granuloma sometimes is referred to as a 'naked tubercle'. Caseation is absent; occasionally, a small area of fibrinoid necrosis may be present. The latter may be distinguished from caseation by the presence of a fine reticulum network which may be visualized by silver staining methods. The histological appearance of sarcoid granuloma remains characteristically similar regardless of the type of tissue involved.

Sarcoid granuloma can be divided into the following stages[1]:

1. *Early*: The early granuloma is composed of loosely arranged epithelioid histiocytes which are derived from macrophages. Giant cells are absent. A peripheral ring of lymphocytes is present; a few lymphocytes may be present in the central portion of the granuloma.
2. *Intermediate*: The granuloma is now well circumscribed and packed with epithelioid cells. Fine reticulum is present throughout the granuloma. Giant cells are present. Apart from the scanty rim of lymphocytes, there are no other inflammatory cells. Eosinophils and plasma cells are usually absent. If the vicinity of a 'sarcoid granuloma' displays a dense chronic inflammatory cell infiltration, think of some other disease entity such as hypersensitivity pneumonitis.
3. *Late*: Complete hyalinization and fibrosis are the features of the end-stage granulomatous process. It is difficult to make a diagnosis of sarcoidosis at this stage (*see Figure 5.1c*).

Components of a sarcoid granuloma

Epithelioid cell

This is a large cell of about 20 μm in size. It is derived from the circulating monocyte. The cell has pale eosinophilic cytoplasm with round or oval nuclei. The function of the epithelioid cell is primarily secretory.

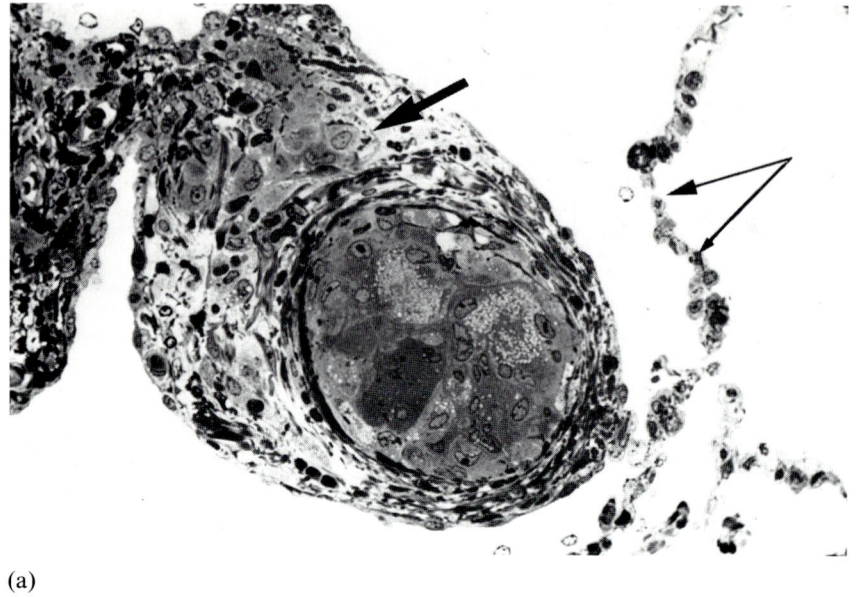

(a)

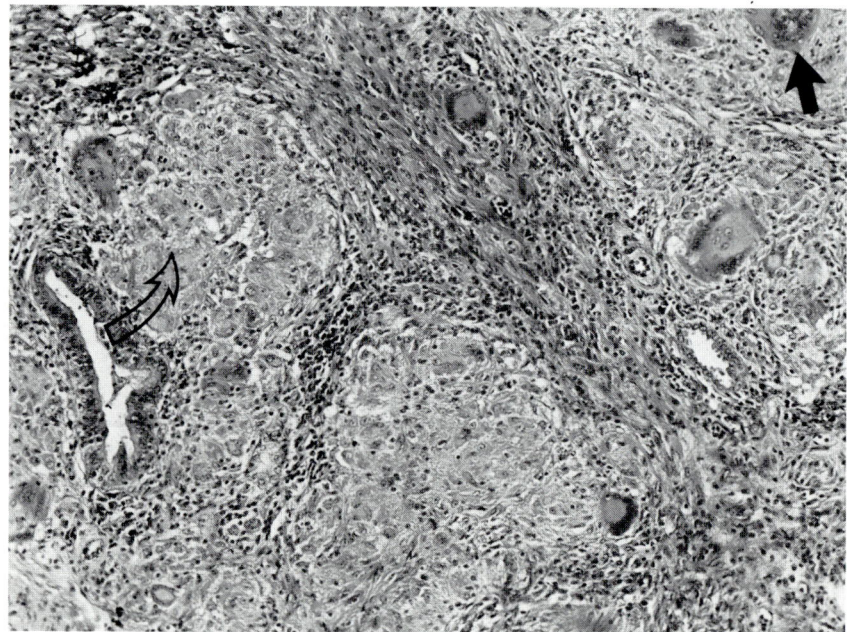

(b)

Figure 5.1

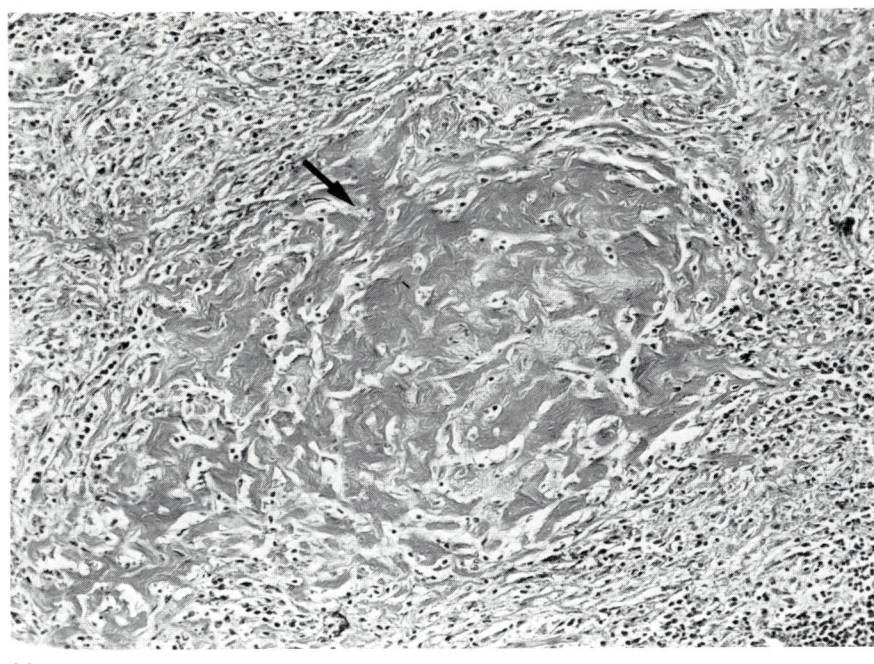

(c)

Figure 5.1(a) Epoxy section (1 μm) of a transbronchial lung biopsy specimen showing three features of a sarcoidosis: (1) delicate alveolar lining showing no evidence of diffuse alveolitis (thin arrow); (2) round, discrete granuloma packed with active epithelioid cells (vacuolated structures) and a few giant cells; and (3) surrounding rim of the granuloma with a very few lymphocytes. Note the presence of epitheliod cells (thick arrow). (Reproduced by courtesy of Dr Russell F. Sherwin, University of Southern California School of Medicine, Los Angeles.) *(b)* Round sarcoid granulomas with compact epithelioid cells (open arrow), scanty rim of lymphocytes and multinucleate giant cells (closed arrow). ((*a*) and (*b*), Haematoxylin and eosin. × 200.) *(c) LATE* stage sarcoid granuloma depicting hyalinization. (Haematoxylin and eosin. × 300.) (Reproduced from Sharma, O.P. (1975) *Sarcoidosis: A Clinical Approach* (Springfield, Il.: Charles C. Thomas), by kind permission of publishers.)

Giant cell

The giant cell is formed from fusion of epithelioid cells. The size of a giant cell varies from 150 to 300 μm. Most of the giant cells are of foreign body or Langhan's type and may contain inclusion bodies which represent metabolic end products.

Lymphocytes

The lymphocytes that surround the granuloma are derived from the circulating pool. Monocytes, macrophages and fibroblasts are also present, in varying amounts, in the cellular cuff that circles the granuloma.

Schaumann bodies or conchoidal bodies

Schaumann bodies were described by Jorge Schaumann in 1941. They are found in a giant cell and occasionally may be extracellular. They consist of concentric, basophilic

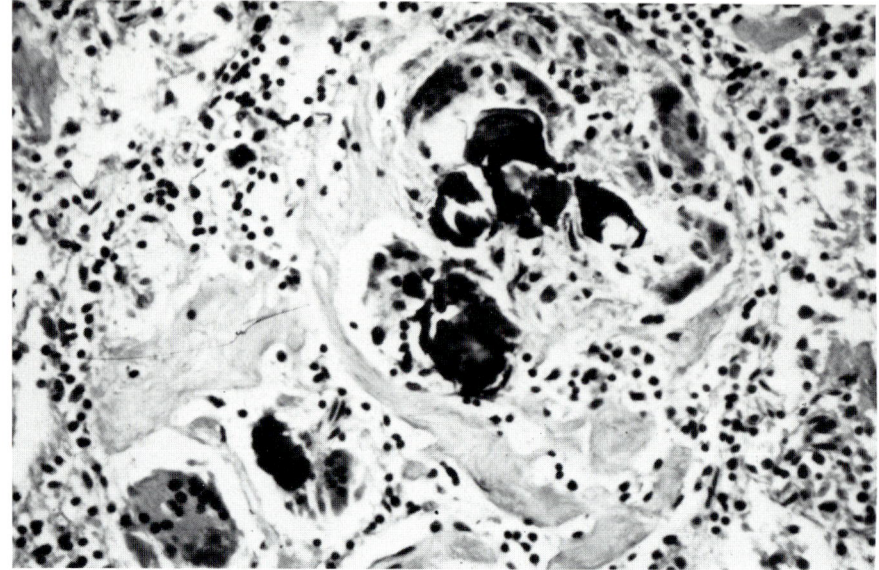
(a)

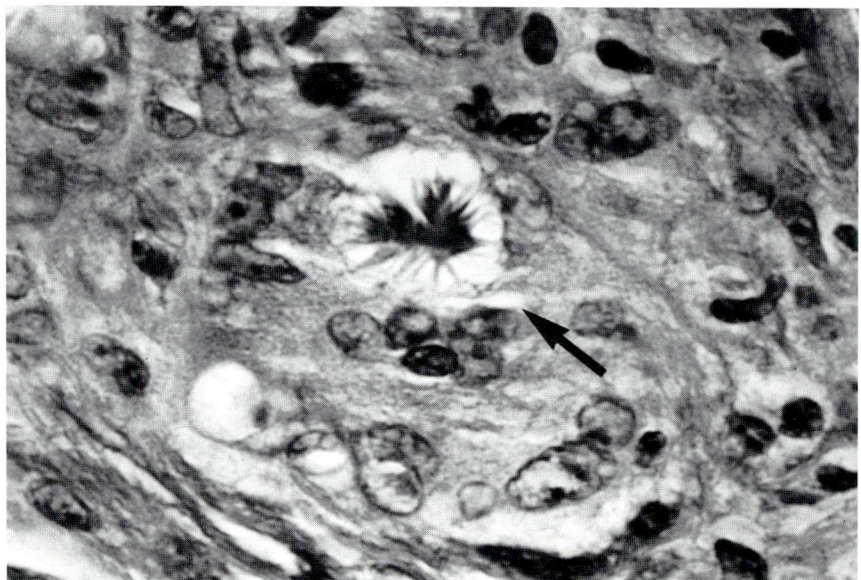
(b)
Figure 5.2

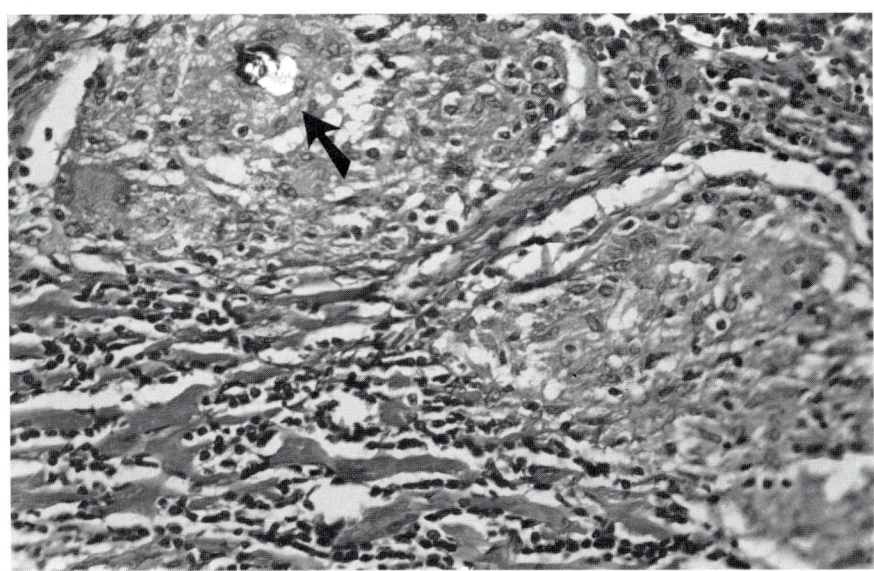

(c)

Figure 5.2(a) Schaumann bodies in a sarcoid granuloma. (Haematoxylin and eosin. × 300.) (Reproduced by courtesy of Dr Russell F. Sherwin and Dr Valda M. Richters, Department of Pathology, University of Southern California School of Medicine, Los Angeles.) (*b*) Asteroid inclusion body (arrowed) in a giant cell. (Haematoxylin and eosin. × 300.) (*c*) Crystalline inclusions in a sarcoid granuloma. (Haematoxylin and eosin. × 225.) ((*b*) and (*c*) reproduced from Sharma, O.P. (1975) *Sarcoidosis: A Clinical Approach* (Springfield, Il.: Charles C. Thomas), by kind permission of publishers.)

lamellae which are made up of calcium phosphate or carbonate iron. Conchoidal bodies are not specific to sarcoidosis for they have been found in berylliosis, tuberculosis and lymphogranuloma inguinale (*see Figure 5.2a*).

Asteroid (stellate) bodies

Asteroid bodies are usually found inside the giant cells. They vary in size from 10 to 25 µm, and are star shaped with a central core surrounded by radiating curved spines (*see Figure 5.2b*). Asteroid bodies are organic protein structures, possibly lipoproteins. Like Schaumann bodies, asteroid inclusions are not specific to sarcoidosis for they have been found in foreign body reaction, tuberculosis, and acute and chronic inflammation and repair.

Residual bodies

Residual bodies are cytoplasmic granules in epithelioid and giant cells of a sarcoid granuloma. They are considered to be the products of activated lysosomes.

Cytoplasmic vacuoles

These are also called centrospheres—they are usually foamy structures which may be located either centrally or peripherally in a giant cell.

Crystalline inclusions

Crystalline inclusions consist of doubly refractile material which varies in size from 1 to 20 µm. The crystals are usually irregular in shape but may be round. Williams showed that the inclusion is made of calcium carbonate in the form of calcite (*see Figure 5.2c*).

Alveolitis of sarcoidosis

The alveolitis of sarcoidosis is defined as the accumulation of inflammatory and immune-effector cells in the interstitium and alveolar areas of lung[2]. Lymphocytes, monocytes and macrophages are the principal cells in sarcoid alveolitis. The alveolitis, most likely, represents an initial alveolar injury and precedes the granuloma formation. It should be noted, however, that the alveolitis is not always a feature and the diagnosis of sarcoidosis depends on the demonstration of non-caseating granulomas.

Electron microscopy

Electron microscopy studies of the sarcoid granuloma show two zones. The central zone consists of epithelioid cells, histiocytes and giant cells. Lymphocytes are usually absent. Epithelioid cells are densely packed with a large number of mitochondria, rough endoplasmic reticulum, Golgi complexes and a number of cytoplasmic vacuoles. The giant cells have an ultrastructure similar to epithelioid cells, but they also contain large numbers of small dense bodies and a few or none of the clear vacuoles. Asteroid bodies are made up of fibrillar structures resembling collagen. The peripheral portion of the granuloma is loosely arranged, has fewer interdigitations and has more lymphocytes (*see Figure 5.3*)[3].

Natural history of a sarcoid granuloma

Clinical, histological and radiological data clearly show that sarcoid granulomas can resolve spontaneously, leaving no scar. They can also persist for a long time with little or no fibrosis, still capable of spontaneous resolution. Granulomas that persist for more than a year or two show peripheral hyalinization and some fibrosis. In late stages, complete hyalinization and fibrosis result in tissue scarring.

Pathogenesis

Functional disturbances and physiological abnormalities reflect the organ involvement by the disease and are due to 'interference of organ function by the granulomata or fibrosis'.

The pulmonary granulomas have a predilection for peribronchial, subpleural and interlobular septal connective tissue. Although the involvement of blood vessels occurs in 42–92% of all cases, clinical pulmonary hypertension is uncommon. Extensive pulmonary involvement, if progressive, results in fibrosis and cor pulmonale. Aspergilloma may occur in the cystic spaces of end-stage pulmonary sarcoidosis[4].

Almost any organ can be involved by sarcoidosis. Glaucoma, cataract and blindness are secondary to fibrosis of the uveal tract; kidney involvement may lead to uraemia and renal failure; and the granulomatous involvement of the myocardium may lead to

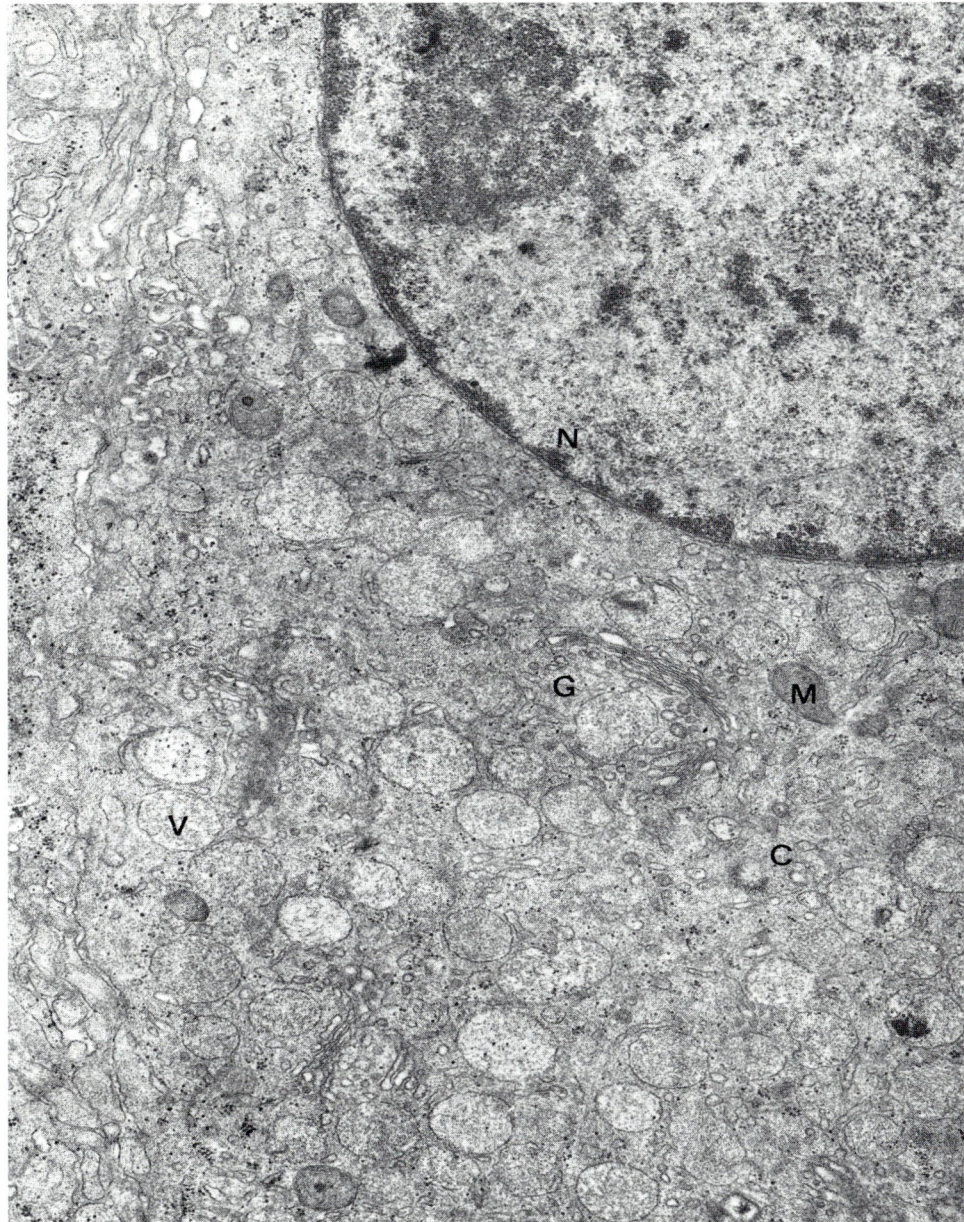

Figure 5.3(a) Electron-microscopic view of an epithelioid cell from a sarcoid granuloma showing a nucleus with narrow rim of dense chromatin (N), many large Golgi complexes (G), numerous lightly stained vesicles (V), mitochondria (M) and centriole (C). (Original magnification × 25 333, reduced to four-fifths in reproduction.)

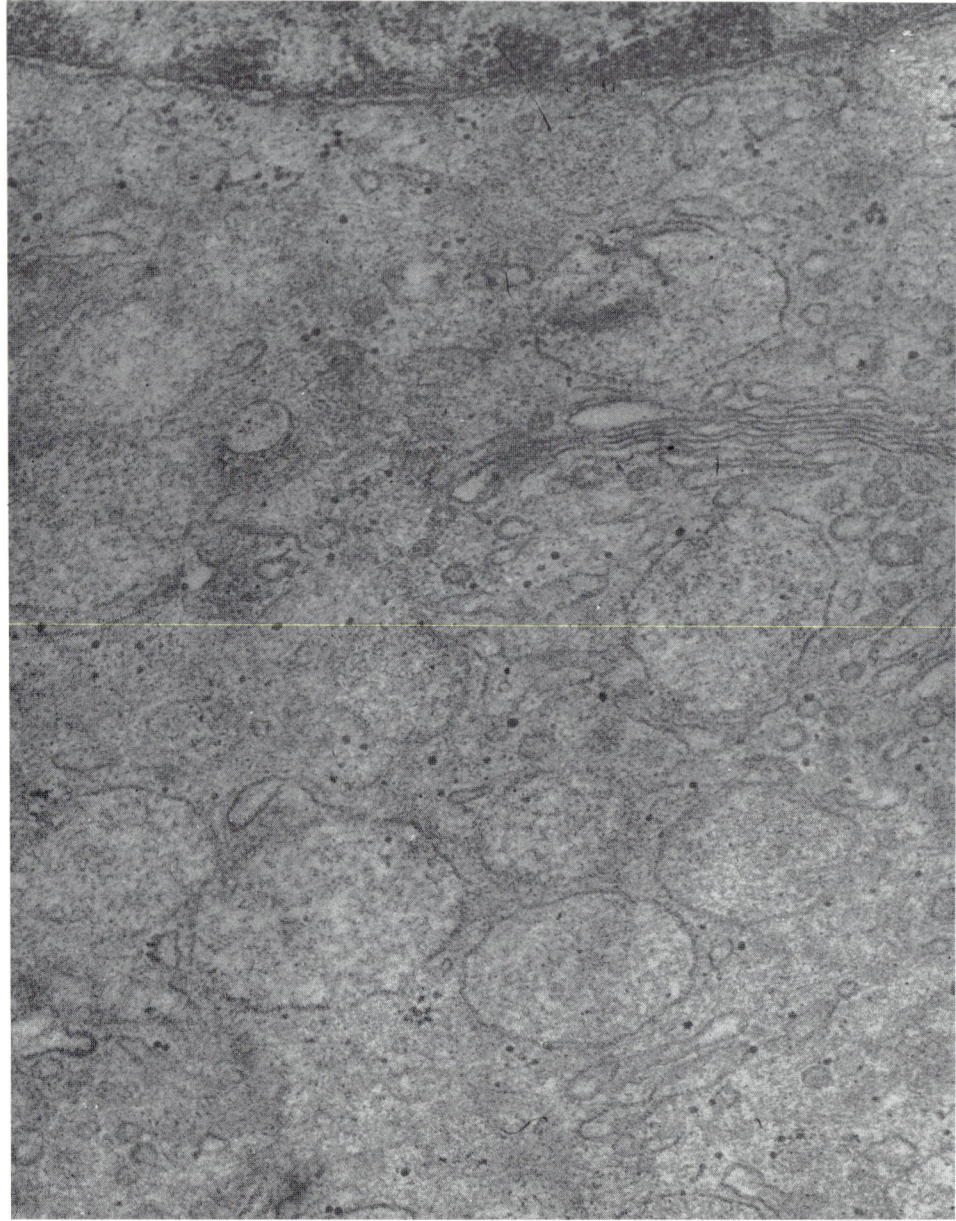

Figure 5.3(b) A higher electron-microscopic magnification showing a nucleus, Golgi complexes and vesicles. (Original magnification × 66 666, reduced to four-fifths in reproduction. (*a*) and (*b*) reproduced by courtesy of Dr William Jones Williams, Cardiff, UK.)

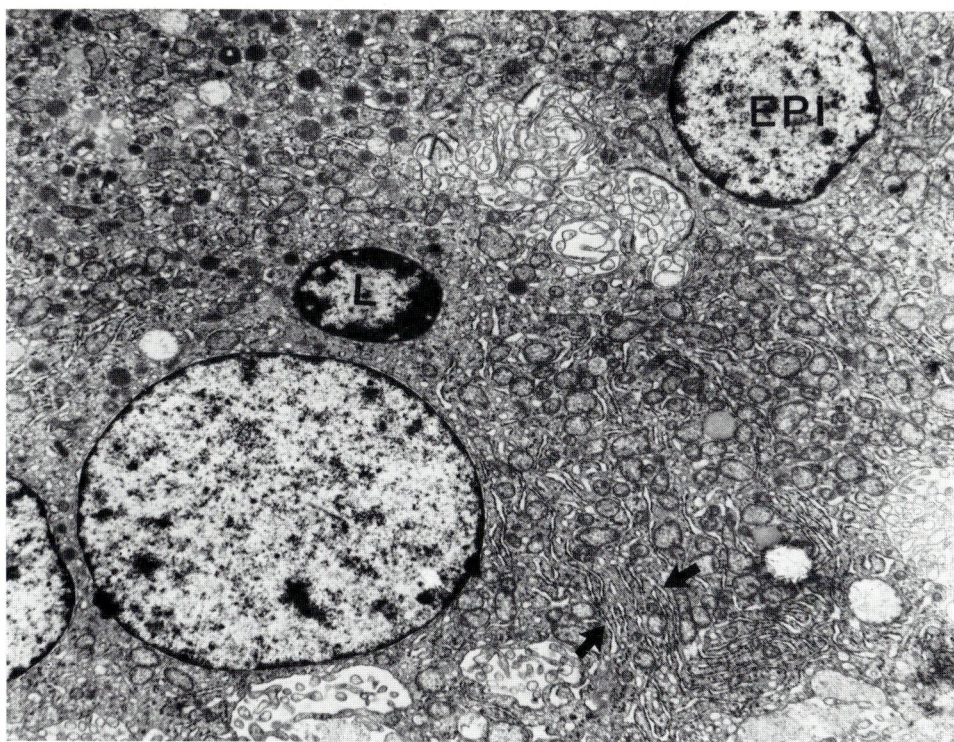

Figure 5.3(c) A low-power electron-microscopic view (× 9 900, reduced to three-fifths in reproduction) showing interdigitating microvilli (arrows) indicating highly active epithelioid–macrophage system. (Reproduced by courtesy of Drs Russel F. Sherwin and Valda Richters, University of Southern California School of Medicine, Los Angeles.)

rhythm disturbances and heart failure. In lymph nodes, the granulomas may replace the whole gland structure. Bones and joints are also affected. Cystic changes in bones are due to collections of sarcoid granulomas surrounded by a zone of osteoclastic reabsorption. Crippling arthritis is uncommon. Sarcoid granulomas may be found in meninges, brain substance, hypothalamus, pituitary gland, spinal cord, and cranial and peripheral nerves. Adrenals, peritoneum and pericardium are rarely affected by sarcoidosis.

Differential diagnosis of sarcoid granuloma

The granulomatous response similar to that of sarcoidosis is found in many other conditions.

Bacterial infections

Tuberculosis

Granulomas have caseation. Acid-fast stains and culture of the biopsied tissue are needed to confirm the diagnosis.

Leprosy

The granulomas usually have little or no caseation. Leprabacilli are scant or absent and cannot be cultured or transmitted to animals. The diagnosis thus depends on the clinical evidence of the disease.

Brucellosis

Granulomas are small and poorly formed. The diagnosis depends on occupational history, and clinical, bacteriological or serological grounds.

Spirochaete

Granulomas of syphilis have plasma-cell infiltration and coagulative necrosis.

Viral infections

Cat scratch disease

The granulomas are usually larger than those of sarcoidosis and show prominent stellate necrosis.

Fungal diseases

Coccidioidomycosis

This fungal disease which is endemic in the South-west United States may produce clinical, histological and radiologic changes similar to that of sarcoidosis. The diagnosis is based on the epidemiological information, special stains and serology (*see Plate 5.1*). Histoplasmosis, cryptococcosis, and blastomycosis may simulate sarcoidosis.

Parasites

Granulomatous reaction similar to sarcoidosis occurs in toxoplasmosis, leishmaniasis, ascariasis and schistosomiasis. Rupture of an hydatid cyst has been reported to produce a granulomatous inflammation.

Minerals

Beryllium

Beryllium produces non-caseating granulomas indistinguishable from those of sarcoidosis. The diagnosis depends on the occupational history, finding of beryllium in the tissues, and lymphocyte transformation in response to beryllium.

Talc (magnesium silicate)

Talc granulomatosis is a common lung disease found in drug addicts. Birefringent particles are present in the granuloma (*see Plate 5.1*).

Colour Plate Section

Plate 3.1
Skin lesions in sarcoidosis.

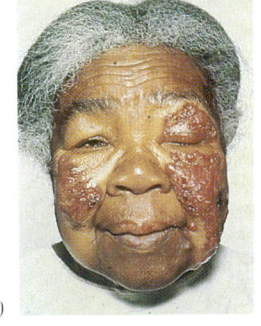
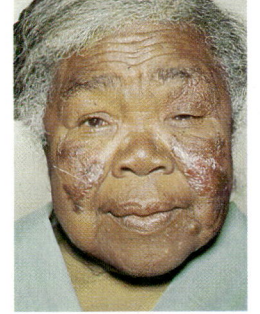

(a/b) Chronic ulcerating lupus pernio-like lesion. (a) Before corticosteroid and chloroquine therapy. (b) Nine months after therapy.

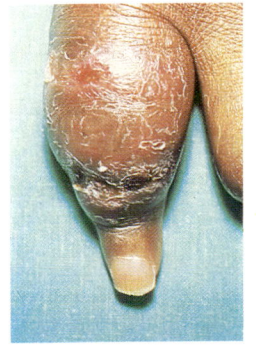
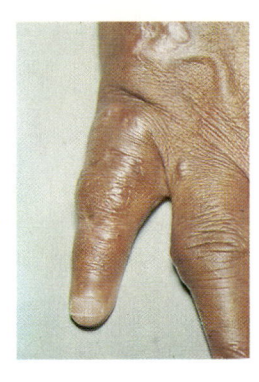

(c/d) Swelling of the digit: A biopsy of the indurated lesion showed non-caseating granuloma: before (c) and after (d) therapy.

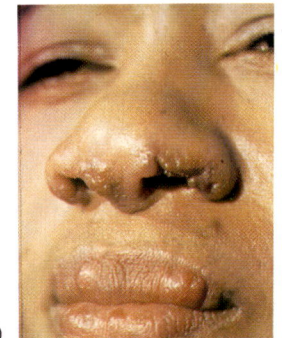
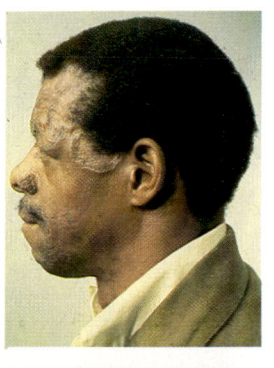

(e) Lupus pernio involving the nose and nasal mucosa.
(f) Chronic skin plaques, the lesion markedly regressed with chloroquine therapy.

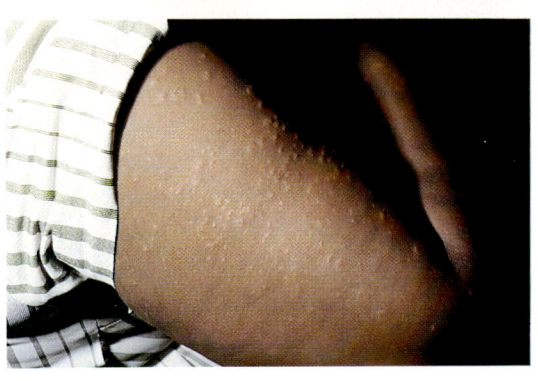

Maculopapular (flat-top) rash in a woman with stage II sarcoidosis.

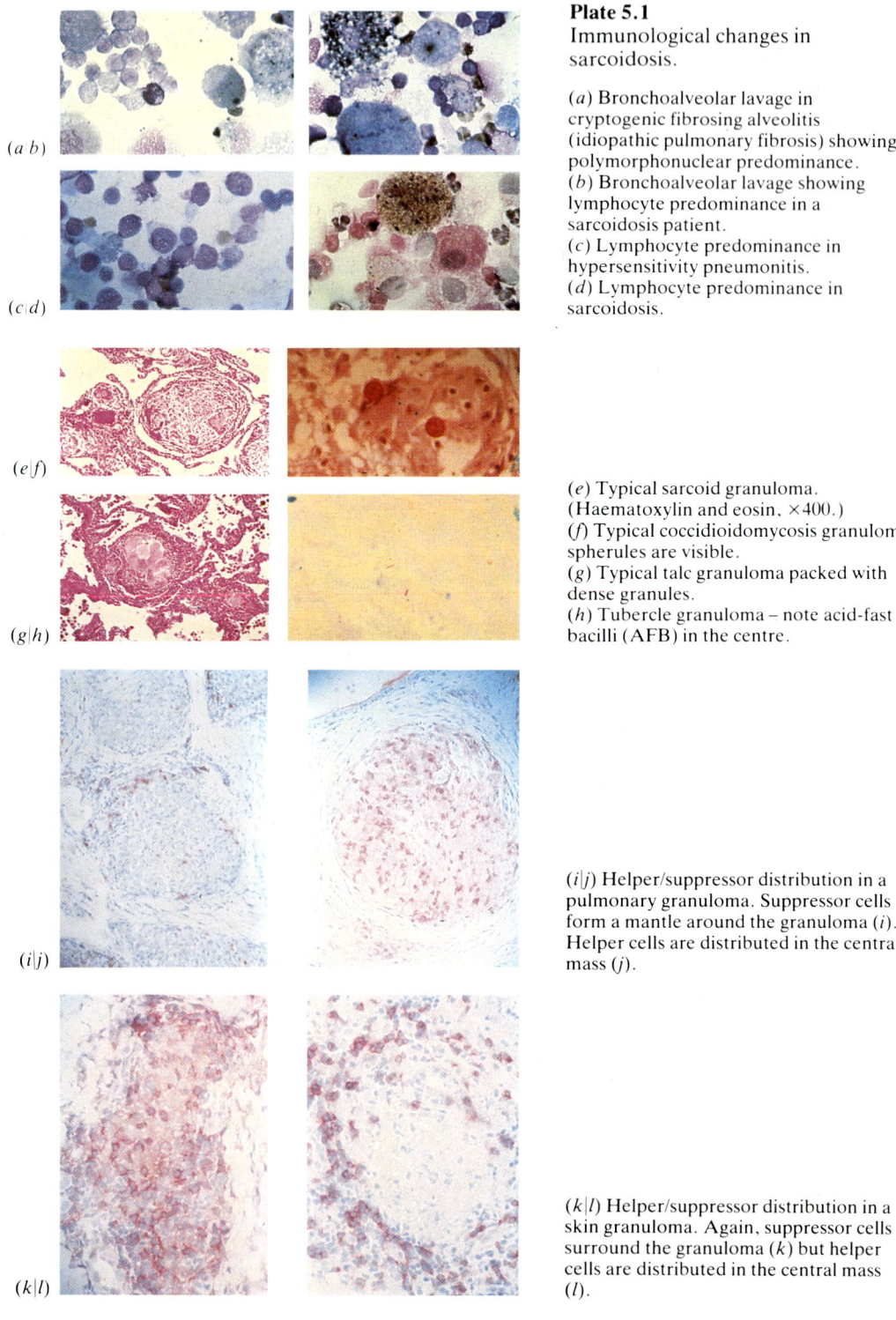

Plate 5.1
Immunological changes in sarcoidosis.

(a) Bronchoalveolar lavage in cryptogenic fibrosing alveolitis (idiopathic pulmonary fibrosis) showing polymorphonuclear predominance.
(b) Bronchoalveolar lavage showing lymphocyte predominance in a sarcoidosis patient.
(c) Lymphocyte predominance in hypersensitivity pneumonitis.
(d) Lymphocyte predominance in sarcoidosis.

(e) Typical sarcoid granuloma. (Haematoxylin and eosin, ×400.)
(f) Typical coccidioidomycosis granuloma spherules are visible.
(g) Typical talc granuloma packed with dense granules.
(h) Tubercle granuloma – note acid-fast bacilli (AFB) in the centre.

(i|j) Helper/suppressor distribution in a pulmonary granuloma. Suppressor cells form a mantle around the granuloma (i). Helper cells are distributed in the central mass (j).

(k|l) Helper/suppressor distribution in a skin granuloma. Again, suppressor cells surround the granuloma (k) but helper cells are distributed in the central mass (l).

Colour Plate Section

Plate 3.1
Skin lesions in sarcoidosis.

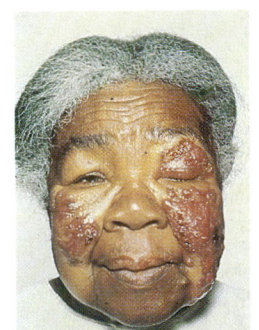
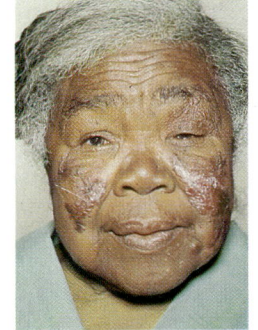

(a|b) Chronic ulcerating lupus pernio-like lesion. (a) Before corticosteroid and chloroquine therapy. (b) Nine months after therapy.

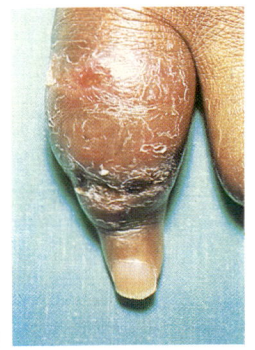
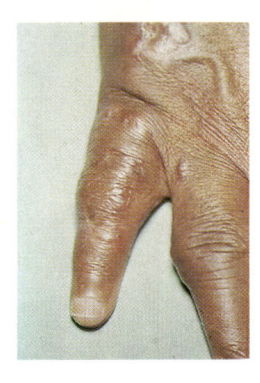

(c|d) Swelling of the digit: A biopsy of the indurated lesion showed non-caseating granuloma: before (c) and after (d) therapy.

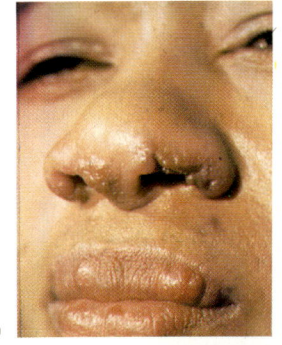
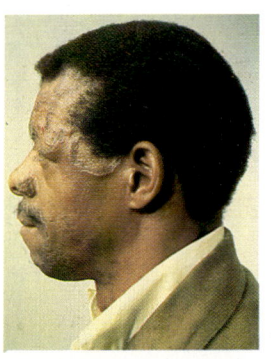

(e) Lupus pernio involving the nose and nasal mucosa.
(f) Chronic skin plaques, the lesion markedly regressed with chloroquine therapy.

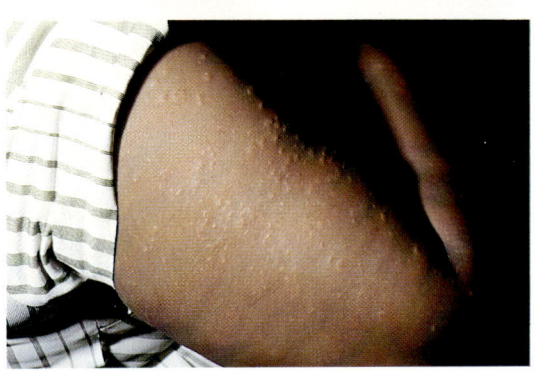

Maculopapular (flat-top) rash in a woman with stage II sarcoidosis.

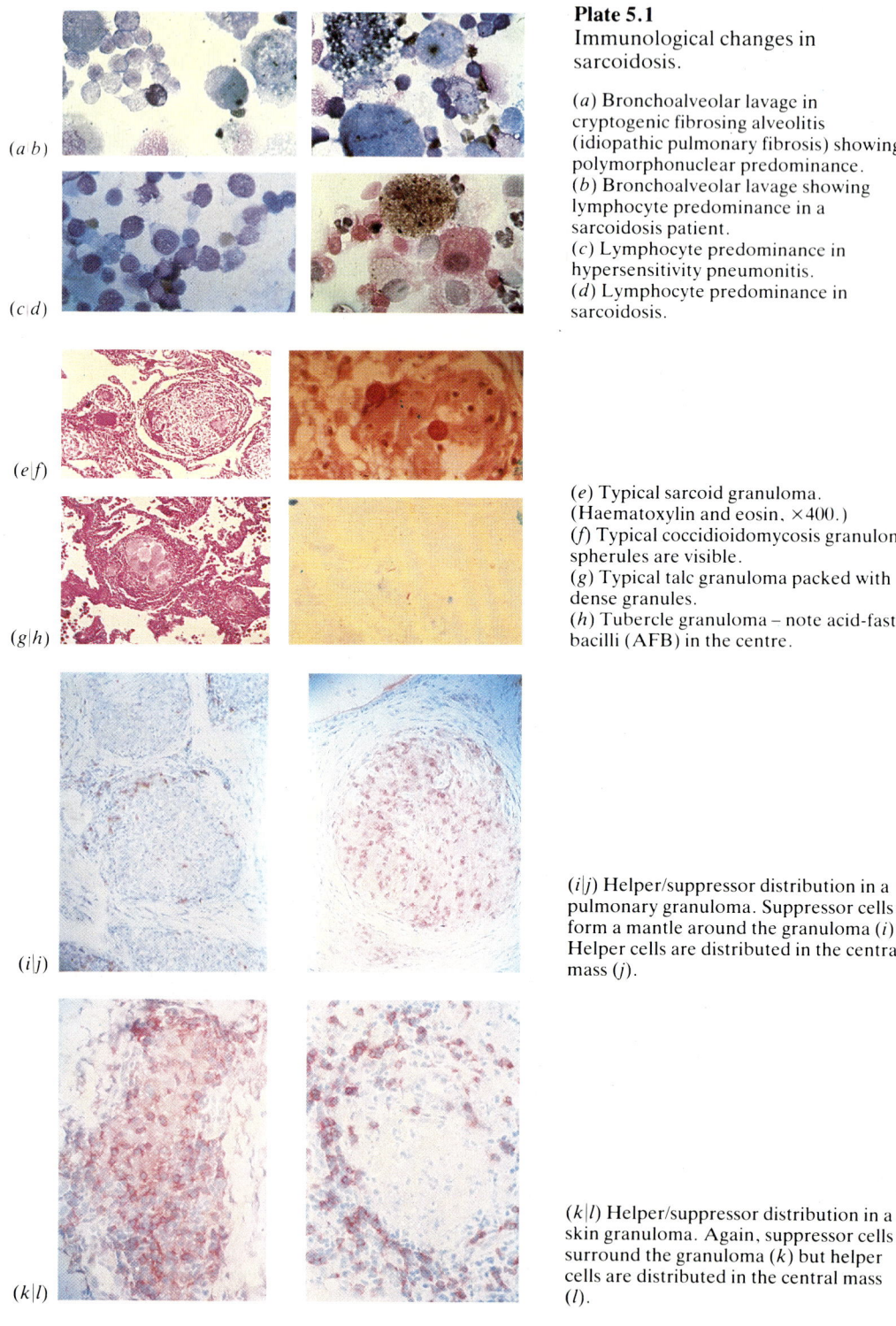

Plate 5.1
Immunological changes in sarcoidosis.

(a) Bronchoalveolar lavage in cryptogenic fibrosing alveolitis (idiopathic pulmonary fibrosis) showing polymorphonuclear predominance.
(b) Bronchoalveolar lavage showing lymphocyte predominance in a sarcoidosis patient.
(c) Lymphocyte predominance in hypersensitivity pneumonitis.
(d) Lymphocyte predominance in sarcoidosis.

(e) Typical sarcoid granuloma. (Haematoxylin and eosin, ×400.)
(f) Typical coccidioidomycosis granuloma spherules are visible.
(g) Typical talc granuloma packed with dense granules.
(h) Tubercle granuloma – note acid-fast bacilli (AFB) in the centre.

(i|j) Helper/suppressor distribution in a pulmonary granuloma. Suppressor cells form a mantle around the granuloma (i). Helper cells are distributed in the central mass (j).

(k|l) Helper/suppressor distribution in a skin granuloma. Again, suppressor cells surround the granuloma (k) but helper cells are distributed in the central mass (l).

Plate 9.1
Eye lesions in sarcoidosis.

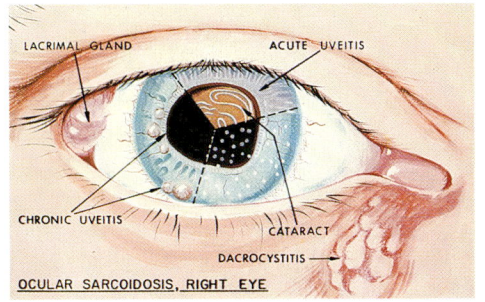

(a) Ocular sarcoidosis: common manifestation.

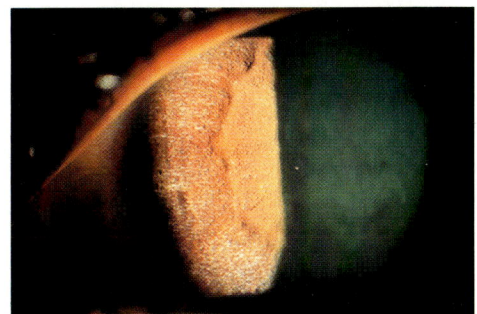

(b) Uveitis (slit-lamp examination).

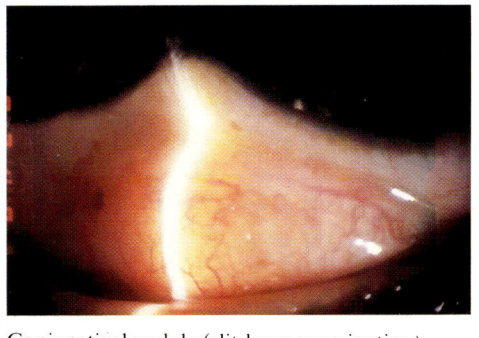

(c) Conjunctival nodule (slit-lamp examination).

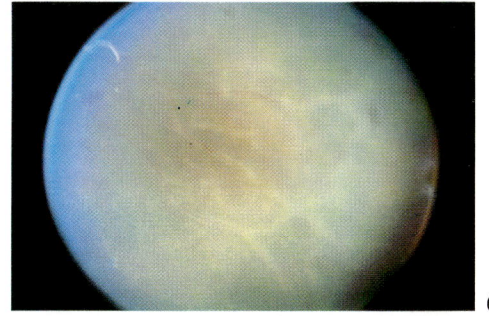

(d) Retinal sarcoid nodule.

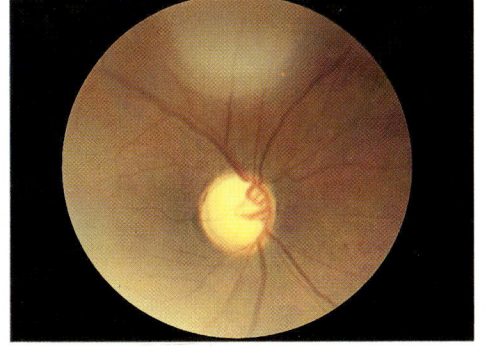

(e) Optic atrophy.

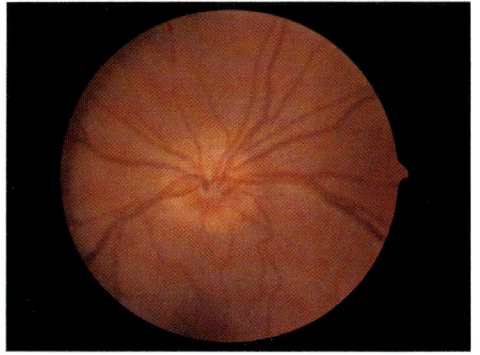

(f) Papilloedema.

Plate 19.1
Some clinical features of sarcoidosis.

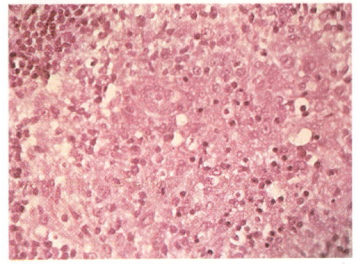

(a)

(b)

(a) Typical laryngeal sarcoidosis involving the false cords and the epiglottis in a 21-year-old woman. The lesion opened up with corticosteroids.
(b) Non-caseating granuloma in the laryngeal lesion shown in (a). (Haematoxylin and eosin, ×300.)

(c/d/e) Sarcoidosis of the spleen: gross (c); cut surface (d) and microscopic section (e) showing granuloma with calcium deposits. (Original magnification ×300.)

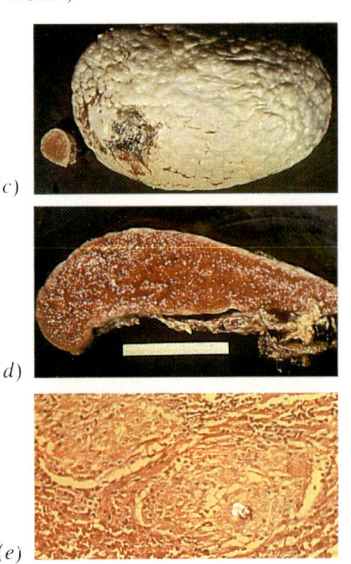

(c)

(d)

(e)

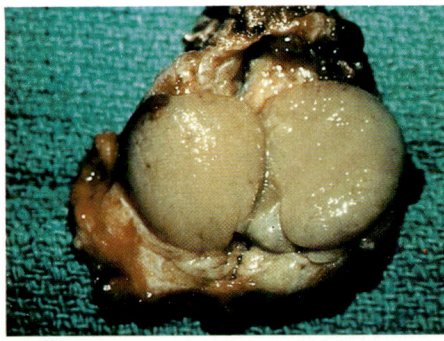

(f)

Parotid involvement in sarcoidosis. Note fine tuberculoid granulomas on the cut surface.

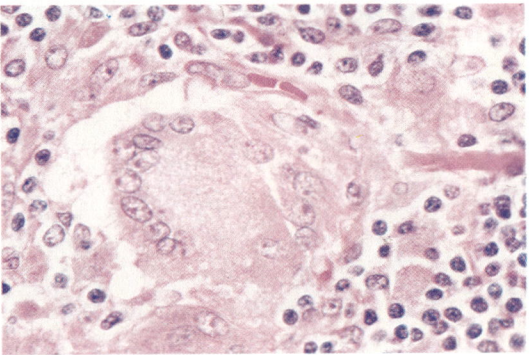

(g)

Giant cell within a non-caseating granuloma. A giant cell is sitting within the lesion. (Haematoxylin and eosin, ×600.)

Silica, zirconium

Epithelioid granulomas on the skin and lungs can be produced by silica.

Organic antigens (extrinsic allergic alveolitis)

A granulomatous hypersensitivity pneumonitis results from inhalation of a variety of organic dusts. There are certain differences betwen the granulomatous reaction caused by sarcoidosis and the one observed in extrinsic allergic alveolitis (*see Table 5.1*). The

TABLE 5.1. Histological features of sarcoidosis and hypersensitivity pneumonitis

Features	Sarcoidosis	Hypersensitivity pneumonitis
Alveolitis	Minimal	Extensive
Granulomas:		
Location	Peripheral, submucosal	Centrilobular
Foreign bodies	Absent	Present
Bronchiolitis obliterans	Absent	Present in 50%
Fibrosis (chronic)	Present	Present

diagnosis depends on the history of exposure, the presence of precipitating antibodies, and a positive response to inhalational challenge with the appropriate antigen.

Local sarcoid reactions

The granulomas similar to that of sarcoidosis may occur in lymph nodes draining an area of carcinoma, lymphoma, Crohn's disease and cholecystitis. However, these patients do not display any evidence of multisystem sarcoidosis.

Necrotizing sarcoidal granulomatosis

This condition was first described by Liebow in 1973 in the James Burns Amberson lecture[5]. He reported 11 patients who had sarcoidal granulomas, vasculitis and necrosis. Radiographically, the patients show bilateral non-cavitary ill-defined densities. Hilar adenopathy is usually absent; extrapulmonary involvement is uncommon[6].

References

1. CUNNINGHAM, J.A. (1967) Sarcoidosis. In *Pathology Annual* (ed. Sommers, S.G.), Vol. **2**, p. 31. (New York: Appleton)
2. CRYSTAL, R.G., ROBERTS, W.C., HUNNINGHAKE, G.W., *et al.* (1981) Pulmonary sarcoidosis: A disease characterized and perpetuated by activated lung T lymphocytes. *Ann. Intern. Med.*, **94**, 73.
3. SOLER, P., BASSET, F., BERNAUDIN, J.F. and CHRETIEN, J. (1976) Morphology and distribution of the cells of a sarcoid granuloma: Ultrastructural study of serial sections. *Ann. N.Y. Acad. Sci.*, **278**, 147.
4. CARRINGTON, C.B., GAENSLER, B.A., MIKUS, J.P., *et al.* (1976) Structure and function in sarcoidosis. *Ann. N.Y. Acad. Sci.*, **278**, 265.
5. LIEBOW, A.A. (1973) The James Burns Amberson lecture: Pulmonary angiitis and granulomatosis. *Am. Rev. Resp. Dis.*, **108**, 1.
6. KOSS, M.N., HOCHHOLZER, L., FEIGIN, D.S., *et al.* (1980) Necrotizing sarcoid-like granulomatosis: Clinical pathologic and immunologic findings. *Hum. Pathol.*, **11**, 510.

Chapter 6
Clinical features

Modes of presentation

Sarcoidosis can involve almost any tissue system in the body. Because of its diverse manifestations, the disease presents to clinicians of many different disciplines (*see Table 6.1 and Figure 6.1*). Clinical manifestations depend on the duration of the illness, the site and extent of tissue involvement, and activity of the disease.

TABLE 6.1. Clinical presentation of sarcoidosis for various disciplines*

General practitioner	*Chest physician*	*Ophthalmologist*
Fever, anorexia, weight loss, lymphadenopathy, parotid enlargement, acute arthritis, nasal stuffiness, hoarseness	Dyspnoea, cough, wheezing, abnormal chest X-ray, cor pulmonale, abnormal lung function tests	Iritis, choroiditis, keratoconjunctivitis, glaucoma, cataract, enlarged lacrimal glands, dry eyes
Dermatologist	*Cardiologist*	*Neurologist*
Erythema nodosum, lupus pernio, maculopapular rash, scars, keloids, nodules	Dyspnoea, cardiac failure, heart block, arrhythmias, abnormal ECG, sudden death	Cranial nerve palsies, papilloedema, meningitis, myopathy, peripheral neuropathy, space-occupying lesions
Radiologist	*Rheumatologist*	*Gastroenterologist*
Abnormal chest X-ray— bilateral hilar adenopathy, interstitial fibrosis; bone cysts	Arthritis, bone cysts	Gastric granuloma, splenomegaly
Urologist	*Nephrologist*	*Endocrinologist*
Hypercalciuria	Renal failure	Diabetes insipidus, hypercalcaemia, hyperthyroidism
Haematologist	*Otorhinolaryngologist*	*Hepatologist*
Leucopenia, thrombocytopenia, hypersplenism	Parotid enlargement, hoarseness, nasal stuffiness	Liver granuloma, portal hypertension, abnormal liver function tests

* Reproduced from Sharma, O.P. (1975) *Sarcoidosis: A Clinical Approach*, (Springfield, Il.: Charles C. Thomas), by courtesy of publishers.

Modes of presentation 23

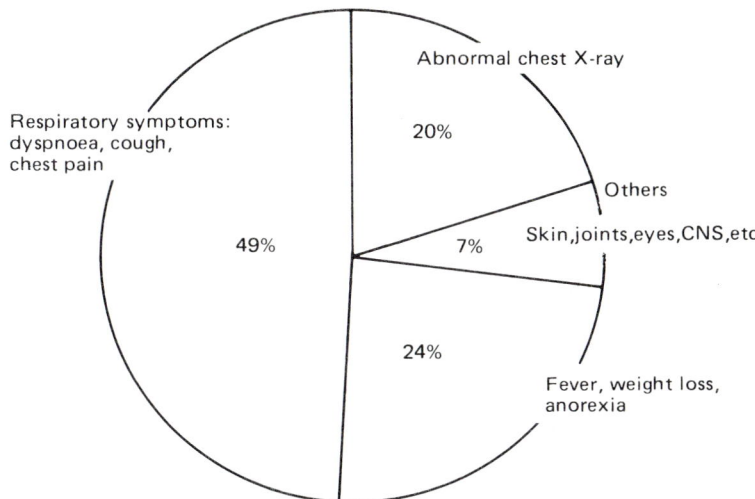

Figure 6.1 Presenting features in sarcoidisis. (Reproduced from Sharma, O.P. (1975) *Sarcoidosis: A Clinical Approach* (Springfield, Il.: Charles C. Thomas) by courtesy of publishers.)

Non-specific constitutional manifestations

About one-third of the patients in my series initially complained of non-specific symptoms of fever, anorexia, fatigue, malaise and weight loss. Fever was generally mild but temperature elevations to 40°C were recorded. Weight loss was generally limited to 5–15 lb (2.3–6.8 kg) during the preceding 10–12 weeks.

These constitutional symptoms indicate a systemic reaction and occur more frequently in Negro than in non-Negro patients. Sixty-two (43%) of 145 patients studied by Mayock *et al.* had one or more of constitutional symptoms; 24% complained of weight loss; and 21% had fever[1]. Sarcoidosis is an important cause of 'fever of unknown origin'[2].

Symptoms related to specific organ systems

Asymptomatic pulmonary sarcoidosis

The intrathoracic involvement may remain asymptomatic during its entire course, the disease being discovered by routine chest radiography. Twenty per cent of the patients in my series were investigated because of an abnormal chest radiograph. Most of these patients were asymptomatic; a few, however, on careful questioning, gave a history of retrosternal chest discomfort. One hundred and twenty-four (40%) of 311 patients studied by Siltzbach at Mount Sinai Hospital, New York, and 119 (22%) of 537 patients reported by James from Royal Northern Hospital, London, were discovered on a routine chest roentgenographic examination[3].

Respiratory symptoms

About 20–50% of patients with sarcoidosis present with respiratory symptoms, including dyspnoea, cough, chest pain and tightness of the chest. The cough is usually dry. Chest pain is confined to the retrosternal area and is generally not more than a vague tightness. Occasionally, the pain may be severe and indistinguishable from the cardiac pain[4]. Haemoptysis is rare. Respiratory symptoms occurred in 73 (48.6%) of 115 of our patients; in 59 (19%) of Siltzbach's series; and in only 49 (9%) of the patients studied by James.

Case 1—Cough as the sole manifestation of sarcoidosis. This 65-year-old woman developed a persistent dry cough over a 2-year period. Initially, her chest radiograph showed an infiltrate in the left upper lobe. Tuberculin and coccidioidin skin tests were negative. Six nebulized sputum cultures did grow acid-fast bacilli. The patient had no other symptoms but agreed to a bronchoscopy which showed non-caseating granuloma. She was given antitussive drugs. Her lung infiltrate persisted for 2 years without any significant change (*see Figure 6.2*). Another bronchoscopy was performed which again showed non-caseating granuloma. Clinical history, laboratory tests and biochemical studies excluded tuberculosis, carcinoma, and other immunological disorders. A diagnosis of sarcoidosis was entertained and she was given prednisone 20 mg once daily.

Case 2—Pain as the prominent symptom of sarcoidosis. A 24-year-old Negro man presented with sharp pain localized to anterior and posterior cervical lymph nodes and the retrosternal area. This pain became intensified after drinking beer. He also complained of weight loss and frequent night sweats. Physical examination showed a diffuse lymphadenopathy. A chest radiograph showed bilateral hilar adenopathy and parenchymal infiltration. Multiple sputum cultures failed to reveal acid-fast bacilli. Cervical lymph-node biopsies showed non-caseating granulomas. Multiple cultures of sputum, urine and gastric washing were normal. He was given prednisone 40 mg once daily which was gradually decreased to 10 mg daily. He became asymptomatic 6 months after treatment was started. After 4 weeks the radiograph showed marked clearing of the infiltrate. He had no more pains and began to consume his usual amount of beer (*see Figure 6.3*).

Extrapulmonary symptoms

Irritation and burning sensation, photophobia, blurring of vision and 'red-eye' result from acute uveitis. The constellation of parotid enlargement, ocular symptoms and facial nerve palsy is called Heerfordt's disease. Less commonly, chronic skin lesions may be the presenting feature of sarcoidosis. Occasionally, polyuria, polydipsia, arthritis, myocardial involvement and unexplained neurological lesions may first call attention to the disease.

Acute (subacute) and chronic sarcoidosis

Patients with sarcoidosis may be divided into two groups: those whose illness has persisted for less than 2 years; and those with chronic disease, with symptoms that have lasted for more than 2 years[5].

Acute (subacute) sarcoidosis

This type of sarcoidosis has an abrupt onset and tends to clear spontaneously. The patients are usually asymptomatic; the condition is frequently diagnosed on routine chest radiographs which frequently show bilateral hilar lymphadenopathy and occasionally diffuse parenchymal infiltration. Erythema nodosum may be present at the onset, especially in Swedish, Irish, Puerto Rican and Mexican women of childbearing years. The chest radiograph clears within a year in over 60% of the patients, and corticosteroids are seldom needed (*see Figure 6.4*).

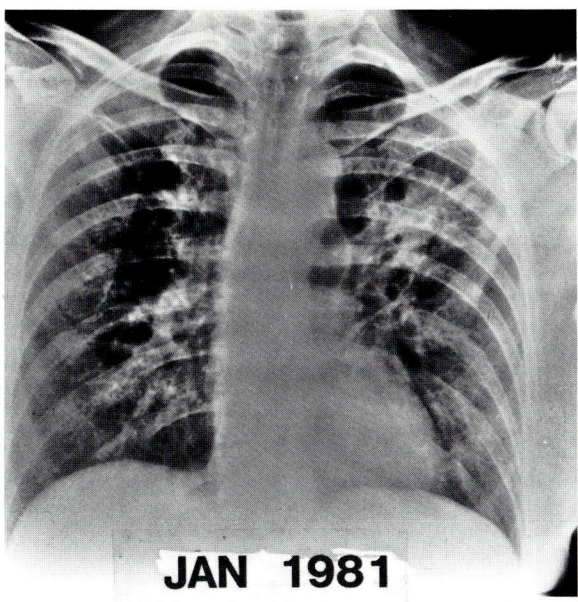

(a)

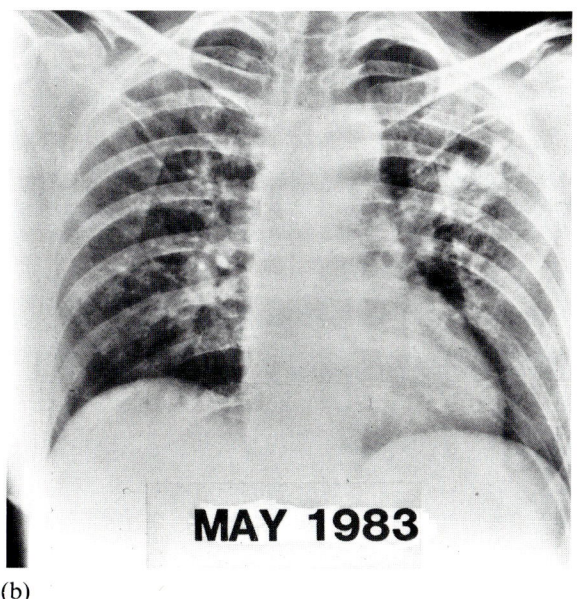

(b)

Figure 6.2(a) Diffuse interstitial and left upper lobe infiltrate in a woman with persistent dry cough. (*b*) After 2 years the infiltrate has remained unchanged. Later, the cough and the infiltrate cleared with prednisone therapy.

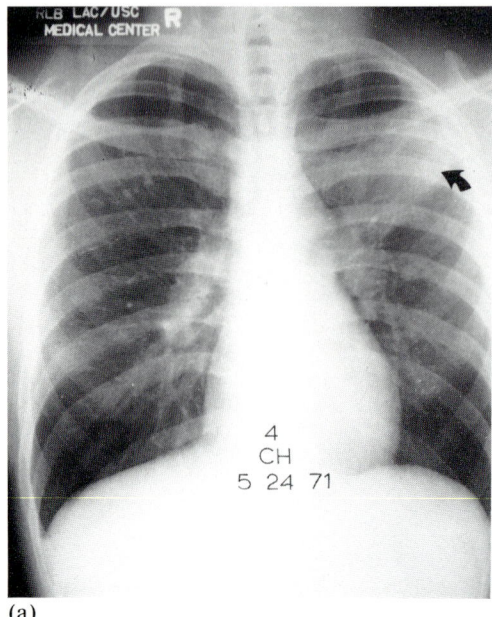

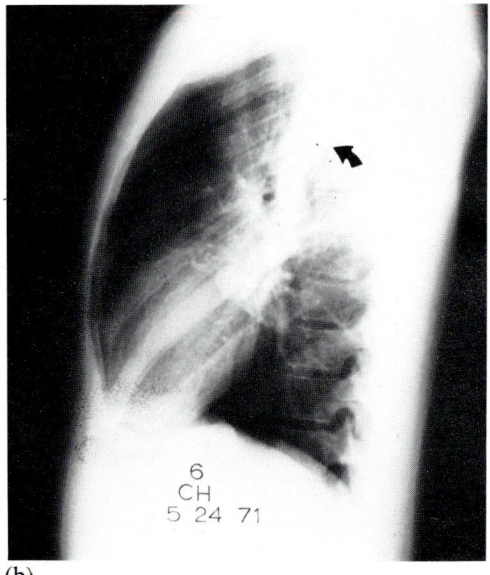

Figure 6.3(a) Posteroanterior radiograph of the chest showing bilateral hilar adenopathy and left upper lobe infiltration (arrow). (*b*) Lateral radiograph showing the infiltrate and loss of volume of apical–posterior segment of the left upper lobe (arrow).

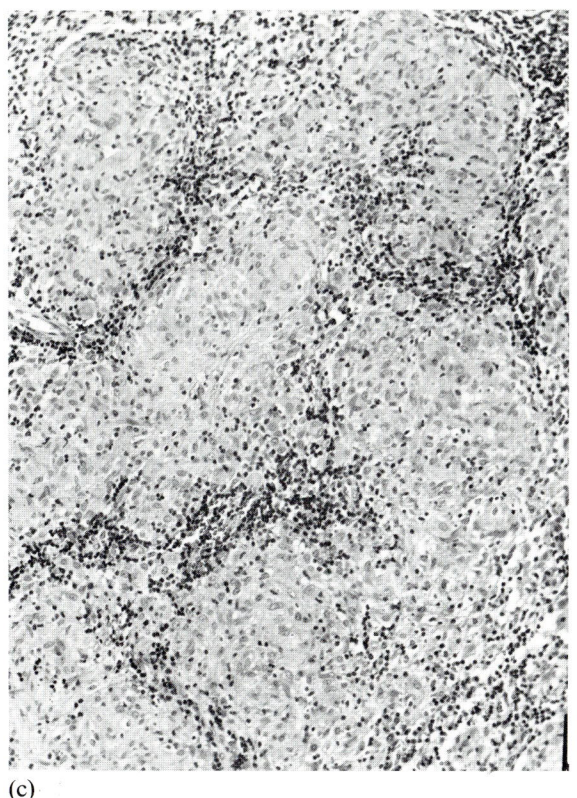

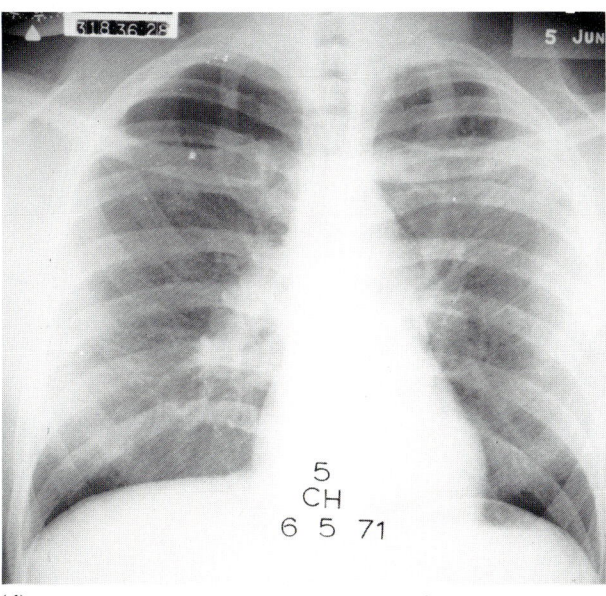

Figure 6.3(c) Cervical lymph-node biopsy showing non-caseating granulomas. (Haematoxylin and eosin. × 125, reduced to seven-tenths in reproduction.) *(d)* Posteroanterior radiograph showing marked clearing of the infiltrate.

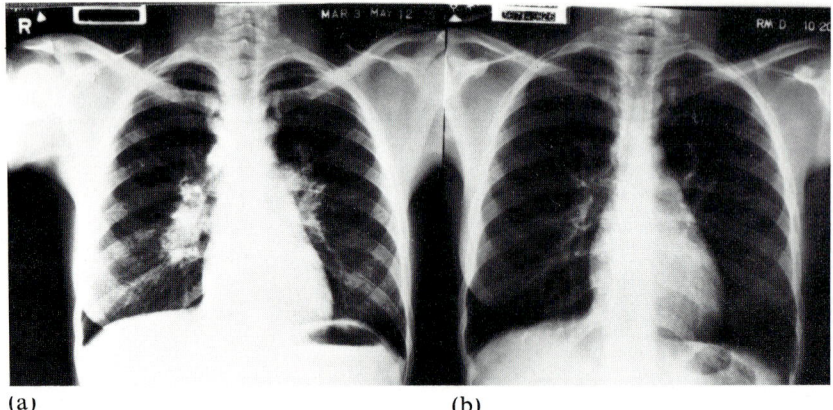

(a) (b)

Figure 6.4(*a*) Bilateral hilar adenopathy and right paratracheal nodes in a young woman. (*b*) After 7 months the chest X-ray film cleared.

Chronic sarcoidosis

Chronic sarcoidosis has a subtle onset and a course that is insidious, progressive and highly variable. In over 90% of patients the chest radiographs show extensive parenchymal infiltration without fibrosis. Lupus pernio, skin plaques, chronic uveitis, glaucoma and persistent parotitis are other frequent findings. Hypercalcaemia and hypercalciuria may lead to nephrocalcinosis and renal failure. Corticosteroids only relieve symptoms and rarely lead to resolution of the structural abnormalities.

References

1. MAYCOCK, R.L., BERTRAND, P., MORRISON, C.E., *et al.* (1963) Manifestations of sarcoidosis: Analysis of 145 patients with a review of nine series selected from the literature. *Am. J. Med.*, **35**, 67.
2. LARSON, E.B., FEATHERSTONE, H.J. and PETERSDORF, R.G. (1982) Fever of undetermined origin: Diagnosis and follow-up of 105 cases 1970–1980. *Medicine*, **61**, 269.
3. JAMES, D.G., NEVILLE, E., SILTZBACH, L.E., *et al.* (1976) A worldwide review of sarcoidosis. *Ann. N.Y. Acad. Sci.*, **278**, 321.
4. HENDRICK, D.J., BLACKWOOD, R.A. and BLACK, J.M. (1976) Chest pain in the presentation of sarcoidosis. *Br. J. Dis. Chest*, **70**, 206.
5. JAMES, D.G. (1961) Clinical concepts of sarcoidosis. *Am. Rev. Resp. Dis.*, **84**, 14.

Chapter 7
Pulmonary sarcoidosis

Common presentations

Lungs are affected in more than 90% of the patients with sarcoidosis. The pulmonary changes on the basis of chest radiograph appearance are conveniently classified into the following broad stages.

Stage 0 (a clear chest radiograph)

5–10% of the patients at the time of initial presentation and during the course of the disease have a normal chest radiograph. Lung function tests, however, may be abnormal. In some of these patients mediastinoscopy and lung biopsy would probably reveal granulomatous inflammation. Four of the 19 patients in stage 0 studied by Marshall and Karlish had a low compliance; one had a significantly reduced carbonmonoxide diffusing capacity[1].

Siltzbach believed that the stage 0 signified a relatively late phase of sarcoidosis; the lung involvement originally present had undergone spontaneous resolution, leaving either chronically florid or fibrosed disease in organs other than the lungs[2]. Others contend that stage 0 represents the earliest phase of the disease.

Bilateral hilar lymphadenopathy (BHL)

This is the earliest abnormality, occurring in more than 50% of all patients with sarcoidosis. Lymph-node enlargement primarily involves the bronchopulmonary, tracheobronchial and paratracheal nodes; there is a translucent space between the enlarged nodes and the cardiovascular margin (*see Figure 7.1*). Because the hilum is better visible on the right the 'space' is clearer on the right side. Hilar adenopathy may be associated with either right paratracheal (25%) or bilateral paratracheal lymphnode enlargement. The 'one-two-three' sign of bilateral hilar and right paratracheal adenopathy is considered classic for the disease. Bilateral paratracheal adenopathy as the sole abnormality, unilateral adenopathy and mediastinal adenopathy are rarely found in sarcoidosis[3].

BHL is the hallmark of acute, early reversible sarcoidosis particularly if associated with erythema nodosum. The differential diagnosis of stage 1 disease includes lymphoma, primary tuberculosis, coccidioidomycosis and metastatic involvement of

30 Pulmonary sarcoidosis

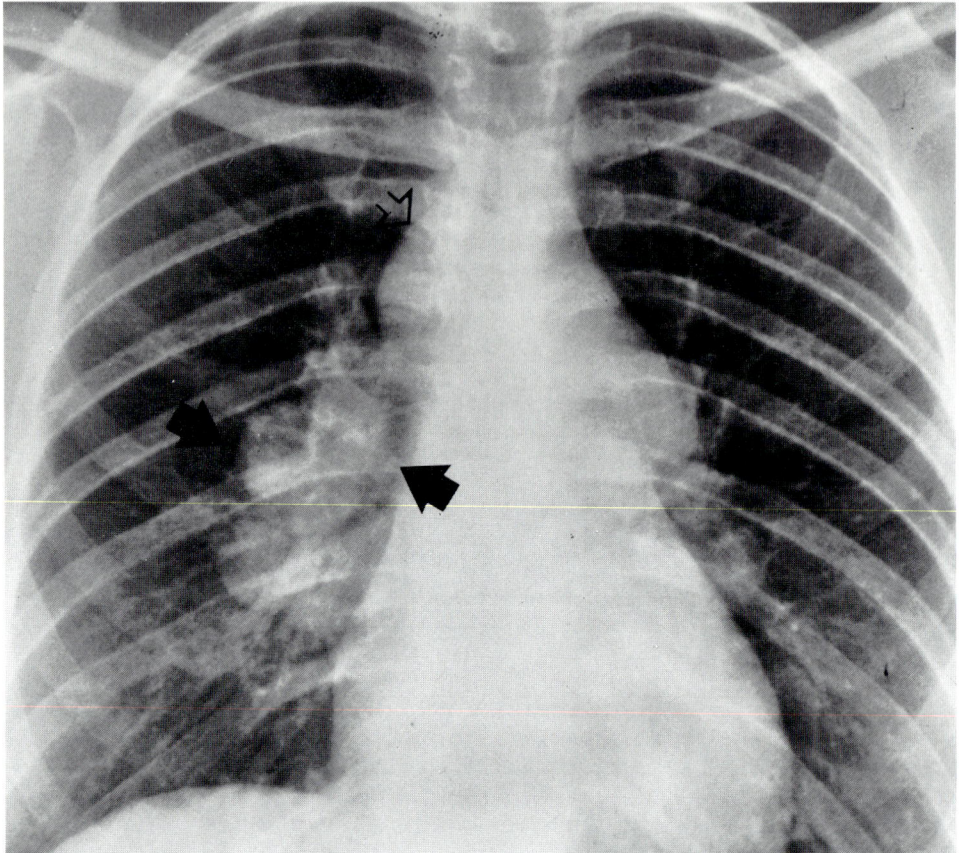

Figure 7.1 Stage I sarcoidosis: bilateral hilar and right paratracheal adenopathy in an asymptomatic patient. Note the translucent space between the right heart margin and the medial border of the right hilar mass (arrow).

nodes due to bronchogenic carcinoma. Some causes of bilateral hilar enlargement are as follows:

1. *Common*—Sarcoidosis, lymphoma, pneumoconiosis, bronchogenic carcinoma, lymph-node metastases, pulmonary hypertension.
2. *Uncommon*—Tuberculosis, histoplasmosis, coccidioidomycosis, phenytoin (Dilantin).
3. *Rare*—Brucellosis, infectious mononucleosis, amyloidosis.

Some causes of unilateral hilar enlargement are:

1. *Common*—Primary tuberculosis, lymphoma, coccidioidomycosis, histoplasmosis, pulmonary valve stenosis, lesion of apical segment of lower lobe.
2. *Uncommon*—Sarcoidosis, amyloidosis, aneurysm of a pulmonary artery, pulmonary embolism, post-stenotic pulmonary artery dilatation.

After analysing 100 patients, Winterbauer *et al.* found that bilateral hilar adenopathy in an asymptomatic patient with a negative physical examination, or in association with erythema nodosum or uveitis, constitute a strong evidence of sarcoidosis. However, bilateral hilar adenopathy in association with anaemia, pleural effusion, anterior mediastinal mass, peripheral lymphadenopathy or hepatosplenomegaly may represent either a neoplasm or lymphoma and need tissue diagnosis[4]. Mediastinal adenopathy in Hodgkin's disease tends to be localized in the anterior and superior mediastinum with a lesser tendency to resemble the 'scalloped' or 'potato' bronchopulmonary nodes due to sarcoidosis (*see Figures 7.2 and 7.3*). Tuberculosis is in the

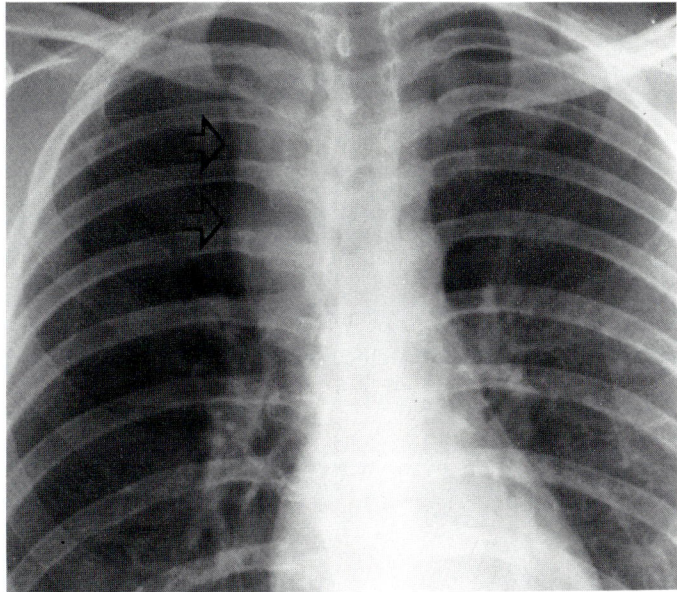

Figure 7.2 Right paratracheal mass (arrows) in a young woman with Hodgkin's disease.

differential diagnosis; however, it should be realized that active tuberculosis was diagnosed in only three out of 397 patients with bilateral hilar adenopathy. In tuberculosis, coccidioidomycosis and neoplasm of the lung the adenitis is usually unilateral (*see Figure 7.4*).

In 60–80% of patients with only bilateral hilar adenopathy, complete or substantial clearing occurs within 2 years. Once the lymph nodes subside spontaneously, they rarely, if ever, enlarge again. About 10% of the patients follow a persistent course. This small group has chronic skin lesions and bone cysts. The remaining 10–15% of the patients with stage I disease may remain stationary or advance only slowly to stage II.

Stage II—bilateral hilar lymphadenopathy and parenchymal infiltration

In 25–30% of the patients, initial chest X-rays show both hilar adenopathy and pulmonary infiltration. As a rule, the parenchymal infiltration is bilateral; rarely, it may be unilateral. The pattern of diffuse parenchymal disease is quite variable, ranging from moderately increased lung marking, through radiographic appearance

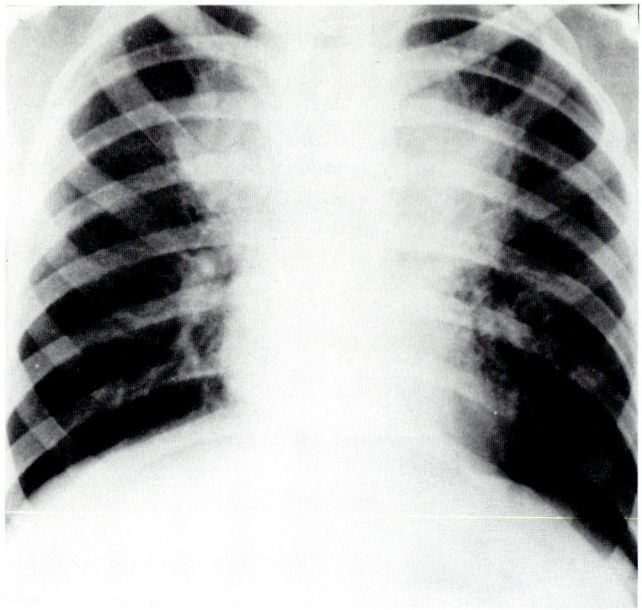

Figure 7.3 Mediastinal mass in a 14-year-old boy with Hodgkin's disease. Hilar adenopathy is not a feature.

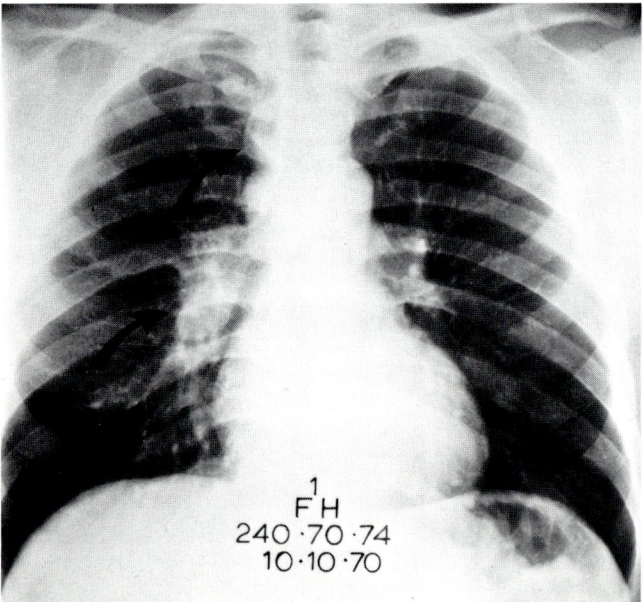

Figure 7.4 Right hilar and right paratracheal adenopathy (arrows) in a young man with primary tuberculosis.

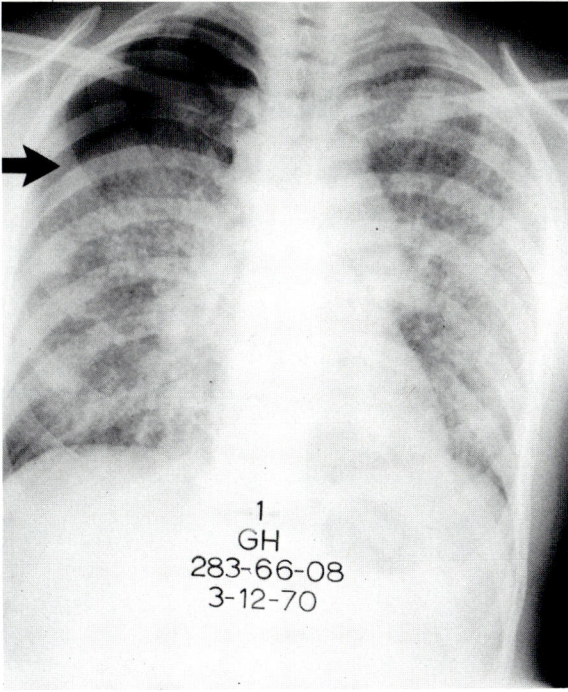

(a)

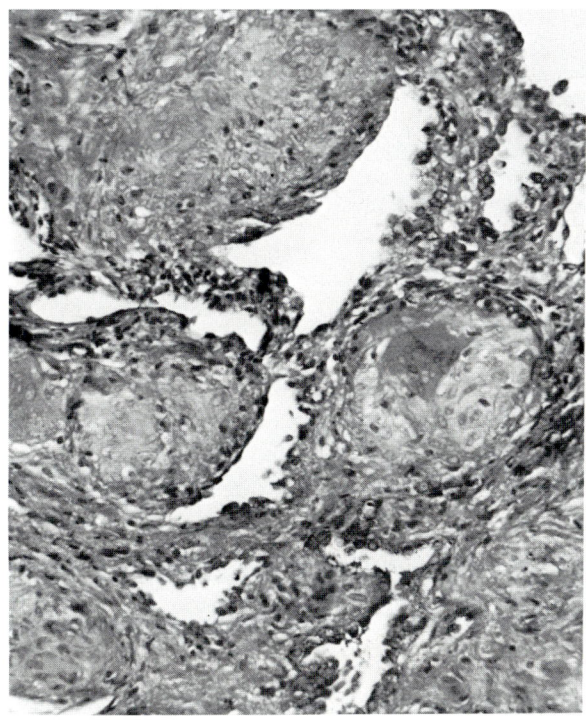

(b)

Figure 7.5(a) Stage II: bilateral hilar and paratracheal adenopathy with diffuse fine nodular infiltrate resembling miliary tuberculosis. Note the right post-bronchial biopsy pneumothorax. (*b*) Non-caseating granuloma in a lung biopsy specimen. (Haematoxylin and eosin. × 100.)

34 Pulmonary sarcoidosis

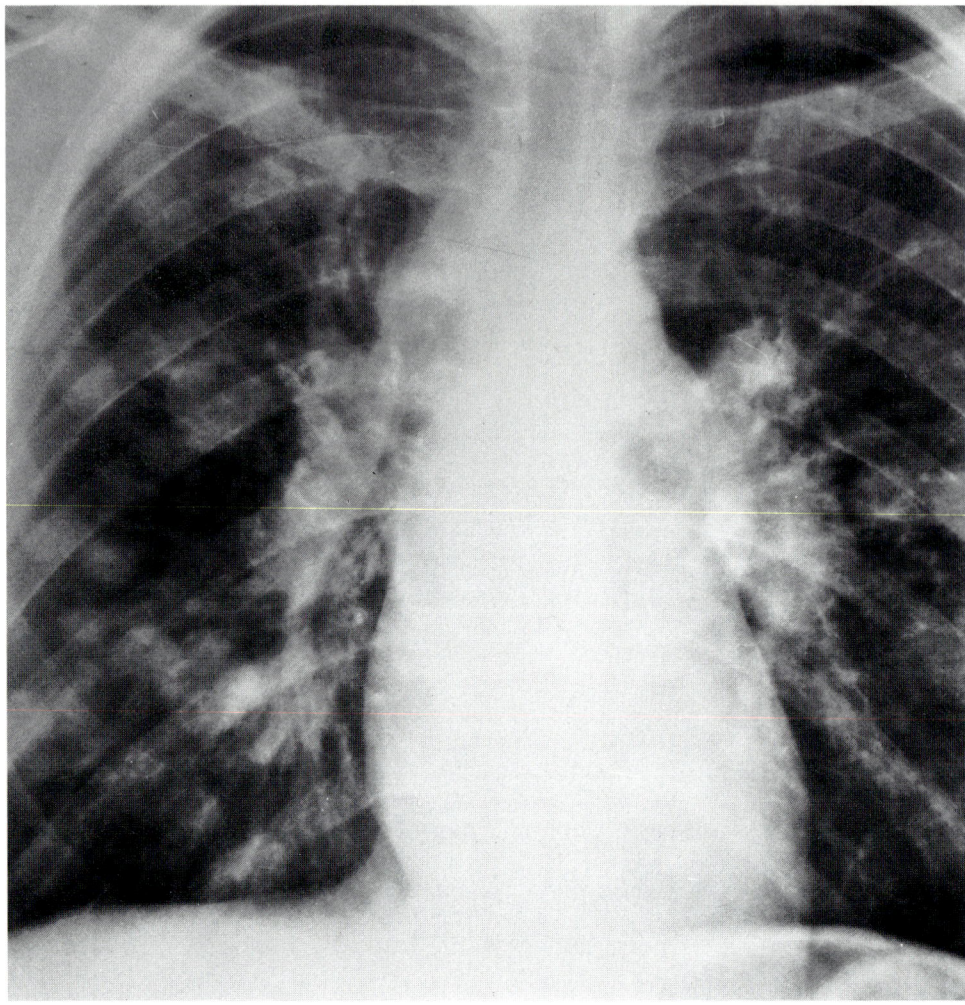

Figure 7.6 Stage II: hilar adenopathy with multiple cannon-balls resembling metastatic neoplasm.

simulating miliary tuberculosis or metastatic neoplasms to extensive interstitial infiltration (*see Figures 7.5–7.7*).

Occasionally, fluffy cotton-wool patches (*see Figure 7.8*) called alveolar sarcoidosis, and multiple cannon-balls scattered over both lungs may occur. The differential diagnosis is as follows:

1. Sarcoidosis.
2. Beryllium lung disease.
3. Silicosis.
4. Tuberculosis.
5. Lymphangitic carcinoma.
6. Coccidioidomycosis.
7. Brucellosis.

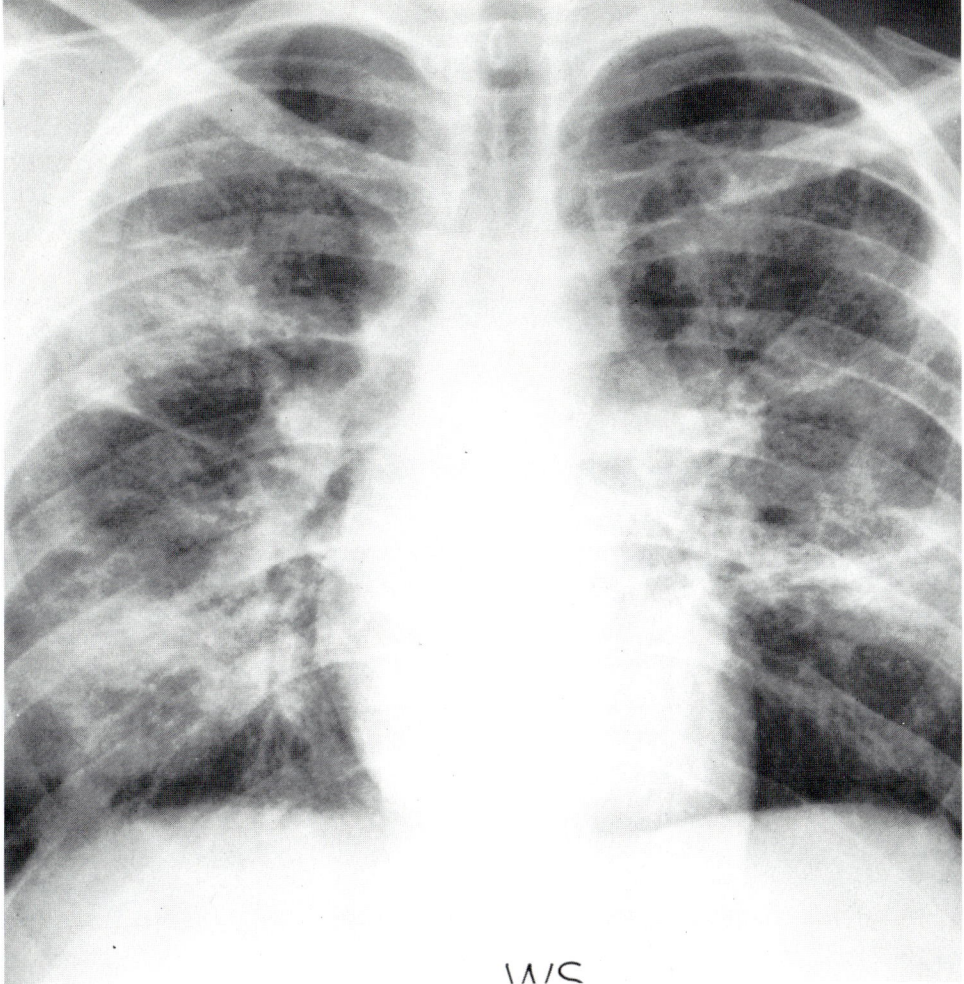

Figure 7.7 Stage II: hilar adenopathy with diffuse interstitial infiltrate, producing a ground-glass haziness.

8. Infectious mononucleosis.
9. Cryptococcosis.

Clinical symptoms in stage II disease are variable and may include fever, weight loss and dyspnoea; some patients remain asymptomatic throughout the course. Symptoms in two-thirds of the patients in stage II eventually resolve; symptoms in the remaining one-third remain stationary or progress to stage III.

Stage III—parenchymal infiltration

About 15% of the patients with sarcoidosis present with a chest X-ray abnormality of widespread parenchymal infiltration without hilar adenopathy. The following three patterns of pulmonary infiltration commonly occur.

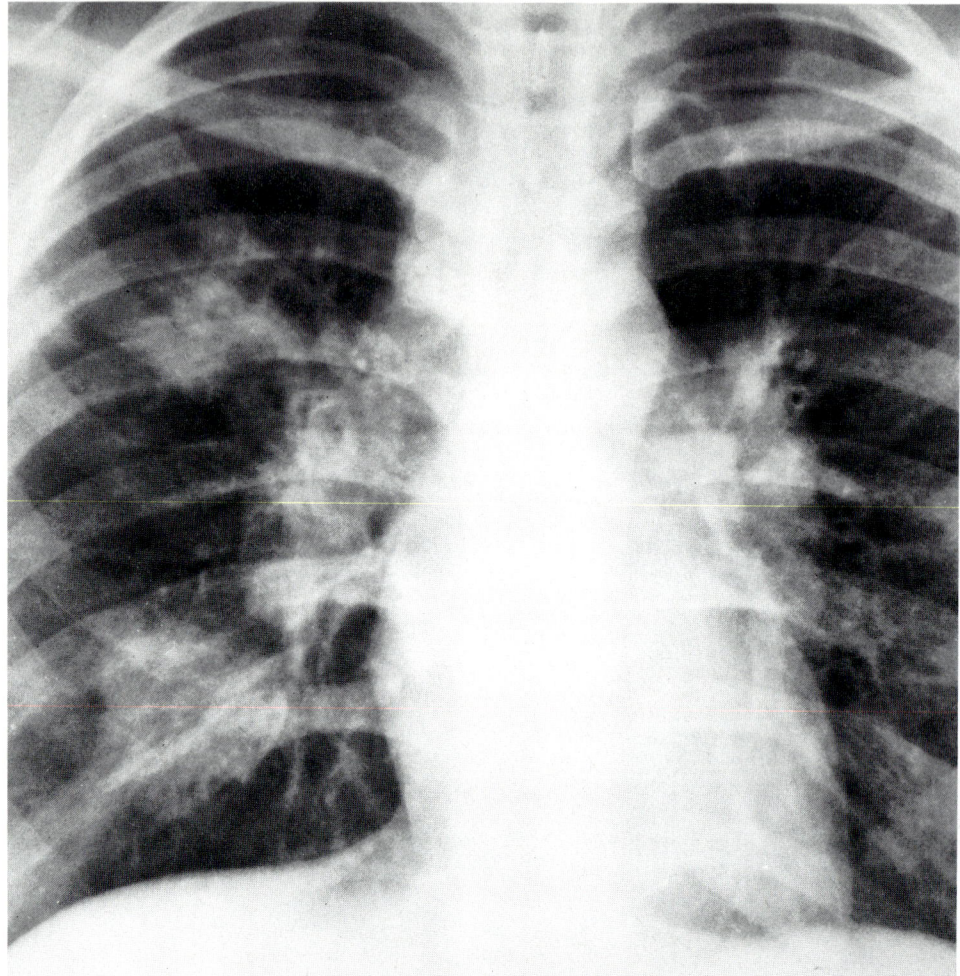

Figure 7.8 Stage II: alveolar sarcoidosis; fluffy cotton-wool patches with bilateral hilar adenopathy.

Reticulonodular

This is the most common parenchymal abnormality and is characterized by a mixture of linear densities and small nodules 3–5 mm in diameter. Rarely, a pure nodular or pure linear pattern may occur. The infiltration is almost always bilateral with a tendency to spare apices or extreme bases (*see Figure 7.9*). Unilateral or localized involvement of the lung parenchyma may also occur (*see Figures 7.10 and 7.11*).

Acinar or alveolar

These shadows consist of coalesced, segmental or lobar infiltrate with fluffy margins. Air bronchograms may be visible. This pattern is most likely due to alveolar filling by inflammatory cells (*see Figure 7.12*).

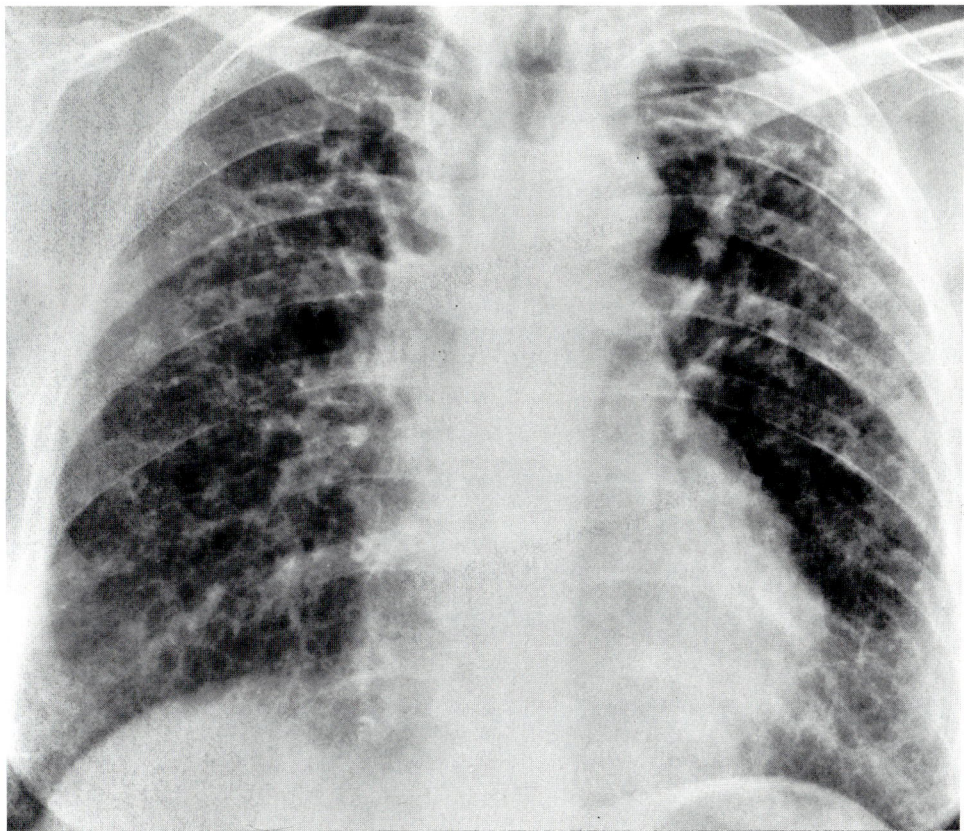

Figure 7.9 Stage III: diffuse linear reticular infiltration.

Nodular

This type of abnormality is discussed on page 51. Dry cough and dyspnoea are the chief symptoms. Occasionally, the cough may be productive of white or yellow sputum. Rarely, haemoptysis may occur. The differential diagnosis at this stage is wide:

1. Fibrosing alveolitis (idiopathic pulmonary fibrosis).
2. Pneumoconiosis.
3. Scleroderma.
4. Rheumatoid lung.
5. Lupus erythematosus.
6. Extrinsic allergic alveolitis.
7. Lymphangitic carcinoma.
8. Tuberculosis (upper lobe disease).
9. Drug reactions.
10. Eosinophilic granuloma.
11. Haemosiderosis.

38 Pulmonary sarcoidosis

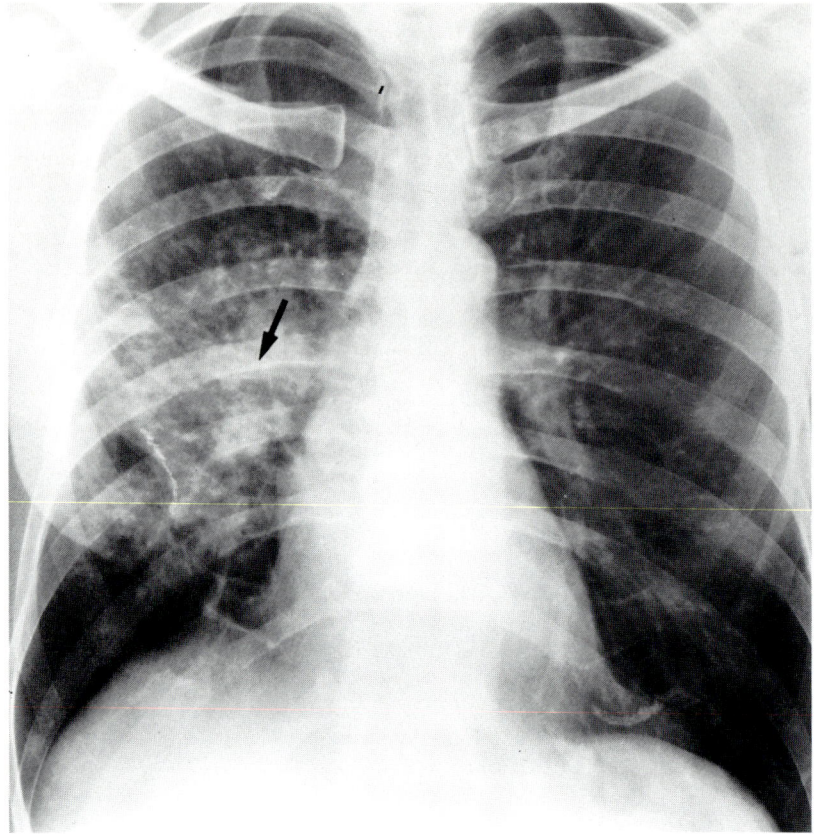

Figure 7.10 Stage III: right mid-lung field infiltrate (arrow) in a middle-aged caucasian business man whose initial presentation was an acute bilateral uveitis. A lung biopsy showed non-caseating granulomas.

Stage IV—irreversible fibrosis/bullae formation

Fibrosis develops in one-fifth of the patients. The lung lesions include irreversible fibrosis with hilar retraction, bullae formation and emphysema (*see Figure 7.13 and 7.14*). The lung retraction usually occurs posteriorly and superiorly. Due to the distortion of the normal pulmonary architecture, the diaphragm becomes 'peaked' or 'tented'. The chest X-ray picture may resemble a number of other conditions, including advanced tuberculosis, silicosis, and chronic non-specific pneumonia. It is conceivable that many patients who are considered to have 'old tuberculosis' on the basis of marked 'upper lobe fibrosis' actually suffer from sarcoidosis. The following case illustrates the point.

A 70-year-old asymptomatic woman was seen for evaluation of progressive pulmonary infiltrate. During the preceding 5 years the patient had been investigated for tuberculosis. Multiple sputum cultures failed to grow acid-fast bacilli. She was given isoniazid and ethambutol but the chest roentgenograms showed worsening of the infiltrate. The patient remained asymptomatic. Physical examination was normal. A

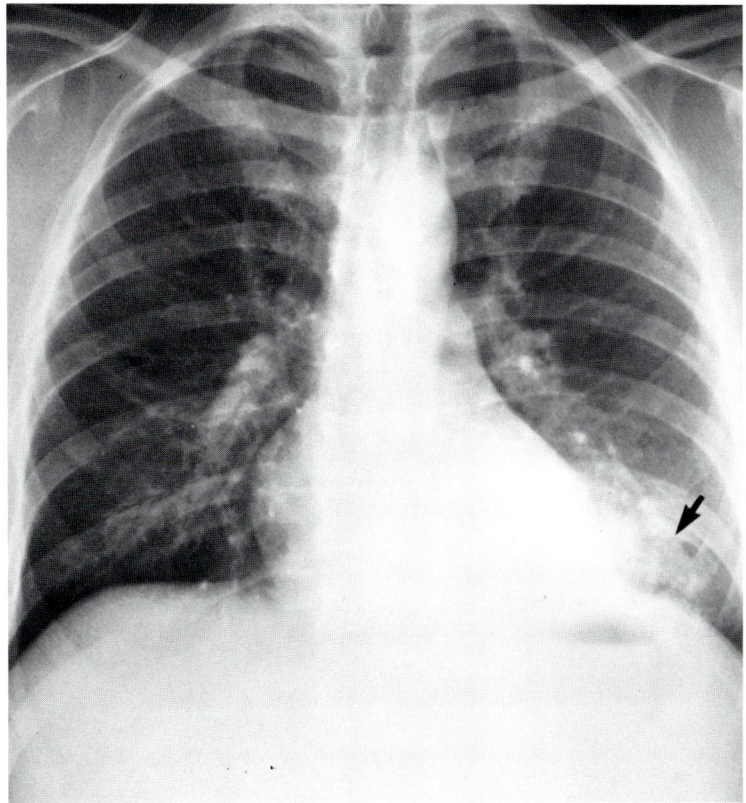

Figure 7.11 Stage III: left lower infiltrate (arrow) in a young Negro man with erythema nodosum and dry cough. A transbronchial biopsy showed non-caseating granulomas. The lesion subsided spontaneously after 6 months.

transbronchial biopsy was performed which showed non-caseating granulomas. Special stains and cultures of the bronchial washings and the lung-biopsy specimens did not show acid-fast bacilli and fungi. She was given prednisone 20 mg once daily. The chest radiograph improved after 3 months of therapy. The prednisone was gradually reduced. After 8 years, the patient remains stable (*see Figures 7.15–7.18*).

Comment — If a chest radiograph abnormality reminds you of diffuse extensive tuberculosis, but sputum cultures and skin tests are repeatedly negative, think of sarcoidosis.

Dyspnoea, cough, and expectoration are the chief symptoms. The patients at this stage suffer from respiratory failure, pneumothorax, and cor pulmonale. Mycetoma (aspergilloma) is the common fungal colonization (*see Figure 7.19*).

40 Pulmonary sarcoidosis

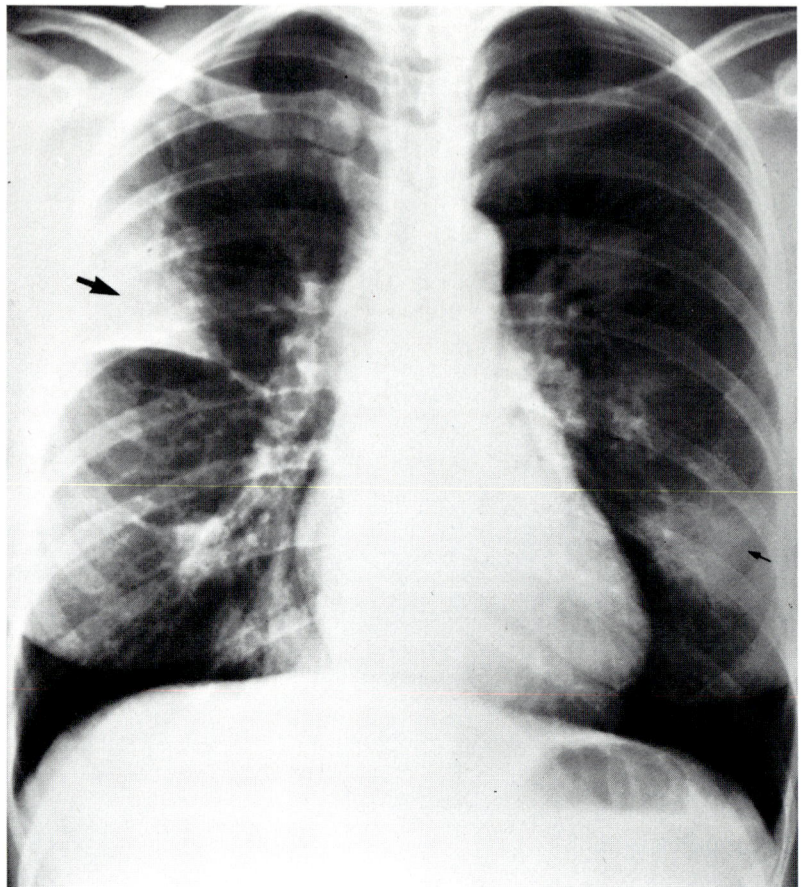

Figure 7.12 Stage III: segmental infiltrate involving the anterior segment of the right upper lobe (arrow) and a fluffy infiltrate in the left lower lobe. The chest radiograph cleared with corticosteroids.

Endobronchial sarcoidosis

The bronchial mucosa is often involved in sarcoidosis. Friedman *et al.* reported that 40% of patients with stage I (bilateral hilar adenopathy) and 70% of patients with stages II and III had non-caseating granulomas in bronchial biopsy specimens[5]. Main, lobar, segmental and subsegmental bronchi may all be involved[6,7]. Gross mucosal abnormalities are uncommon but nodular elevations of 2–3 mm in diameter may be seen during the bronchoscopy. Various patterns, described as 'wart-like excrescences', 'bleb-like elevations' and 'corrugated drain pipe' are unusual. Rarely, the granulomatous involvement may produce narrowing of bronchi with resulting atelectasis and pulmonary infections distal to the obstruction[8]. Occasionally, an isolated endobronchial sarcoid lesion may be the cause of an unexplained pulmonary infiltrate[9].

Although the endobronchial involvement is usually asymptomatic, some patients

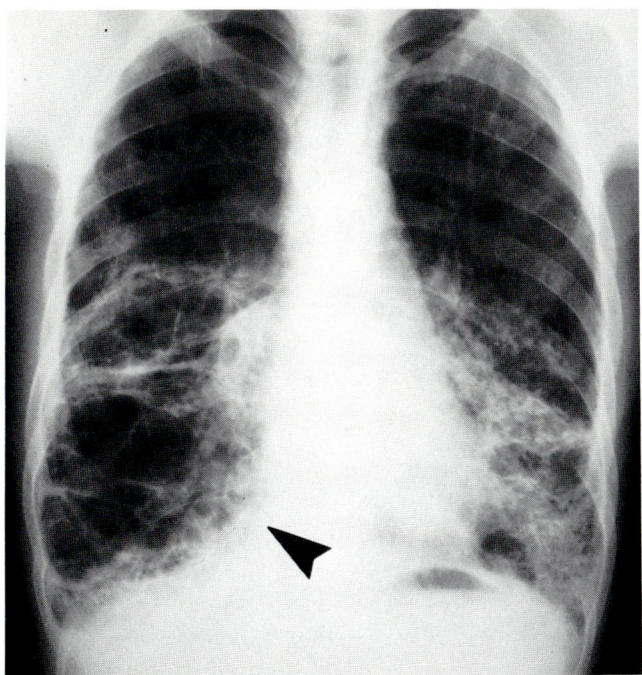

Figure 7.13 Stage IV: extensive fibrosis and bullae formation involving mainly the lower lung fields in a young man who died of cor pulmonale at the age of 32 years.

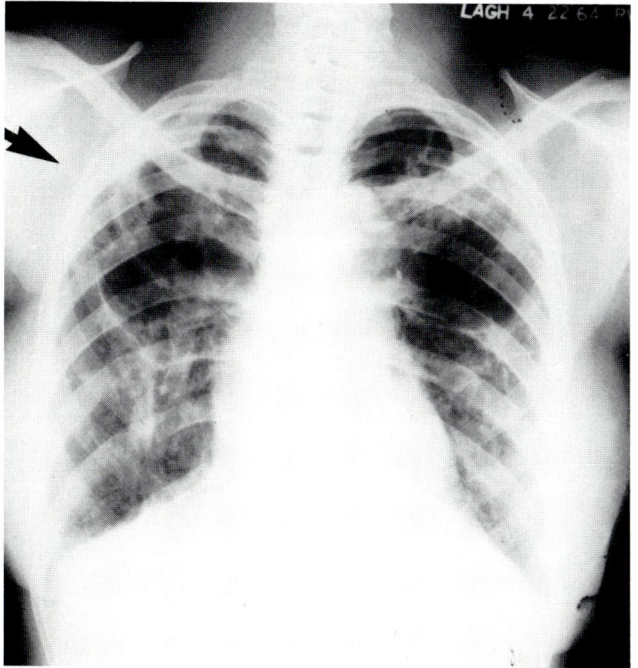

Figure 7.14 Stage IV: fibrosis, retraction of hila and bullae formation (arrow), mainly in the upper lung fields.

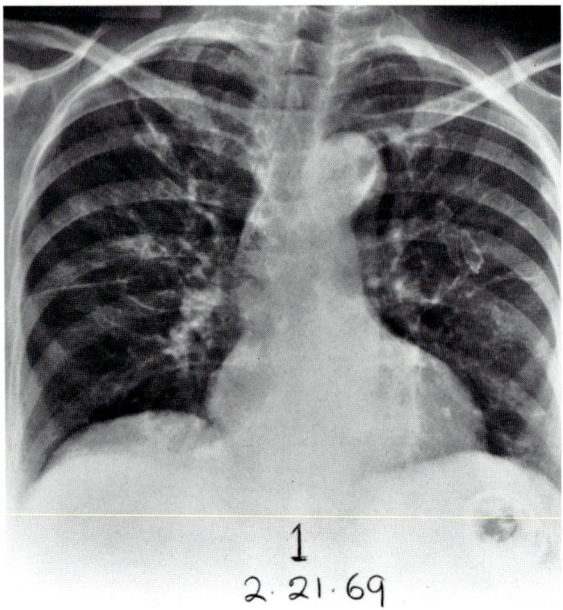

Figure 7.15 Minimal bilateral apical infiltrate. Tuberculin test was negative. There was no evidence of tuberculosis.

may complain of cough, wheezing and haemoptysis. In a patient with sarcoidosis the persistence of a localized pulmonary infiltrate or atelectasis calls for a flexible fibre-optic bronchoscopy. If the biopsy specimen shows non-caseating granulomas, the patient should be treated with corticosteroids.

Pulmonary sarcoidosis: Uncommon presentations

Pleural effusion

Twenty years ago the pleural effusion was considered to be an unusual manifestation of sarcoidosis. The picture, however, changed and during the seventies many excellent papers appeared describing the occurrence of pleural effusion in sarcoidosis[10-14]. About 5% of the patients with sarcoidosis develop a pleural effusion. Solomon *et al.*, using CT scans, found that some degree of pleural disease is present in 35% of sarcoid patients[15]. The effusion may be the initial manifestation of sarcoidosis (*see Figure 7.20*) or may appear any time during the course of the disease. The diagnosis may be delayed if the pleural effusion is the sole radiological manifestation. The effusion may be right sided or left sided; bilateral effusions are uncommon. It may be associated with hilar adenopathy or pulmonary infiltrate (*see Figure 7.21*).

In earlier reports of sarcoid pleural effusion, higher protein concentrations and lymphocytosis were observed. Lymphocytosis was present in seven (70%) of 10 patients; and the pleural fluid protein concentration of $4.0\,\text{g}.100\,\text{ml}^{-1}$ ($40\,\text{g}.\ell^{-1}$) or higher was present in nine (69%) of 13 patients studied by us (*see Table 7.1*). Bloody fluid has also been reported[16].

Most of the effusions clear within 2–3 months, but some progress to chronic pleural

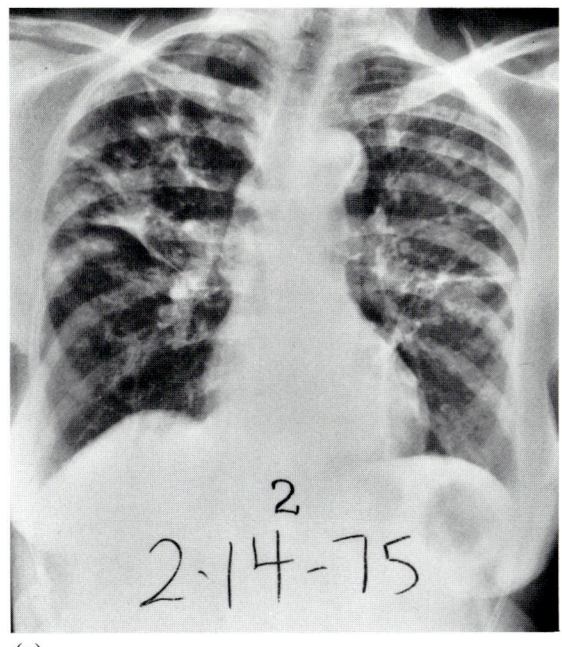
(a)

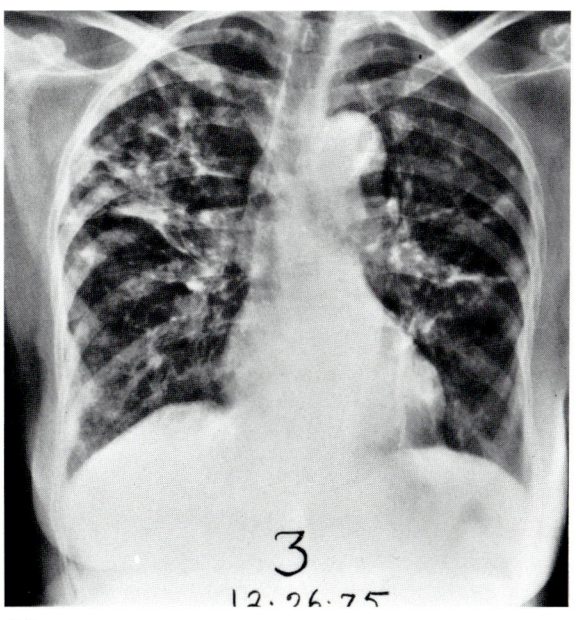
(b)

Figure 7.16(a) The pulmonary infiltration shown in *Figure 7.15* has worsened. No evidence of tuberculosis was found but the patient received isoniazid and ethambutol. (*b*) Pulmonary infiltration worsened on antituberculosis drugs. A transbronchial biopsy showed non-caseating granulomas. There was no evidence of tuberculosis or fungi in tissue cultures.

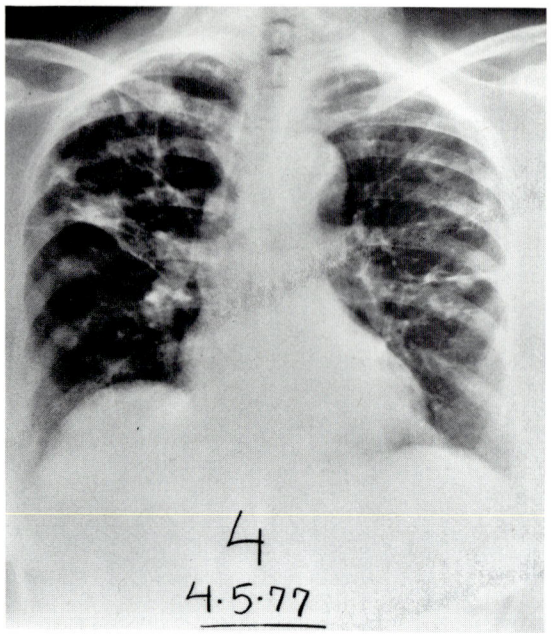

Figure 7.17 Infiltrate shown in *Figures 7.15* and *7.16* cleared with prednisone 20 mg daily.

TABLE 7.1. Pleural fluid: laboratory tests

Patient	Appearance	Amount aspirated (ml)	Specific gravity	Cells	Protein (g.(100ml)$^{-1}$)*	Glucose (mg.(100ml)$^{-1}$)*
1	Cloudy yellow	130	1.020	Lymphocytes	6.5	40
2	Yellow	50	1.016	Lymphocytes	3.8	80
3	Straw coloured	38	1.016	None	4.0	70
4	Serous	170	1.017	None	5.7	68
5	Turbid yellow	25	1.014	Lymphocytes	4.6	85
6	Serosanguinous	60	1.018	Not available	5.6	80
7	Serous	50	1.016	Mononuclears	3.6	60
8	Yellow	60	1.017	None	4.8	68
9	Yellowish	65	1.016	Lymphocytes	4.2	Not done
10	Straw coloured	300	1.018	Lymphocytes	4.8	64
11	Straw coloured	180	1.016	Lymphocytes	4.0	60
12	Yellowish	80		Not available	3.8	Not available
13	Straw coloured	95	1.018	Lymphocytes	5.0	85

* Conversion factors: Glucose, 1 mg.(100 ml)$^{-1}$ = 0.555 mmol.ℓ^{-1}; total protein, 1 g.(100 ml)$^{-1}$ = 10 g.ℓ^{-1}.

thickening. Since the pleural effusion in sarcoidosis is not a common event, one should always exclude tuberculosis, fungal diseases and malignancy by obtaining a tissue biopsy and performing tests for appropriate bacteriological and fungal diseases.

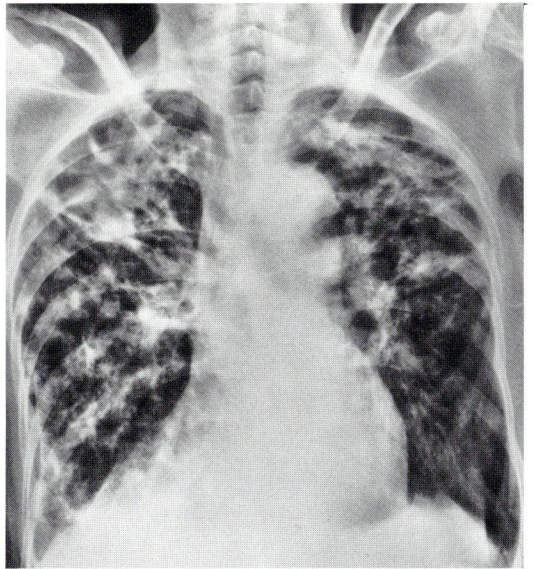

(a)

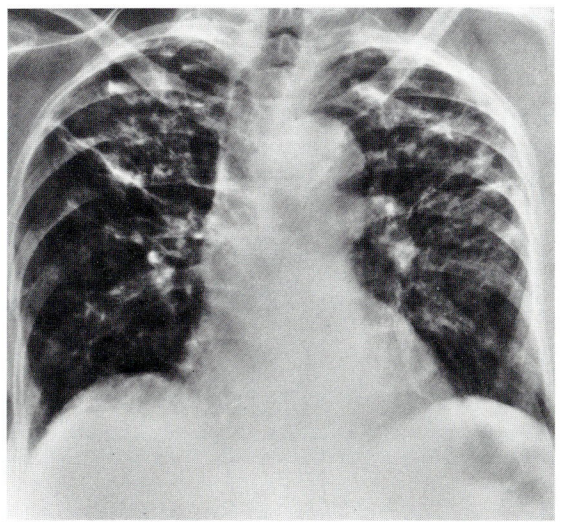

(b)

Figure 7.18(a) Pulmonary changes seen in Figure 7.15 reappeared after prednisone was discontinued. (b) Once again, pulmonary infiltration responded to steroid therapy.

Pneumothorax

The incidence of pneumothorax in sarcoidosis is less than 2%. Whether pneumothorax and sarcoidosis are causally related or are simply two clinical entities occurring independently in the same individual has been the point of some debate. Scadding feels that since both tend to occur in younger people, their association is simply fortuitous[17]. Riley, on the other hand, contends that pneumothorax is directly related to either rupture of a subpleural bleb or necrosis of a subpleural granuloma[18]. Several authors have supported the belief that pneumothorax may result from the rupture of an emphysematous bleb. Because of the rarity of pleural involvement in sarcoidosis,

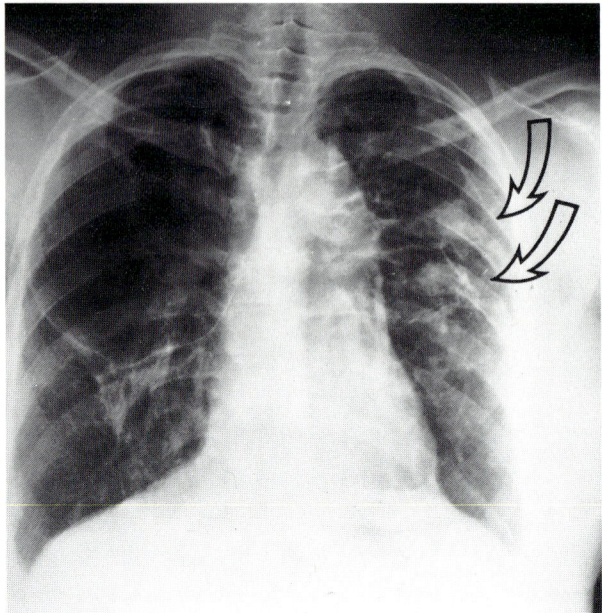

Figure 7.19 Stage IV: extensive fibrosis and bullae formation. Two fungus balls are present in the left upper lobe (arrows).

the theory of subpleural tubercle necrosis leading to pneumothorax has not received much attention.

The patient described below had five episodes of spontaneous pneumothorax involving both lungs. No further episodes occurred following corticosteroid therapy. In this patient a pneumothorax was present at the time of initial presentation, whereas in the other four the pneumothorax appeared during the follow-up period. I believe that in certain cases, necrosis of subpleural tubercles is responsible for pneumothorax in sarcoidosis; therefore, an adequate, early corticosteroid therapy might be beneficial.

Case report—A 35-year-old woman was admitted with severe shortness of breath and right-sided chest pain. The chest radiograph demonstrated a large right pneumothorax, large bullae on the right side and diffuse interstitial fibrosis on the left. A chest tube was inserted. The patient improved and was discharged from the hospital. After 6 weeks, she was readmitted because of dyspnoea. Following demonstration of a right pneumothorax (*see Figure 7.22*), a chest tube was again inserted. Because of a persistent large air leak, plication of the right upper lobe bullae was performed together with biopsy of the lung, pleura and lymph nodes. All specimens showed non-caseating granulomas and were negative on smear and culture for acid-fast bacteria and fungi. The chest tube was removed after a week. On the same day, a left pneumothorax occurred. Ten days later the left chest tube was removed but pneumothorax recurred the following day and the tube was replaced. Five days later a small right pneumothorax occurred and required another tube. Three days later corticosteroids were started. After 2 weeks both chest tubes were taken out and the patient was discharged on prednisone 40 mg. She has been continued on decreasing doses of prednisone for about 1 year. She has had no recurrences of pneumothorax.

I have followed up four other patients for more than 5 years. In none of these patients did pneumothorax develop after steroid therapy (*see Table 7.2*).

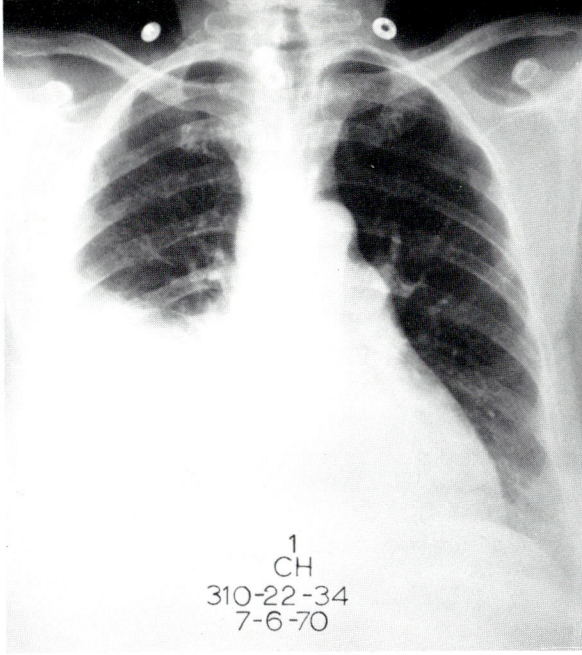

(a)

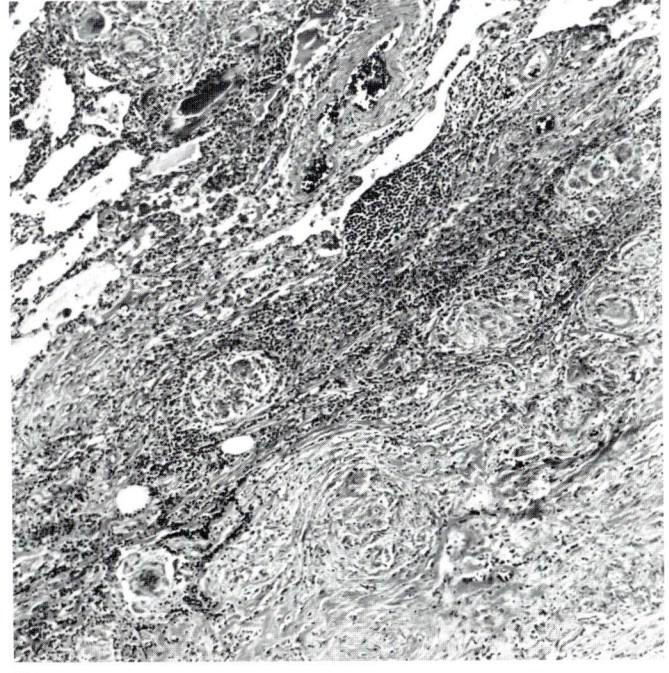

(b)

Figure 7.20(a) Right pleural effusion was the presenting feature of sarcoidosis in this young Negro woman. (*b*) A pleural biopsy specimen showing non-caseating granuloma. Pleural fluid and tissue cultures did not grow acid-fast bacilli or fungi. (Haematoxylin and eosin. × 75, reduced to three-quarters in reproduction.)

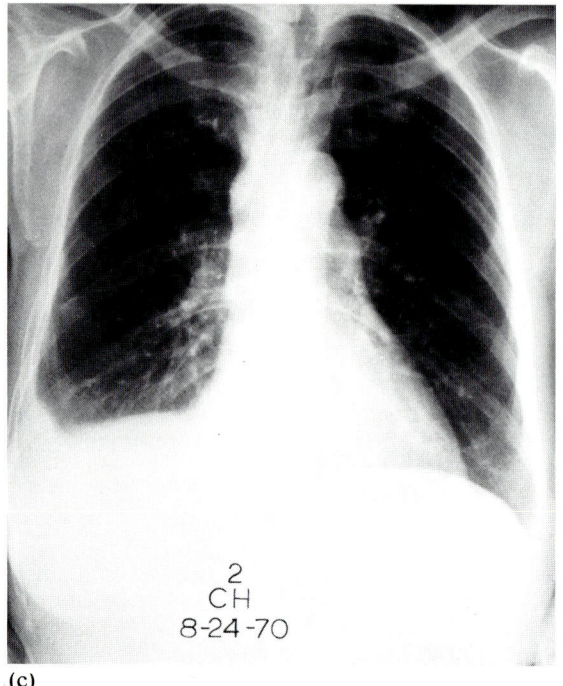
(c)

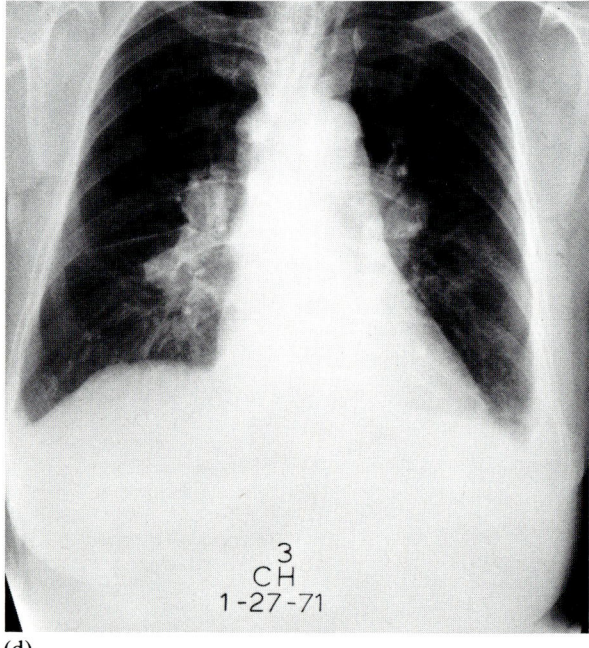
(d)

Figure 7.20(c) The fluid was tapped. (*d*) After 5 months bilateral hilar adenopathy appeared. The patient was asymptomatic.

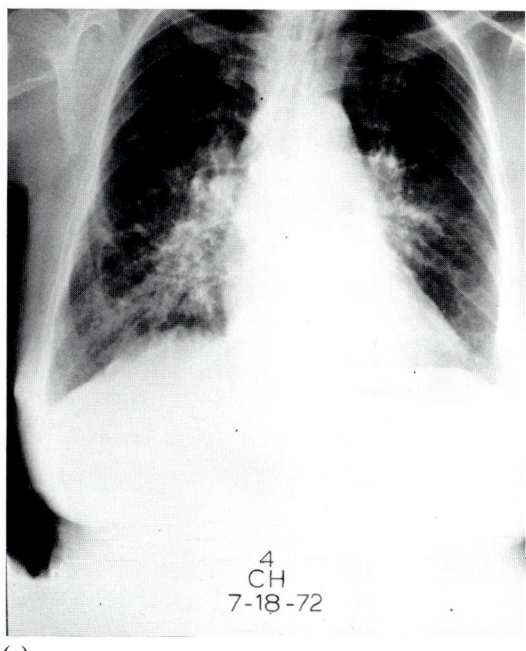

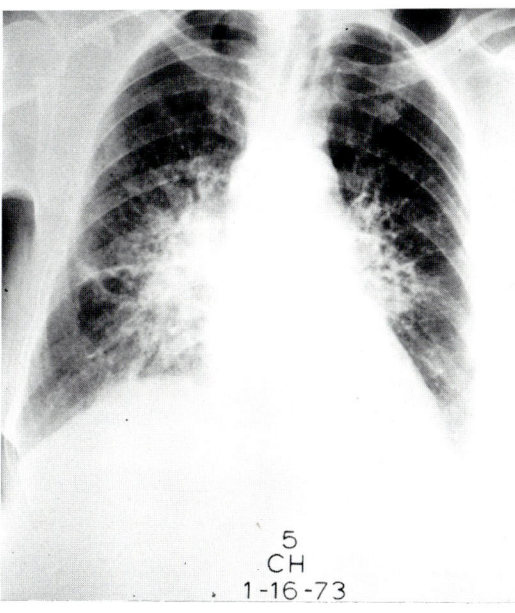

Figure 7.20(e) After 18 months the patient returned with shortness of breath. Hilar nodes have shrunk but bilateral interstitial infiltrate has appeared. There is no pleural effusion. (*f*) The patient was given prednisone. After 6 months the infiltration has progressed slightly.

50 Pulmonary sarcoidosis

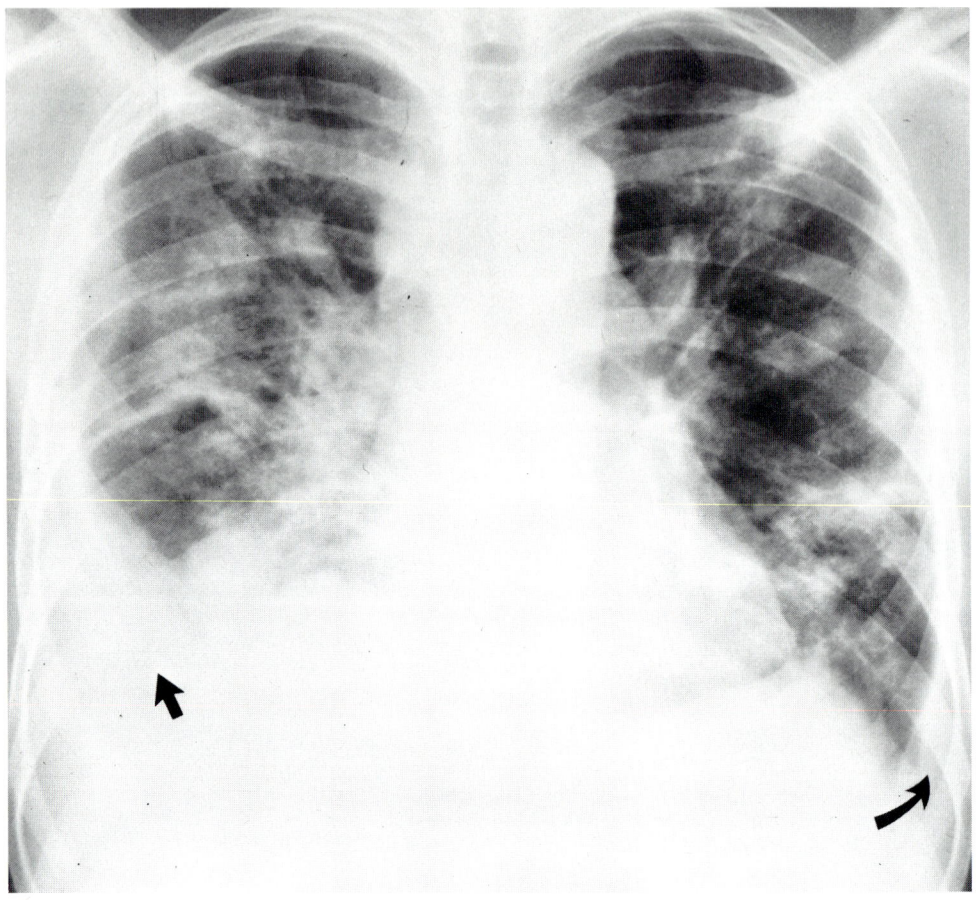

Figure 7.21 Bilateral pleural effusion (arrows) in a Negro man with bilateral hilar adenopathy and multiple pulmonary nodules (state II).

TABLE 7.2. Pneumothorax in sarcoidosis. Summary of four patients with pneumothorax

Patient	Age (years)	Sex	Clinical features	Chest X-ray stage	Pneumothorax	Biopsy	Treatment
1	30	M	Cough, dyspnoea	III	Right side	Mediastinal node	Corticosteroids, chest tube (5-years follow-up)
2	57	F	Dyspnoea, weight loss	III	Right side	Scalene node	Corticosteroids, chest tube (10-year follow-up)
3	34	F	Cough, dyspnoea	III	Right side	Scalene node	Corticosteroids (8-year follow-up)
4	33	F	Chest pain, dyspnoea	III	Left side	Lung	Corticosteroids (5-year follow-up)

Nodular sarcoidosis

Multiple circular or oval pulmonary densities on a chest X-ray most commonly represent neoplastic metastases. Such densities may also be seen in infectious diseases (tuberculosis, histoplasmosis, coccidioidomycosis), immunological disorders (Wegener's granulomatosis, rheumatoid lung), pneumoconiosis, bronchial adenoma, hamartoma and pulmonary A-V malformations. How often do the pulmonary nodules occur in sarcoidosis? The exact incidence is not known but it is less than 5%[19-22]. Nodular lesions were present in 10 of my patients with biopsy-proved sarcoidosis. Clinical and radiological data on these patients are summarized in *Table 7.3*. Several points deserve comment. Eight of the 10 patients were Negro. All were under the age of 40 years at the time of onset. Eight patients had bilateral hilar adenopathy and two

TABLE 7.3. Nodular sarcoidosis: clinical and laboratory findings*

Patient	Age (years), sex	Clinical symptoms	Chest X-ray features	Diagnostic biopsy	Serum globulin $(g.(100\,ml)^{-1})$*
1	31, F	Fever, enlarged parotid and lacrimal glands	BHL, MPN	Hilar node	4.2
2	20, M	Fever, weight loss, night sweats	BHL, MPN	Lung	4.8
3	21, F	Fever, erythema nodosum	BHL, MPN	Lung	4.6
4	38, M	Weight loss, chest pain	MPN	Lung	5.0
5	39, M	Uveitis	BHL, MPN	Conjunctiva	4.2
6	21, F	Cough, weight loss	BHL, MPN	Mediastinal node	4.4
7	22, M	Asymptomatic	BHL, MPN	Lung, mediastinal node	5.2
8	30, F	Fever, erythema nodosum	BHL, MPN	Mediastinal node	6.0
9	25, M	Asymptomatic	MPN	Lung	4.8
10	29, M	Asymptomatic	BHL, MPN	Lung	5.0

* A tuberculin test was negative in all patients.
† Conversion factor: $1\,g.(100\,ml)^{-1} = 10\,g.\ell^{-1}$. Normal range = $3-4\,g.(100\,ml)^{-1}$ $(30-40\,g.\ell^{-1})$.
BHL = Bilateral hilar lymphadenopathy; MPN = Multiple pulmonary nodules.

had pleural effusion. Nodular lesions varied in size from less than 1 cm to 4 cm in diameter. Most of the lesions had well-circumscribed borders but in some there was coalescence and the true margins became indistinct (*see Figure 7.23*). Many of these patients suffered from systemic effect of sarcoidosis—fever, anorexia and weight loss. Initially some of the patients were considered to have either an infection or a malignancy and the diagnosis was established by a transbronchial or an open-lung biopsy. The following case is a good example of nodular sarcoidosis.

Case report—At the age of 28, this man developed chest pain, vague fatigue and weight loss. Physical examination was normal. A chest radiograph showed multiple cannon-balls (*see Figure 7.23*). Tuberculin, histoplasmin and coccidioidin skin tests were negative. An intravenous pyelogram was normal. Microscopic examination of the tissue obtained by scalene node and open-lung biopsy showed non-caseating

52 Pulmonary sarcoidosis

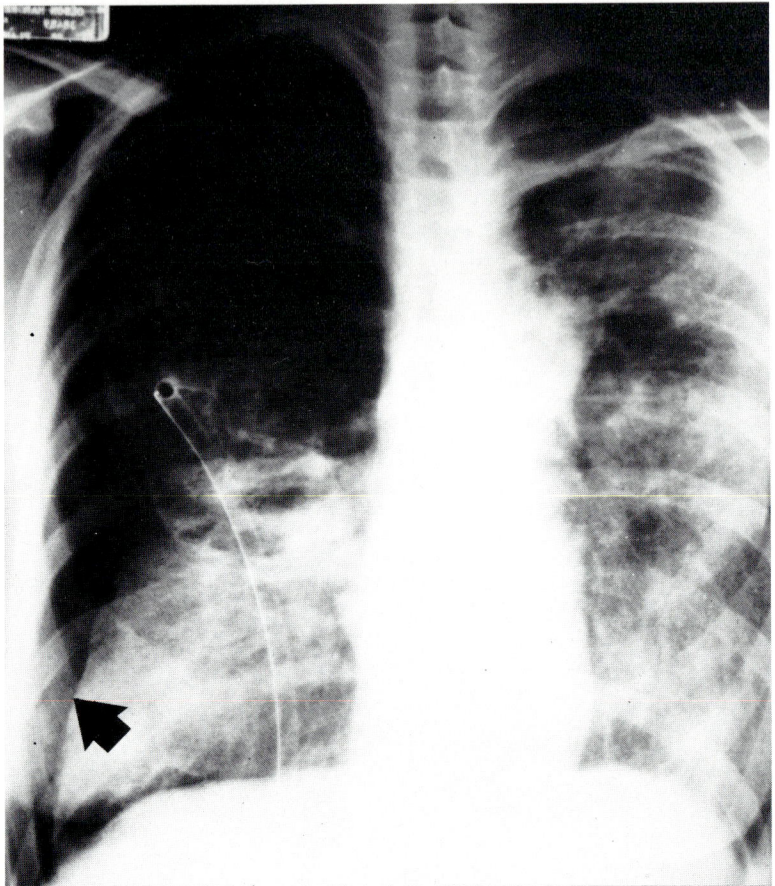

Figure 7.22 Pneumothorax (arrow) in a 35-year-old patient with extensive parenchymal lung disease. (*a*) before and (*b*) after treatment.

granulomas. The patient was given separate courses of corticosteroids and azathioprine. After 4 years his chest radiograph has remained unchanged. He remains asymptomatic.

Cavitary sarcoidosis

There have been only a few reports of cavitation in pulmonary sarcoidosis. Some of these descriptions raise the question whether sarcoidosis was the primary cause of the cavity. Schiffner reviewed 10 patients with cavitary sarcoidosis from the literature and concluded that the true pulmonary cavitation related to necrosis of granulomatous tissue was uncommon[23]. Rohatgi and Schwab described three more patients with primary cavities[24].

Sarcoid cavities usually occur in younger patients. The cavity may be present at the time of initial visit (*see* case report below) or it may develop during the course of the disease. The cavities are usually round; they may be thin or thick walled, solitary or multiple, and range from 3 to 5 cm in diameter. The primary sarcoid cavity is caused

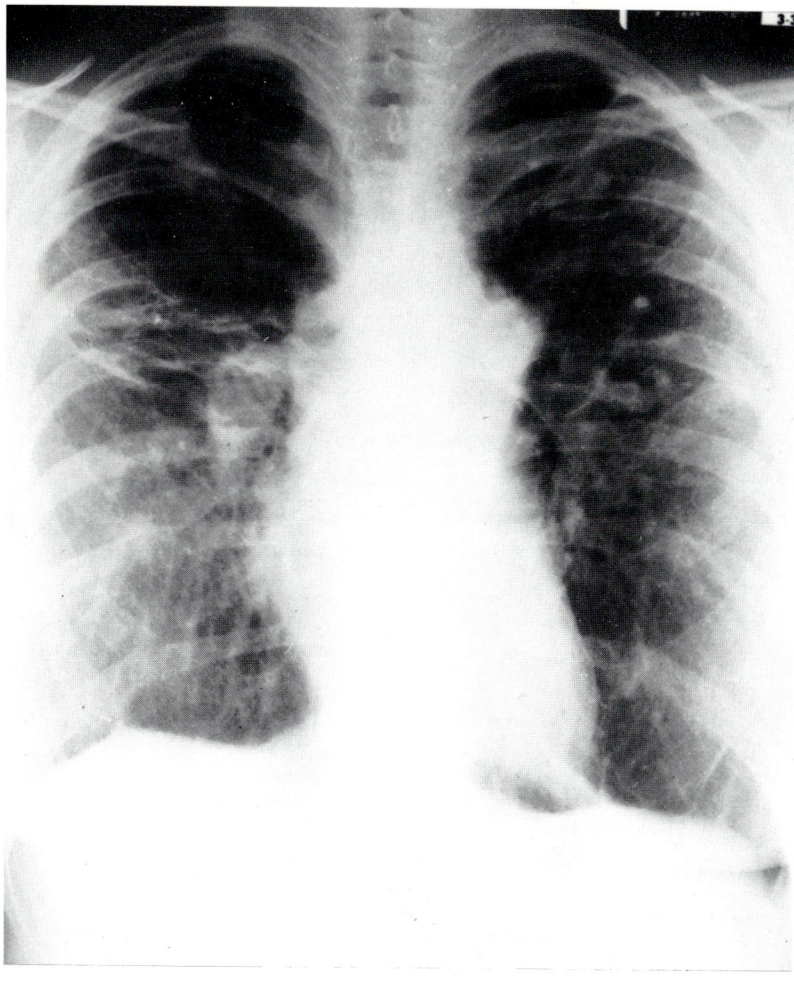

(b)

by necrosis of the granulomatous mass[25]. It must be emphasized that other causes such as mycobacteria, fungi, parasites and pyogenic organisms must be excluded by appropriate laboratory and biopsy studies before the diagnosis of primary sarcoid cavity can be accepted (*see Table 7.4*).

TABLE 7.4. **Diagnosis of sarcoid cavity**

Parameter	Primary	Secondary
Cause	Granulomatous necrosis	Infection (TB, fungi, bacteria)
Size	Less than 5 cm	Greater than 5 cm
Number	Single or multiple	Single
Appearance	Round, thin walled	Thick walled, irregular
Treatment	Corticosteroids	Appropriate antibiotics

54 Pulmonary sarcoidosis

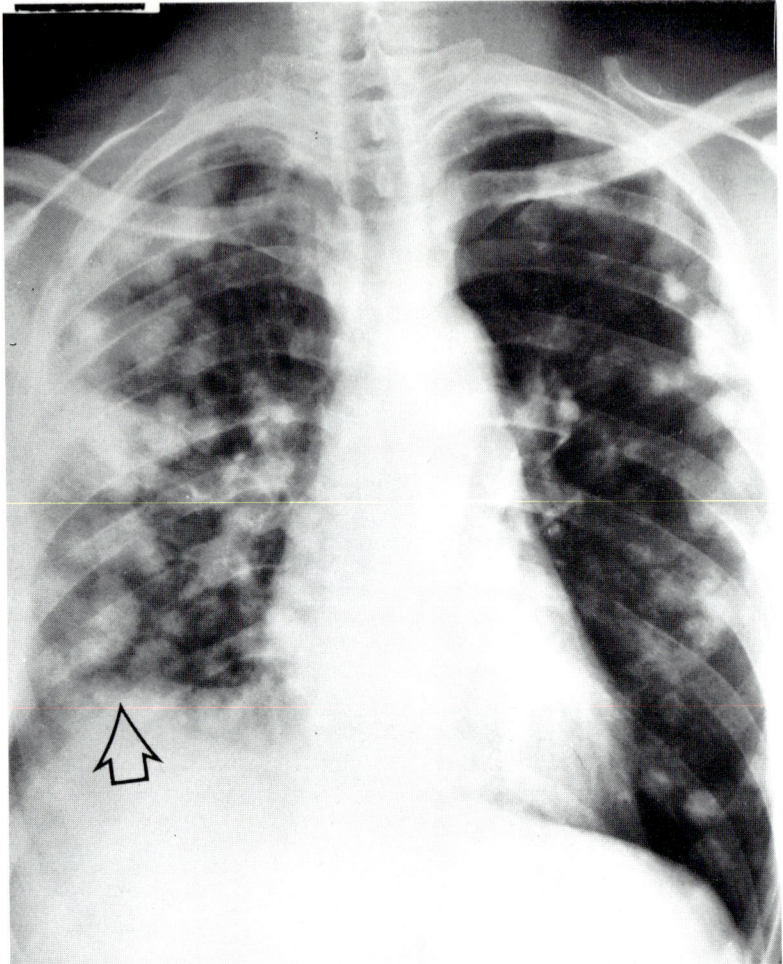

Figure 7.23 Nodular sarcoidosis.

Case report—Dyspnoea, cough, fever and spotty haemoptysis were the main complaints of this 33-year-old Negro man. He had been in good health until 3 months previously. Tuberculin and coccidioidin skin tests were negative. Sputum cultures failed to grow any fungi or acid-fast bacilli. A chest roentgenogram showed diffuse interstitial infiltration with a thin-walled cavity in the right upper lobe (*see Figure 7.24a*). Increased gallium-67 uptake was noted in the lungs and the parotid areas. A transbronchial lung-biopsy specimen showed non-caseating granulomas. He was given corticosteroids. After a few weeks his cavity disappeared, the lung infiltrate diminished and the parotids became smaller (*see Figure 7.24b*). In this patient cavitary sarcoidosis responded to corticosteroids.

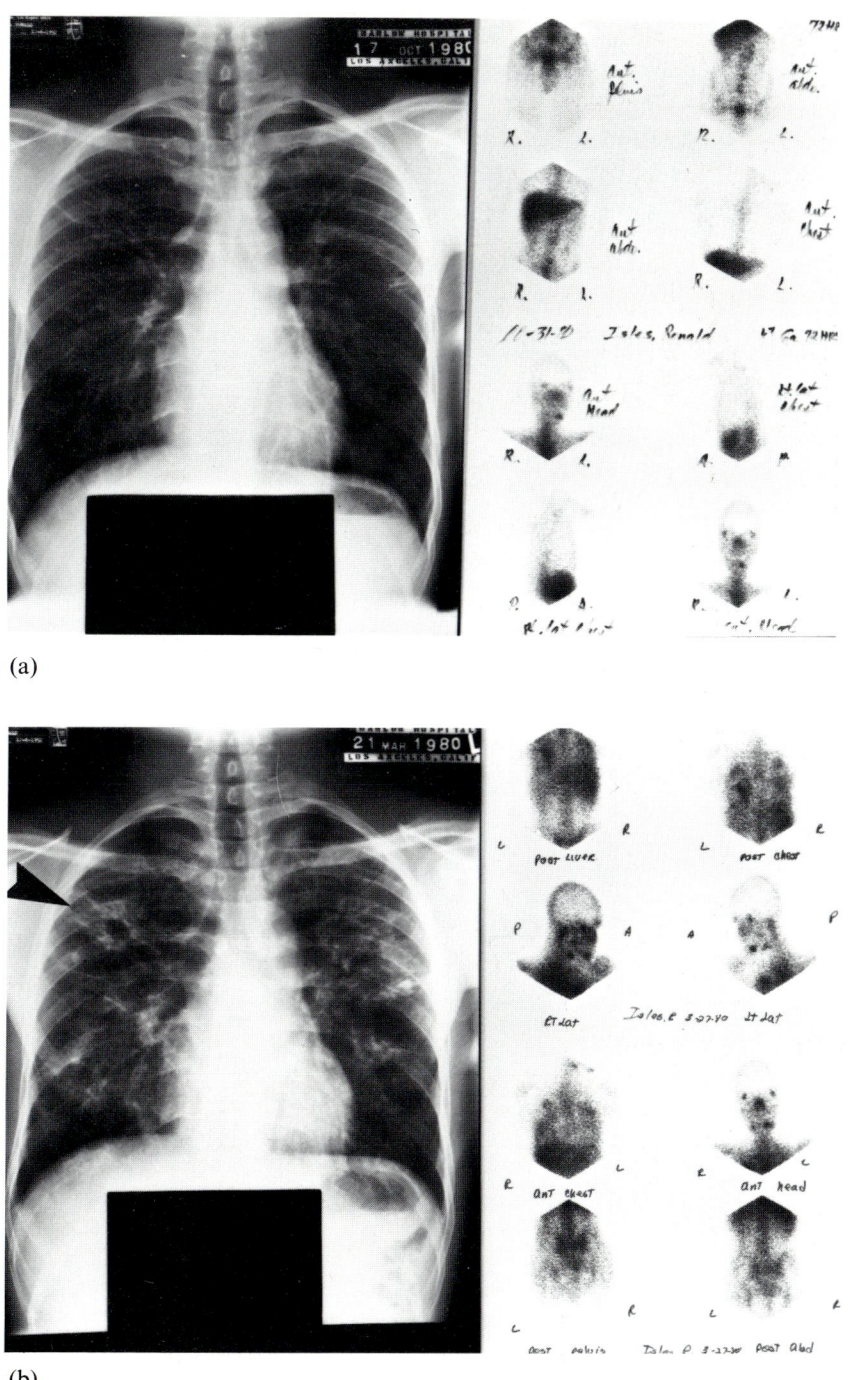

(a)

(b)

Figure 7.24(*a*) Thin-walled cavity and diffuse pulmonary infiltration in a 33-year-old man. Increased gallium-67 uptake is noticed in the lungs, salivary and lacrimal glands. (*b*) After 6 months of therapy the pulmonary infiltration regressed and salivary glands were smaller.

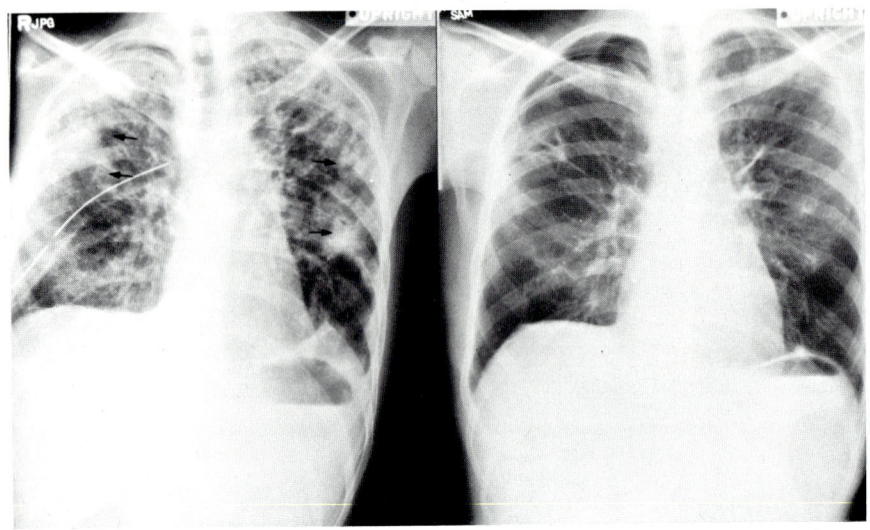

(a)   (b)

Figure 7.25 Chronic eosinophilic pneumonia before (*a*) and after (*b*) therapy.

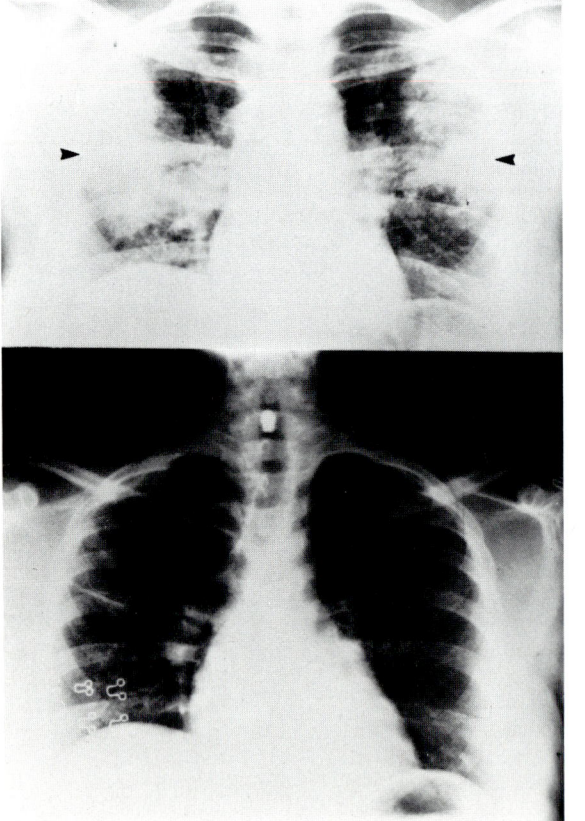

(a)

(b)

Figure 7.26 Hilar adenopathy and peripheral lung densities in a 31-year-old woman with sarcoidosis. (*a*) Before and (*b*) after corticosteroid therapy.

Peripheral infiltration with eosinophilia

The chest X-ray picture of dense pulmonary infiltrate occupying peripheral areas of the lungs is considered typical of chronic eosinophilic pneumonia (*see Figure 7.25*). Lung biopsy specimens show intra-alveolar exudate consisting of eosinophils, lymphocytes, macrophages and occasional histiocytic giant cells.

Three patients with multisystem sarcoidosis showed chest radiographic evidence of peripheral pulmonary infiltrates; two of the three had mild eosinophilia in peripheral blood. Lung biopsy specimens in all the three patients showed non-caseating granulomas; two had a positive Kveim–Siltzbach test.

Case report—A 31-year-old woman came to the hospital with 'redness' and 'blurry' vision of both eyes, fever and swollen parotid and lacrimal glands. A chest radiograph showed bilateral peripheral densities. She was given prednisone 30 mg daily. Her chest X-ray cleared within 10-weeks (*see Figure 7.26*). Thus sarcoidosis should be added to the list of causes of peripheral infiltration with eosinophilia syndrome (*see Figure 7.27*).

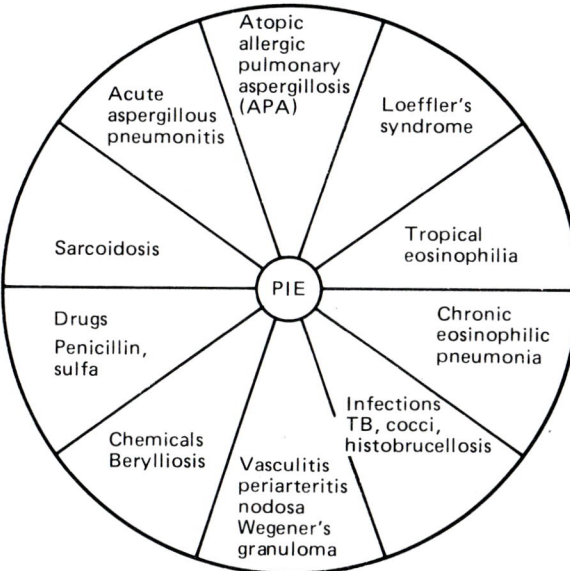

Figure 7.27 Causes of pulmonary infiltration with eosinophilia (PIE) syndrome.

Calcification

Calcification of the hilar lymph nodes occurs in about 5–10% of patients (*see Figure 7.28*). It occurs in chronic disease and is associated with extensive pulmonary fibrosis. Parenchymal calcification is rare. The differential diagnosis usually consists of tuberculosis, histoplasmosis, and healed varicella pneumonia. Occasionally, egg-shell calcification—a characteristic finding of silicosis—may also be found in sarcoidosis[26]. The use of CT scans will unearth more cases of calcification in sarcoidosis, because the technique is more sensitive in detecting minimal calcific deposits than conventional

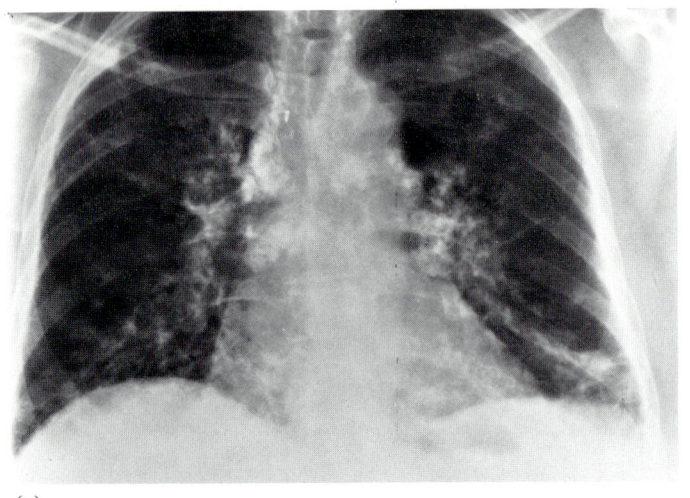

(a)

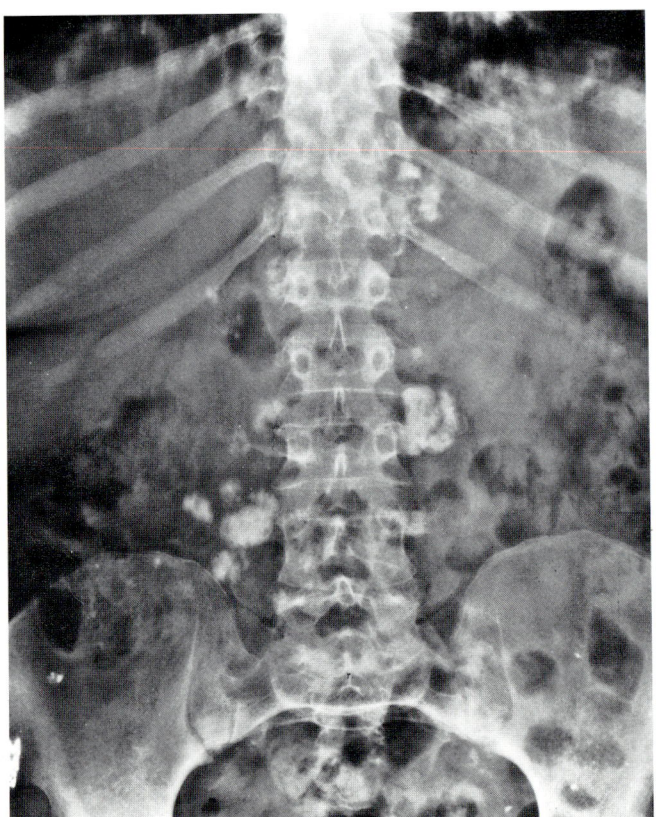

(b)

Figure 7.28

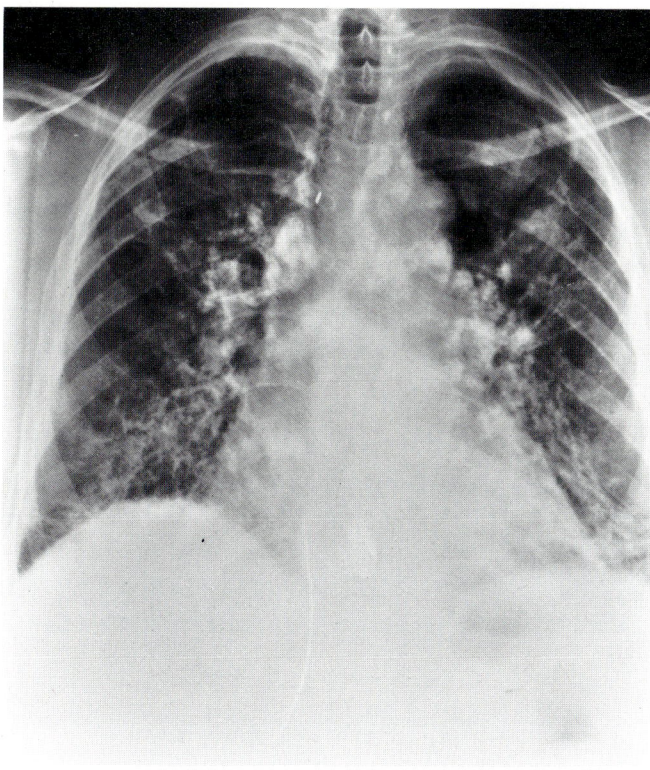

(c)

Figure 7.28 Hilar (*a*) and abdominal (*b*) lymph-node calcification in a 55-year-old woman. After 5 years (*c*) hilar calcification had increased.

chest radiography[27]. Extensive calcification of the soft tissue has also been reported (*see Figure 7.29*). Some causes of hilar calcification are as follows:

1. *Common*—Tuberculosis, silicosis, histoplasmosis, sarcoidosis, lymphoma after radiotherapy.
2. *Uncommon*—Pulmonary arteries (thromboembolism), idiopathic.

Some causes of diffuse pulmonary calcification are:

1. *Common*—Histoplasmosis, chicken-pox pneumonia, pneumoconiosis (silicosis, tin, barium), tuberculosis, costochondral calcification.
2. *Uncommon*—Alveolar microlithiasis, metastases (chondro- or osteosarcoma), pentastomiasis, amyloidosis, hyperparathyroidism (vitamin-D intoxication).

Lung functions

Lung volumes

Extensive physiological studies have demonstrated functional changes characteristic of 'restrictive impairment'[28]. Vital capacity, residual volume, and total lung capacity are reduced. The ratio of the forced expiratory volume in 1 second (FEV_1) to vital

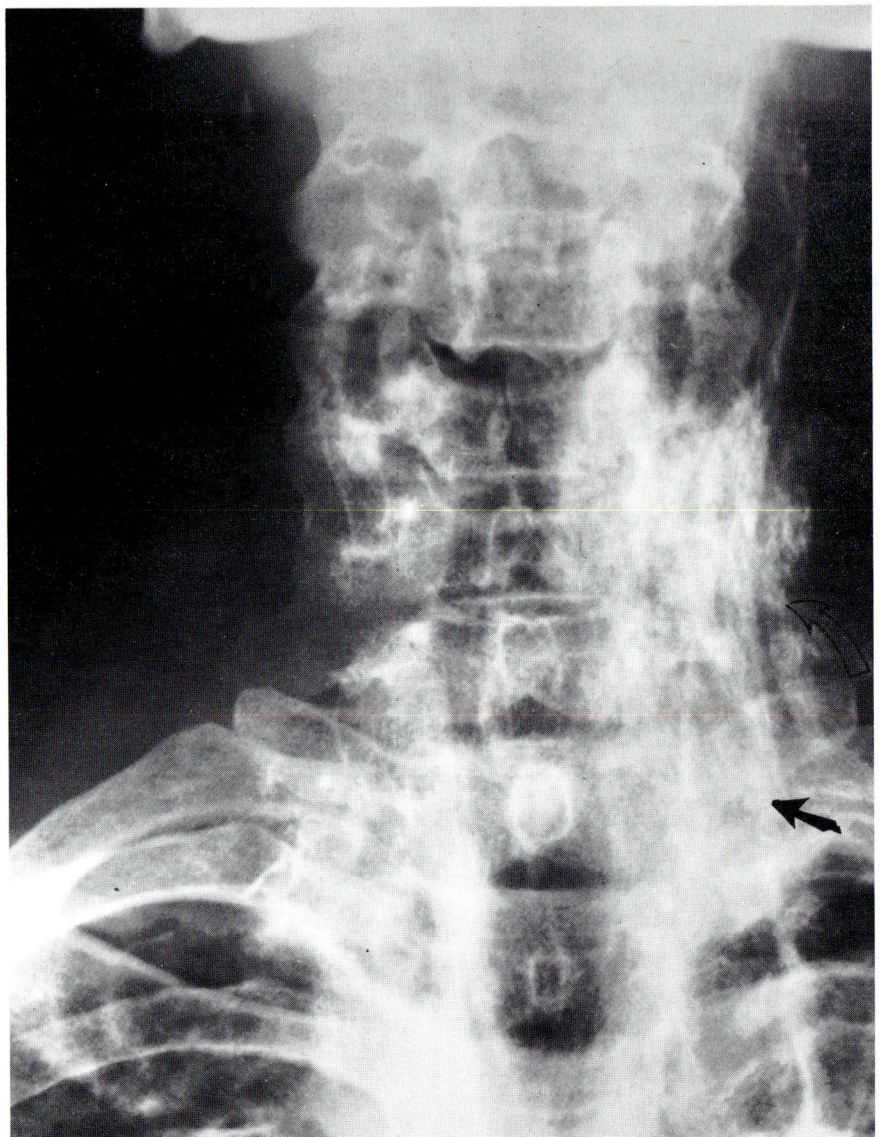

Figure 7.29 Calcification (arrowed) of soft tissues in the neck in a 65-year-old woman with long-standing sarcoidosis. She also has nephrocalcinosis and nephrolithiasis.

capacity is usually normal or increased. As the lungs become stiff, lung compliance is decreased. Hypoxaemia and a wide alveolar arterial oxygen difference, particularly during exercise, result from a ventilation ($\dot{V}$)-perfusion ($\dot{Q}$) mismatch. The disruption of the gas-exchanging units results in the diffusing capacity impairment.

Although sarcoidosis is frequently associated with reduction of lung volumes, the loss of diffusing capacity remains the most common lung function abnormality in sarcoidosis. The diffusing capacity is reduced even in patients with hilar adenopathy without any associated parenchymal infiltrate (stage I). Seventeen of the 18 patients in stage I sarcoidosis, in one study, had a low diffusing capacity[29]. Poe et al.[30] and Huang et al.[31] observed granulomas and alveolitis in patients with apparently normal chest radiographs. This widespread granulomatous infiltration with or without fibrosis is responsible for the low diffusing capacity. As the disease becomes more visible on the chest roentgenogram, impairment of diffusing capacity and vital capacity becomes more common[32]. The pulmonary function abnormality, however, does not always correlate with the degree of parenchymal involvement present on a chest roentgenogram.

Airway obstruction

Levinson and associates examined the airway function in 18 patients with sarcoidosis. They measured static and dynamic pulmonary volumes, diffusing capacity, static transpulmonary pressures, closing volumes and frequency dependence of compliance. The function of the airway was abnormal in every patient by at least one of these tests[33]. Using flow-volume curves and the nitrogen wash-out method, Miller et al. demonstrated the common occurrence of airway obstruction in sarcoidosis. Even in patients with stage I disease, some reduction of expiratory flow rate is common. Eight of 18 such patients studied by Sharma et al. had reduction of expiratory flow and five patients had increased airway resistance. Thus, airways obstruction is a relatively common manifestation of sarcoidosis[34].

The dysfunction of airways—large and small—may result either from endobronchial granulomas and bronchiolitis or from the disruption of the supporting structure around terminal and respiratory bronchioles. It is also possible that mediator-induced smooth-muscle constriction may play a role. Results of studies by Bechtel et al. show increased methacholine responsiveness in 10 out of 20 patients with sarcoidosis[35]. Histamine concentrations in lavage fluid from patients with sarcoidosis are increased.

Patients with diffuse airway involvement tend to have significant dyspnoea, dry cough and wheezing, and the disease tends to be extensive and persistent[36]. Localized endobronchial obstruction may cause atelectasis and bullae formation.

Pulmonary hypertension and ventilation–perfusion relationship

Severe pulmonary hypertension and cor pulmonale occurs in about 5% of sarcoidosis patients with chronic pulmonary disease. Sometimes, pulmonary hypertension may primarily be due to pulmonary arteritis, as sarcoid granuloma frequently involve the pulmonary vasculature[37-39]. Emirgil, Sobol and Herbert have demonstrated that the pulmonary hypertension in sarcoidosis is mostly due to interstitial lung disease rather than pulmonary vasculitis[40].

Lung function abnormalities due to ventilation–perfusion impairment include widening of the alveolar-arterial (A-a) oxygen tension difference which can be demonstrated in all stages of sarcoidosis. In addition to the wide A-a oxygen difference, the physiological deadspace and the total ventilation are increased. In sarcoidosis, there is no correlation between the blood gas abnormalities and the severity of pulmonary hypertension.

Control of ventilation

Resting hyperventilation is frequently present in sarcoidosis. The mechanisms responsible for increased respiratory drive include stimulation of vagally mediated mechanoreceptors in the lungs or chest-wall reflex stimuli in the diseased lung[41].

References

1. MARSHALL, R. and KARLISH, A.J. (1961) Lung function in sarcoidosis. *Thorax*, **26**, 402.
2. SILTZBACH, L.E. (1967) Sarcoidosis: Clinical features and management. *Med. Clin. N. Am.*, **51**, 483.
3. TSOU, E., ROMANO, M.C. and KERWIN, D.W. (1980) Sarcoidosis of anterior mediastinal nodes and uterine cervix. Three unusual sites in the same patient. *Am. Rev. Resp. Dis.*, **122**, 333.
4. WINTERBAUER, R.H., BELIC, M. and MOORES, K.D. (1973) A clinical interpretation of bilateral hilar adenopathy. *Ann. Intern. Med.* **78**, 65.
5. FRIEDMAN, O.H., BLAUGRUND, S.M. and SILTZBACH, L.E. (1963) Biopsy of the bronchial wall as an aid in diagnosis of sarcoidosis. *J. Am. Med. Assoc.*, **108**, 846.
6. KALIBIAN, V.V. (1957) Bronchial involvement in pulmonary sarcoidosis. *Thorax*, **12**, 18.
7. HONEY, M. and JEPSON, E. (1957) Multiple bronchostenoses due to sarcoidosis: Report of two cases. *Br. Med. J.*, **ii**, 1330.
8. OLSSON, T., BJORNSTAD-PETTERSON, H. and STJERNBERG, N.L. (1979) Bronchostenosis due to sarcoidosis: A cause of atelectasis and airway obstruction simulating pulmonary neoplasm and chronic obstructive pulmonary disease. *Chest*, **75**, 663.
9. CORSELLO, B.F., LOHAUS, G.H. and FUNAHASHI, A. (1983) Endobronchial mass lesion due to sarcoidosis: Complete resolution with corticosteroids. *Thorax*, **38**, 157.
10. HAHN, R. (1971) Unusual forms of sarcoidosis. *Southern Med. J.*, **64**, 541.
11. NELSON, D.G. and LOUDON, R.G. (1973) Sarcoidosis with pleural involvement. *Am. Rev. Resp. Dis.*, **108**, 647.
12. SHARMA, O.P. and GORDONSON, J. (1975) Pleural effusion in sarcoidosis: A report of six cases. *Thorax*, **35**, 95.
13. NELSON, D.G. and LOUDON, R.G. (1973) Sarcoidosis with pleural involvement. *Am. Rev. Resp. Dis.*, **108**, 647.
14. SHARMA, O.P. (1977) Sarcoidosis: unusual pulmonary manifestations. *Postgrad. Med. J.*, **61**, 67.
15. SOLOMON, A., KREEL, L., MCNICOL, M. and JOHNSON, N. (1979) Computed tomography in pulmonary sarcoidosis. *J. Comp. Axial Tomogr.*, **3**, 754.
16. DEVUYST, P., DETROYER, A. and YERNAULT, J.C. (1979) Bloody pleural effusion in a patient with sarcoidosis. *Chest*, **76**, 607.
17. SCADDING, J.G. (1967) *Sarcoidosis*. (London: Eyre and Spottiswoode)
18. RILEY, E.A. (1950) Boeck's sarcoid: A review based upon a clinical study of 52 cases. *Am. Rev. Tuberc.*, **62**, 231.
19. FELSON, B. (1958) Uncommon roentgen patterns of pulmonary sarcoidosis. *Dis. Chest*, **34**, 357.
20. FREUNDLICH, I.M., LIBSCHITZ, H.I., GLASSMAN, L.M., *et al.* (1970) Sarcoidosis, typical and atypical manifestations and complications. *Clin. Radiol.*, **21**, 376.
21. ONAL, E., LORATA, M. and LOURENCE, R.V. (1977) Nodular pulmonary sarcoidosis: Clinical roentgenographic and physiologic course in five patients. *Chest*, **72**, 296.
22. SHARMA, O.P., HEWLETT, R. and GORDONSON, J. (1973) Nodular sarcoidosis: an unusual radiographic appearance. *Chest*, **64**, 189.
23. SCHIFFNER, R.O. and SHARMA, O.P. (1977) Acute pulmonary cavitation in sarcoidosis. *West. J. Med.*, **127**, 346.
24. ROHATGI, P.K. and SCHWAB, L.E. (1980) Primary acute cavitation in sarcoidosis. *Am. J. Radiol.*, **134**, 1199.
25. SCADDING, J.G. and LENNOX, B. (1950) Sarcoidosis with lung cavitation. *Postgrad. Med. J.*, **26**, 494.
26. MCLOUD, T.C., PUTNAM, C.E. and PASCUAL, R. (1976) Egg-shell calcification with systemic sarcoidosis. *Chest*, **66**, 515.
27. DUNBAR, R.D. (1978) Sarcoidosis and its radiologic manifestations, CRC. *Crit. Rev. Diag. Imag.*, **Dec**, 185.
28. SVANBORG, N. (1961) Studies on the cardiopulmonary function in sarcoidosis. *Acta Med. Scand.*, **170** (Suppl. 366), 119.
29. SHARMA, O.P., COLP, C. and WILLIAMS, M.H., Jr. (1966) Pulmonary function studies in patients with bilateral sarcoidosis of hilar lymph nodes. *Arch. Intern. Med.*, **117**, 436.
30. POE, R.H., ISRAEL, R.H., UTELL, M.J., *et al.* (1979) Probability of a positive transbronchial biopsy result in sarcoidosis. *Arch. Intern. Med.*, **139**, 761.
31. HUANG, C.T., HEURICH, A.E., ROSEN, Y., *et al.* (1979) Pulmonary sarcoidosis: Roentgenographic, functional and pathologic correlations. *Respiration*, **37**, 337.
32. MILLER, A., TEIRSTEIN, A.S., JACKLER, I., *et al.* (1974) Airway function in chronic pulmonary sarcoidosis with fibrosis. *Am. Rev. Respir. Dis.*, **109**, 179.
33. LEVINSON, R.S., METZGER, L.F., STANLEY, N.N., *et al.* (1977) Airway function in sarcoidosis. *Am. J. Med.*, **62**, 51.

34. KANEKO, K. and SHARMA, O.P. (1977) Airway obstruction in pulmonary sarcoidosis. *Bull. Eur. Physiopathol. Respir.*, **13,** 231.
35. BECHTEL, J., STARR, T., DANTZKER, D., *et al.* (1981) Airway hyperactivity in patients with sarcoidosis. *Am. Rev. Respir. Dis.*, **124,** 759.
36. DUTTON, R.E., RENZI, P.M., LOPEZ-MAJANO, *et al.* (1982) Airway function in sarcoidosis: smokers versus nonsmokers. *Respiration*, **43,** 164.
37. CARRINGTON, C.B., GAENSLER, E.A., MIKUS, J.P., *et al.* (1976) Structure and function in sarcoidosis. In *Proceedings of the VIIth International Conference on Sarcoidosis* (ed. Siltzbach, L.E.). *Ann. N.Y. Acad. Sci.*, **278,** 365.
38. ROSEN, Y., VULENTIN, J.C., PERSCHUNK, L.P., *et al.* (1979) Sarcoidosis from the pathologist's vantage point. *Pathol. Ann.*, **14,** 405.
39. BATTESTI, J.P., GEORGES, R., BASSET, F., *et al.* (1978) Chronic cor pulmonale in pulmonary sarcoidosis. *Thorax*, **33,** 76.
40. EMIRGIL, C., SOBOL, B.J. and HERBERT, W.H. (1971) The lesser circulation in pulmonary fibrosis secondary to sarcoidosis and its relationship to respiratory function. *Chest*, **60,** 371.
41. WILLIAMS, M.H., Jr. (1983) Pulmonary function in sarcoidosis. In *Sarcoidosis and Other Granulomatous Lung Disease* (ed. Fanburg, B.L.). *Lung Biology in Health and Disease*, Vol. **20,** p. 70. (New York: Marcel Dekker)

Chapter 8
Cutaneous involvement

Skin involvement occurs in about one-quarter of patients with sarcoidosis. The lesions are both specific and non-specific. The specific lesions are lupus pernio, plaques, maculopapular eruption, subcutaneous nodules and scars. The important non-specific lesion is erythema nodosum. Alopecia, erythrodermas and ulcerative and vesicular lesions are rare.

Lupus pernio

In 1889, Ernest Besnier coined the term lupus pernio in describing one of his patients with persistent skin lesions. 'Here is a man of 34 who presents with similar lesions of the face and arms, but which are not recognized or described. Those on the face look superficially like lupus erythematosus. I propose the name lupus pernio or purple lupus. They resemble but are not identical to Hutchinson's lupus[1]'.

Lupus pernio is the most characteristic of all sarcoid skin lesions. It is a chronic, persistent bluish indurated lesion with a predilection for nose, cheeks, ears and lips (*see Figure 8.1*). The nose lesion is often associated with granulomatous infiltration of the nasal mucosa. Occasionally, nasal septum may be destroyed. Lupus pernio is seen commonly in women with a long-standing disease, and it is associated with extensive pulmonary infiltration and fibrosis, chronic uveitis and bone changes. The last lesions occur in 10–20% of patients. Bone changes rarely occur in the absence of skin lesions[2]. Bulbous and sausage-shaped fingers in a patient with lupus pernio point towards underlying bone cysts (*see Figure 8.2*). Occasionally, nails become dystrophic, distorted and brittle (*see Figure 8.3*).

Five out of six patients with lupus pernio in my series had extensive pulmonary infiltration; the sixth had a normal chest reoentgenogram. Bone cysts were present in 50% of the patients. All six were anergic, hyperglobulinaemia was noted in four, and one patient had hypercalcaemia. The duration of lupus pernio ranged from $2\frac{1}{2}$ to 19 years. Five patients received corticosteroids. The skin lesions cleared in one patient; none of the five showed clearing of their chest radiograph abnormality. Chloroquine produced marked regression of the chest lesion after 6 months of therapy[3].

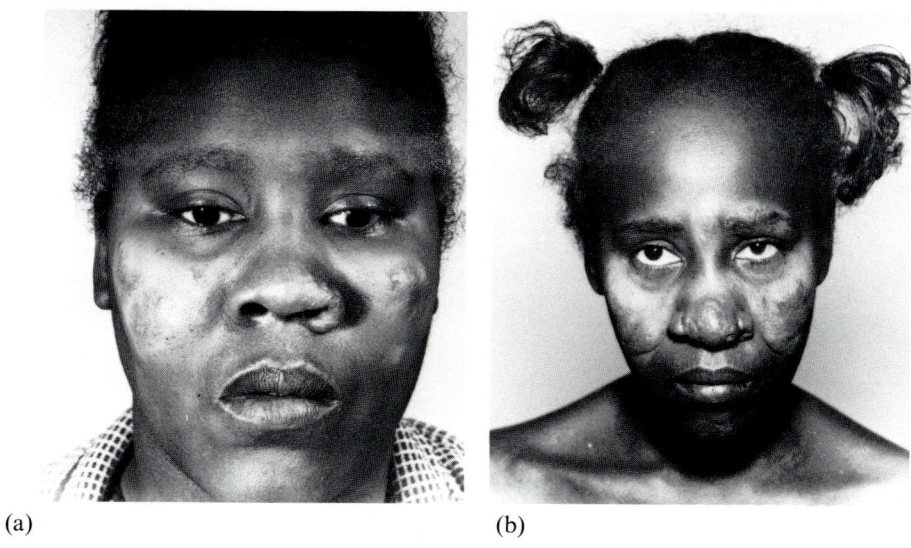
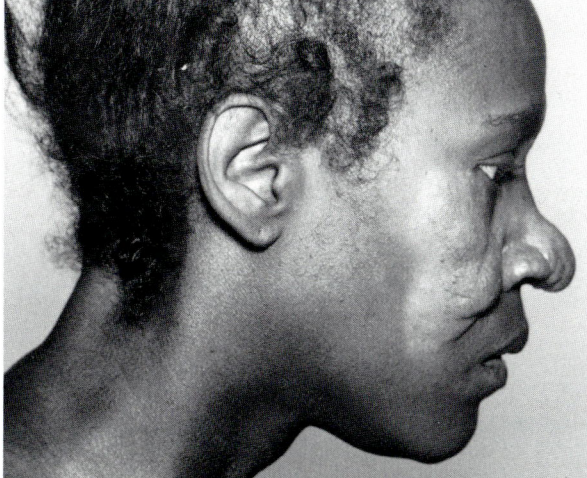

Figure 8.1 Development of lupus pernio over 20 years.

Skin plaques

Skin plaques, like lupus pernio, are chronic, persistent, purple, elevated patches, commonly located on the limbs, face and buttocks. The centre of the plaque is usually pale and atrophic, whereas the periphery is indurated, elevated and dark (*see Figure 8.4*). The distribution of the plaques is often symmetrical. James has reported the frequent occurrence of lymphadenopathy and splenomegaly associated with plaques as opposed to lupus pernio where bone and eye lesions are common[4]. In the presence of telangiectatic vessels the lesions are called angiolupoid.

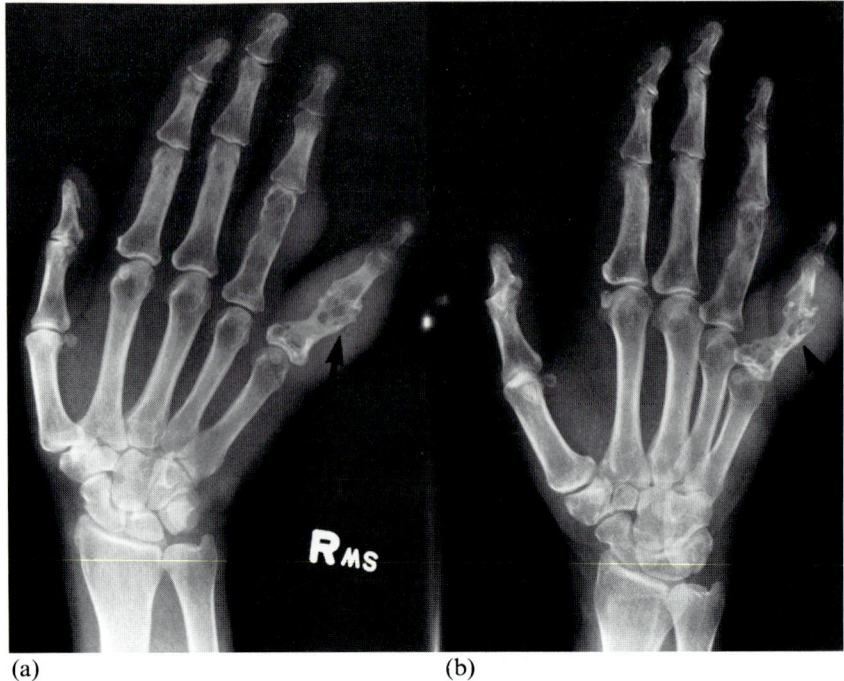

Figure 8.2 Bone cysts (arrows) and sausage-shaped fingers in a patient with lupus pernio.

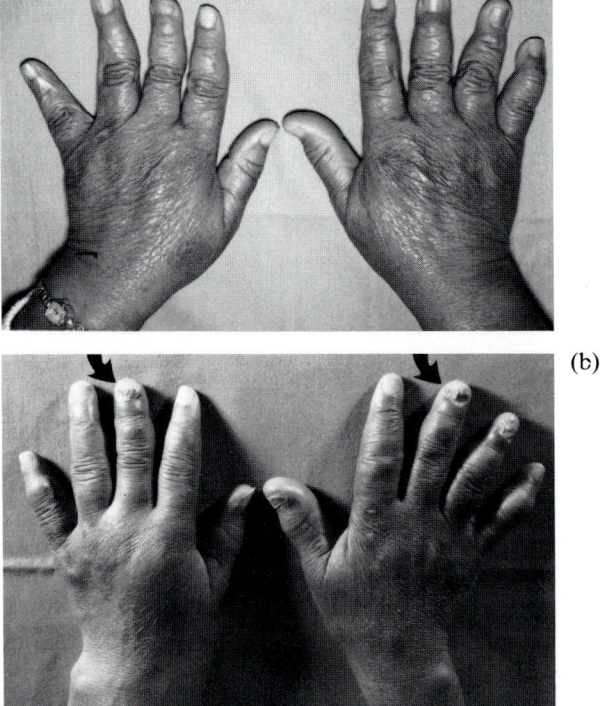

Figure 8.3 (*a*) Dystrophic, distorted and brittle nails in a 53-year-old woman with chronic skin and bone lesions. (*b*) Six months after chloroquine therapy nails have become normal.

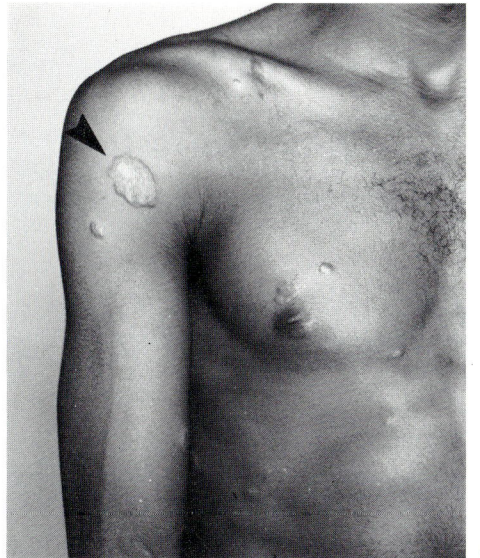

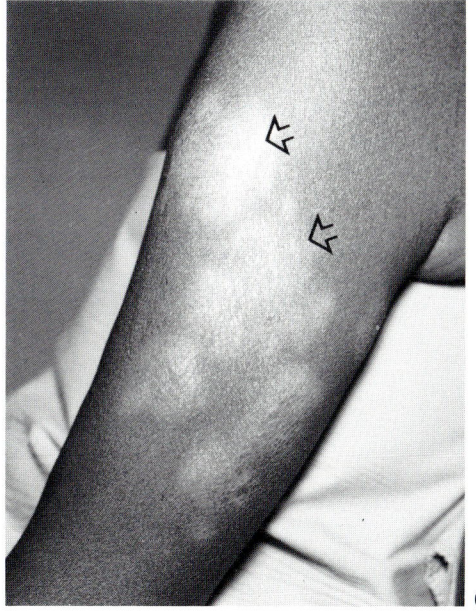

Figure 8.4 Skin plaques (arrows) on the arms (*a,b*).

Maculopapular eruptions

Maculopapular eruptions characteristically occur on the face, in the nasolabial folds, on the lids, around the orbits and on the nape and the upper back. The lesions are elevated and have a distinct flat top with a waxy translucent appearance and vary

68   Cutaneous involvement

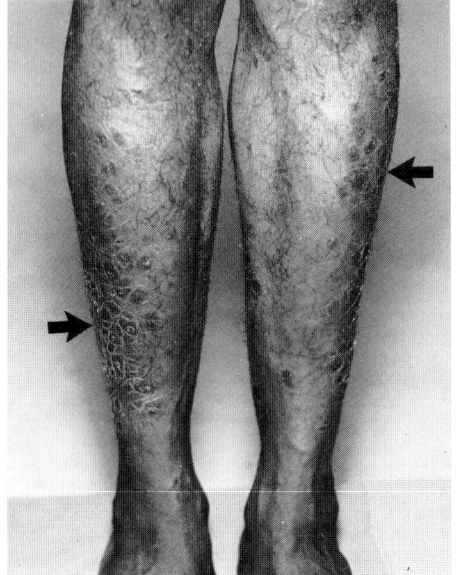

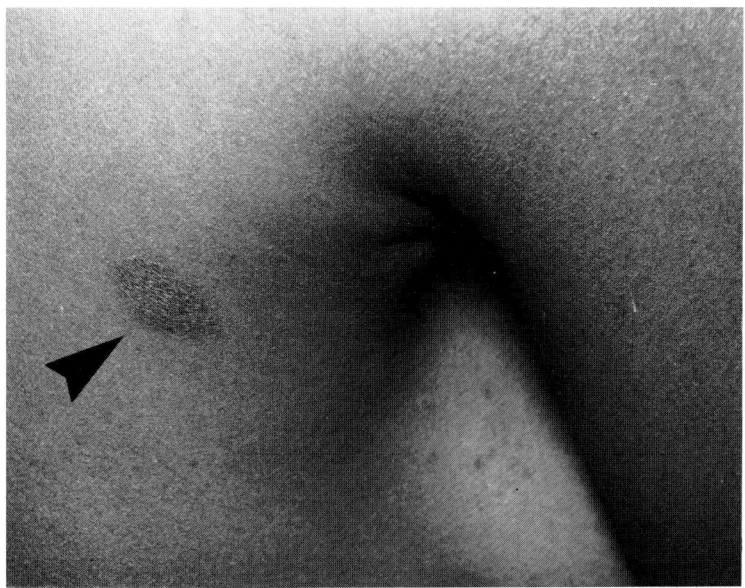

Figure 8.4 (cont.) Skin plaques (arrows) on the legs (*c*), back (*d*).

from 2 to 6 mm in diameter. The eruption is usually associated with peripheral lymphadenopathy and splenomegaly. The intrathoracic involvement is at an earlier stage of development, for bilateral hilar adenopathy with or without parenchymal infiltration was seen in 60% of the patients with maculopapular eruptions. The maculopapular lesions are the commonest skin manifestation of sarcoidosis in Negro patients (*see Figure 8.5*).

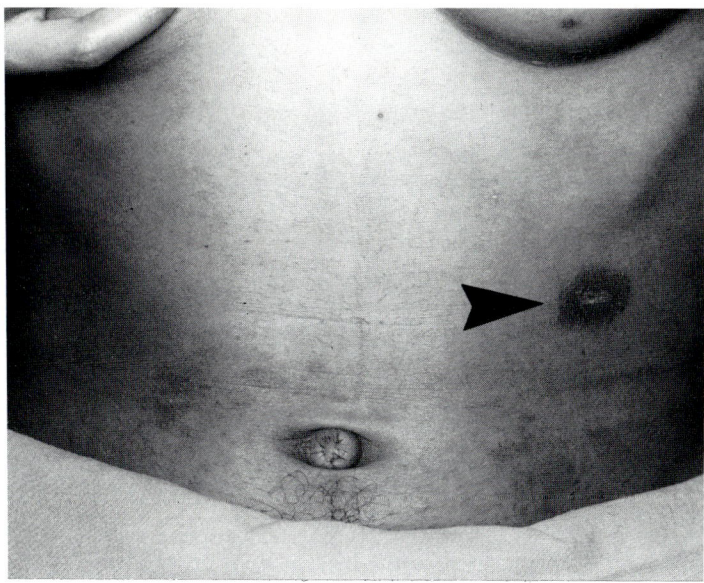

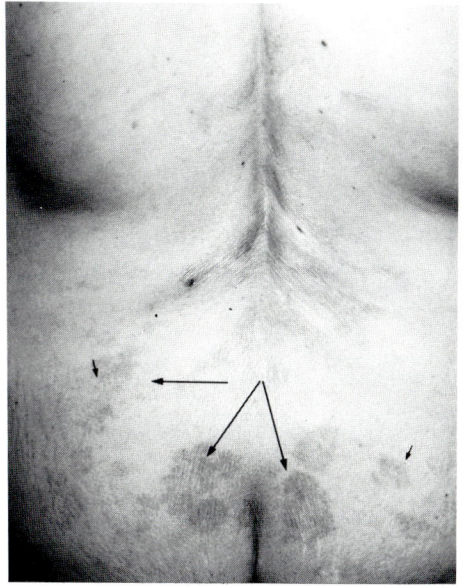

Figure 8.4 (cont.) Skin plaques (arrows) on the abdominal wall (*e*) and buttocks (*f*).

Subcutaneous nodules

Subcutaneous nodules are called Darier–Roussy sarcoid. The nodules arise in deep dermis and subcutaneous tissue and have a predilection for trunk and extremities. Nodules appeared in two of my patients in association with erythema nodosum and bilateral hilar adenopathy. The nodules are painless and biopsy shows non-caseating granulomas.

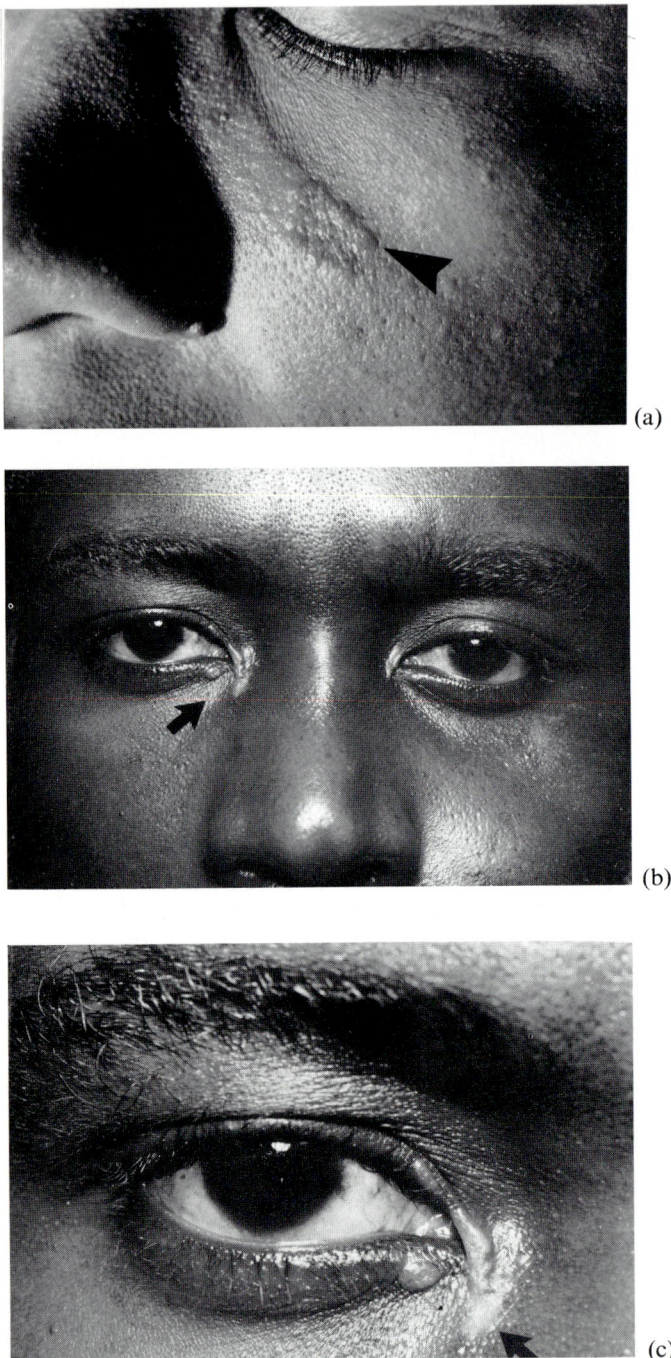

Figure 8.5 Maculopapular eruptions (arrows) on the face (*a*), around the orbit (*b,c*), at the back of the elbows (*d*), on the wrist (*e*) and on the knee (*f*).

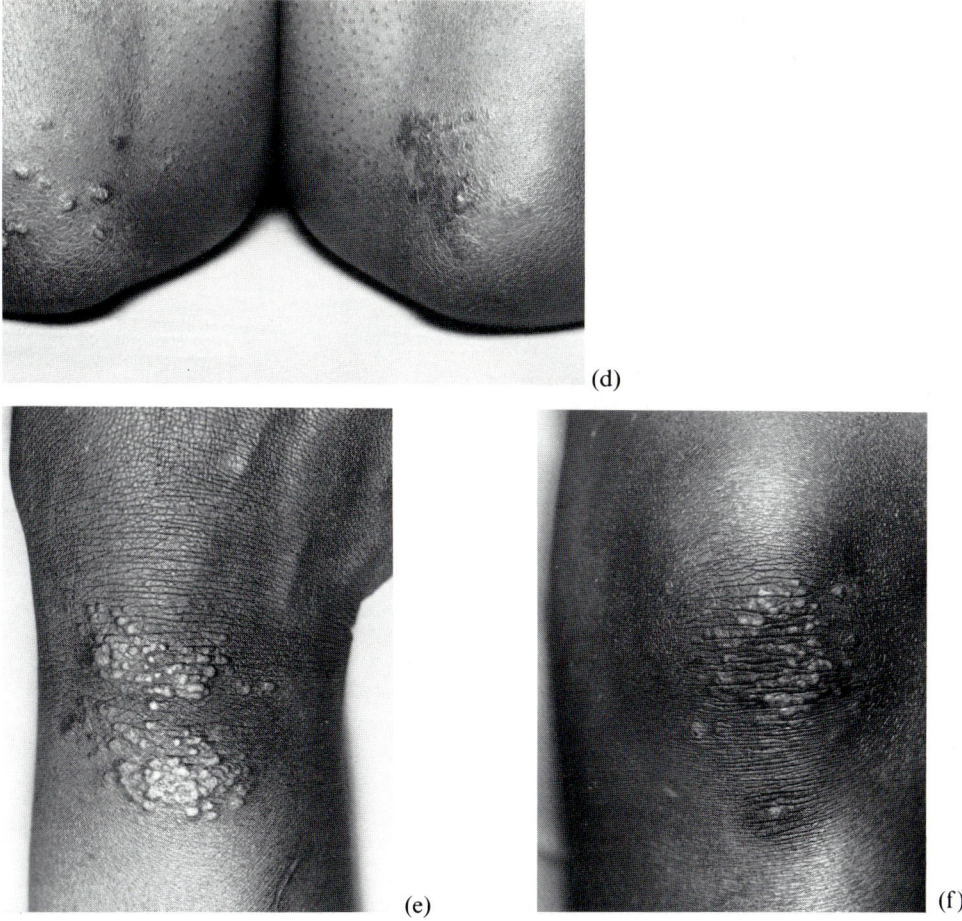

Figure 8.5 (cont.)

Scars

Old atrophic, surgical or traumatic scars may become purple, oedematous, and, rarely, tender either at the time of initial presentation or during reactivation of the disease. Vaccination and acne scars and keloids are all subject to these changes. Biopsy samples of these scars show non-caseating granulomas (*see Figure 8.6*).

Erythema nodosum

Erythema nodosum is a hypersensitivity reaction which results from exposure to the following bacterial, fungal and chemical antigens.

Infections
  Primary tuberculosis
  Coccidioidomycosis
  Histoplasmosis

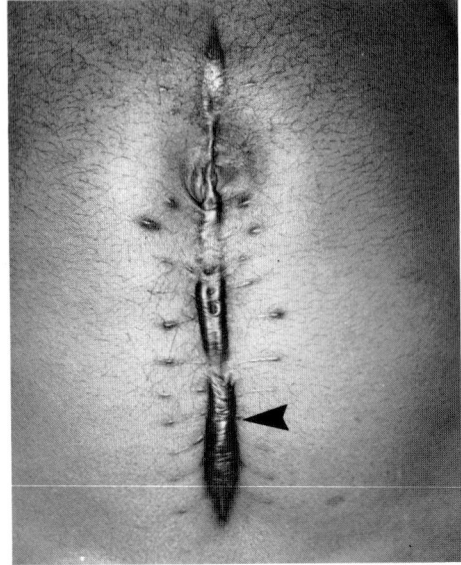

(a)

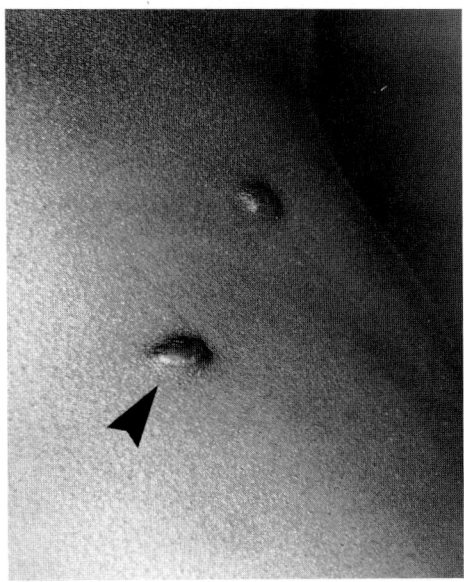

(b)

Figure 8.6 Scar sarcoid lesions (arrows) on an old surgical suture line (*a*) and on acne scars (*b*).

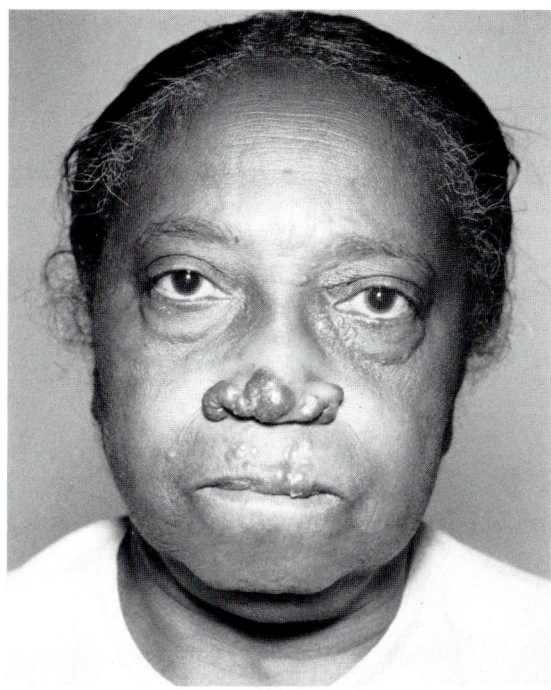

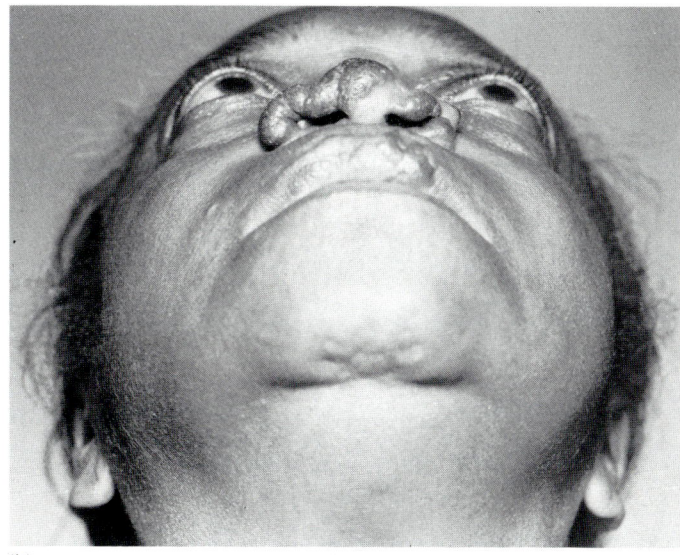

Figure 8.7 Lupus pernio (*a,b*).

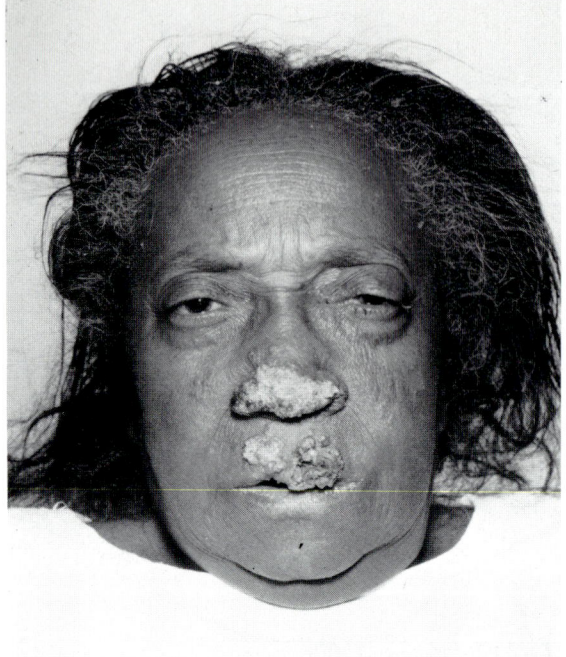

(c)

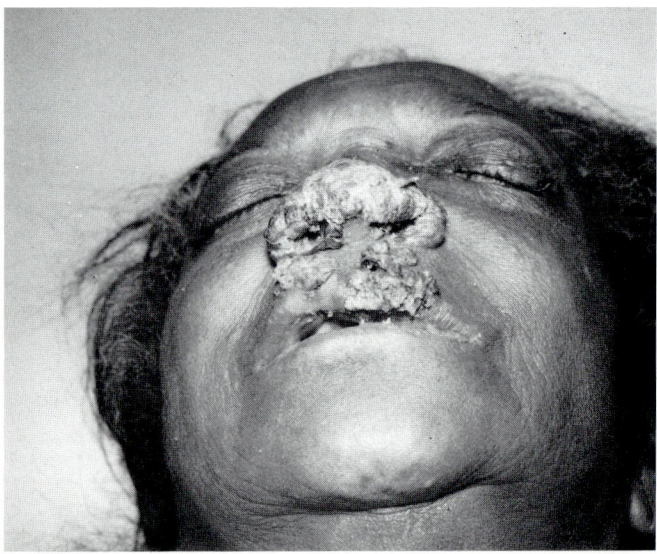

(d)

Fig 8.7 (cont.) Ulcerated after 2 years (*c,d*). The patient was not on any therapy.

β-Haemolytic streptococcal infections
  Brucellosis
  Psittacosis
  Lymphogranuloma venereum
  Leprosy
Drugs
  Penicillin
  Sulphonamides
  Bromides
  Iodides
  Oral contraceptives
Immunological disorders
  Sarcoidosis
Miscellaneous
  Ulcerative colitis
  Regional enteritis

Erythema nodosum is the most common non-specific cutaneous manifestation of sarcoidosis. It occurs much more frequently in Europe than in North America. It is more frequent amongst Puerto Ricans living in New York and Irish immigrants in London. Erythema nodosum is the hallmark of acute sarcoidosis. It occurs predominantly in women of childbearing age. Systemic manifestation such as fever, malaise and polyarthralgia occur in about 50% of patients having erythema nodosum.

In nine of 14 patients with erythema nodosum in a predominantly Negro series, a chest radiograph showed bilateral hilar adenopathy. However, in non-Negro patients, as many as 90% with erythema nodosum have stage I sarcoidosis. The constitutional symptoms usually subside within an average period of 4–6 weeks. More than 80% of patients show complete resolution of chest radiograph abnormality in less than 2 years. Usually, patients with erythema nodosum do not need corticosteroid therapy because of such a high rate of spontaneous resolution.

Other lesions

Alopecia may result if the granulomatous lesions affect the scalp. Psoriasiform sarcoid lesions or violaceous or brownish plaque are seen on the trunk and extremities in American Negroes. Generalized skin rash resembling exfoliative dermatitis has also been reported. An ichthyosis-like picture has been observed in a biopsy-proven sarcoid patient. Lupus pernio and subcutaneous nodules may rarely ulcerate (*see Figure 8.7*)[5]. Pruritus is uncommon. However, I have studied a patient with maculopapular rash whose initial complaint was a severe pruritus[6].

References

1. BESNIER, E. (1889) Lupus pernio de la face. *Ann. Derm. Syph.*, **10**, 333.
2. JAMES, D.G. (1981) Lupus pernio. In *Sarcoidosis* (eds. Chretien, J., Marsa, J. and Saltiel, J.C.), pp. 168–72). (Paris: Pergamon Press)
3. SHARMA, O.P. (1972) Cutaneous sarcoidosis: Clinical features and management. *Chest*, **61**, 320.
4. JAMES, D.G. (1959) Dermatological aspects of sarcoidosis. *Q.J. Med.*, **28**, 109.
5. SCHIFFNER, J. and SHARMA, O.P. (1977) Ulcerative sarcoidosis. *Arch. Dermatol.*, **113**, 676.
6. FONG, W.Y. and SHARMA, O.P. (1975) Pruritic maculopapular eruption in sarcoidosis. *Arch. Dermatol.*, **111**, 362.

Chapter 9
Ocular sarcoidosis

Any structure of the eye may be involved in sarcoidosis. Ocular changes occur in about one-quarter of the patients; but the incidence varies considerably, depending on racial composition of the series and whether a thorough eye evaluation, including a slit-lamp examination, was performed. Eye lesions are noted more frequently in Negro patients. Of the 72 patients examined by Longcope and Freiman, 64% showed some evidence of ocular involvement[1]. The lower incidence of eye involvement in some series presumably may be due to inclusion only of the patients with symptomatic lesions since the ocular disease may remain asymptomatic and only be discovered by routine slit-lamp examination (*see Plate 9.1*).

Uveitis

The most common of the eye lesions in sarcoidosis is granulomatous uveitis, which may be subacute or chronic. Of the 442 patients studied by James, 89 (22%) had uveitis as a presenting feature[2]. Thirty-nine (14%) of Scadding's 275 patients had uveitis at some stage of their disease[3]. Crick, Hoyle and Smellie performed a thorough eye examination in 185 patients; 61 (33%) showed evidence of uveitis[4].

Subacute uveitis

Subacute uveitis or iridocyclitis presents suddenly with watering and redness of eyes, cloudy vision and photophobia. Circumcorneal ciliary congestion is present; pupils are irregular; and 'mutton fat' KPs (keratic precipitates) may be prominent in the anterior chamber. The aqueous humor may be turbid. Nodules on the iris occur rarely. The patient may have other manifestations of early sarcoidosis, including erythema nodosum and bilateral hilar lymphadenopathy. Association of uveitis, parotid enlargement and the seventh cranial nerve is known as Heerfordt's syndrome. Acute iridocyclitis tends to clear spontaneously. The prognosis is good.

Chronic uveitis

Chronic uveitis, on the other hand, develops slowly and may lead to adhesions between the iris and the lens, glaucoma, cataract formation and blindness. Ciliary congestion is absent; KPs (keratic precipitates) are present in the anterior chamber. The patient usually complains of pain and blurred vision. Other manifestations of chronic sarcoidosis including persistent skin plaques, lupus pernio, interstitial fibrosis and bone cysts accompany chronic uveitis. The prognosis is poor.

Posterior uveitis (choroidoretinitis)

Posterior uveitis is much more common than is generally realized because it may be difficult to diagnose in the presence of anterior uveitis. Evidence of posterior uveitis, on careful eye examination, was present in 40 (66%) of 61 patients of Crick et al.[4] and 11 (25%) of James' 442 patients[2]. Examination of fundi may reveal choroiditis, white waxy choroidal nodules, periphlebitis, retinal oedema and retinal degeneration. Blurring of vision may be the only symptom. The posterior uveitis constitutes an absolute indication for systemic corticosteroid therapy.

Conjunctivitis and conjunctival follicles

Conjunctival involvement is the second most common ocular finding in sarcoidosis. Phlyctenular or non-specific conjunctivitis occurred in 14 (3%) of the patients in one series; eight of these had erythema nodosum and bilateral hilar lymphadenopathy. The lesion was bilateral in all but four patients. Bornstein, Frank and Radner obtained a positive conjunctival biopsy result in 25% of 64 patients with sarcoidosis[5].

Conjunctival follicles are tiny, translucent, pale yellow nodules occurring commonly in the fornices, palpebral conjunctiva, and occasionally in the bulbar conjunctiva. Crick, Hoyle and Mather observed conjunctival follicles in 79 (56%) of 139 patients; in 20 of these, biopsy revealed non-caseating granulomas[6]. Follicular collections usually subside spontaneously. Irritation is the symptom that brings the patient to the physician. Corticosteroids are indicated in a symptomatic patient.

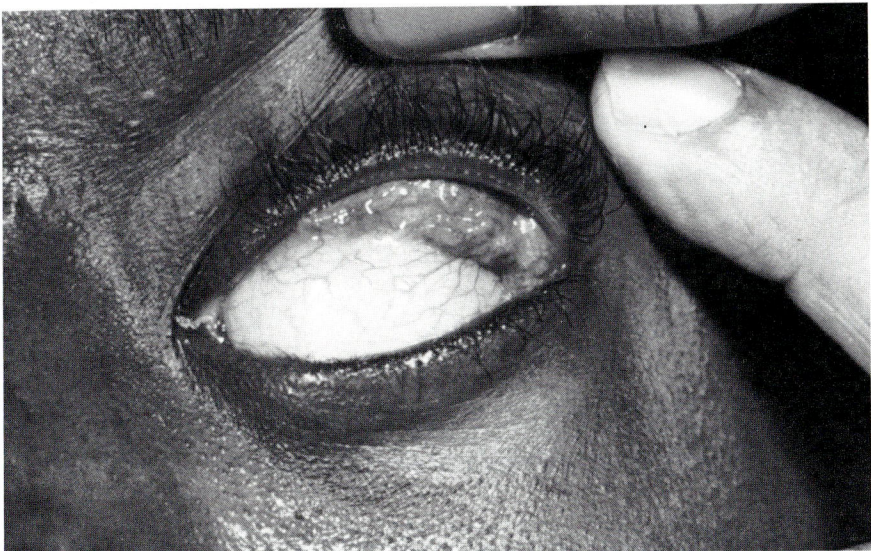

Figure 9.1 Sarcoid nodules involving the left lacrimal gland.

Keratoconjunctivitis sicca

Granulomatous infiltration of the lacrimal glands may produce deficiency of tears which results in dry, sore eyes. Incidence of keratoconjunctivitis sicca in sarcoidosis is about 4–5%. Asymptomatic lacrimal dysfunction is more frequent because in the absence of dry eyes a decrease in lacrimal secretions can be demonstrated by Schrimer's test. There is no correlation between lacrimal gland dysfunction and other serious eye lesions (see Figure 9.1).

Miscellaneous lesions

Other rare manifestations of sarcoidosis are periphlebitis retinae with retinal haemorrhages and retinitis proliferans, cataract, band keratopathy, proptosis and exophthalmos[7].

Diagnosis of ocular sarcoid

Diagnosis of ocular sarcoidosis is relatively easy if the typical eye lesions—including the granulomatous uveitis, conjunctival follicles and lacrimal gland enlargement—are associated with bilateral hilar adenopathy, erythema nodosum, peripheral lymphadenopathy and depression of delayed-type hypersensitivity. When the eye lesions occur in the absence of clinical features of sarcoidosis, conjunctival and lacrimal

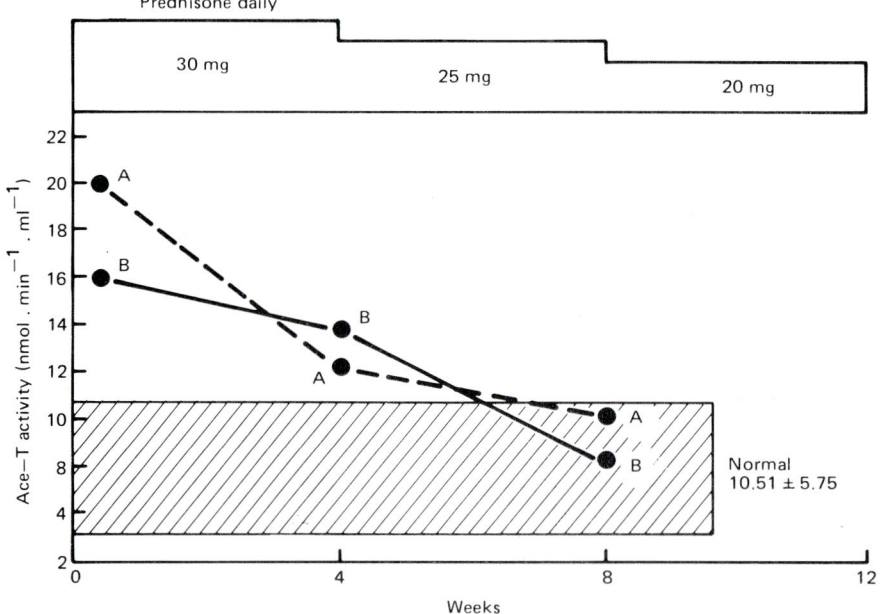

Figure 9.2 Effect of corticosteroids on angiotensin converting enzyme (ACE-T) activity in tears in two patients with ocular sarcoidosis. (Reproduced from Sharma, O.P. (1983) *Arch. Ophthalmol.*, **101**, 559, by courtesy of publishers.)

biopsies are required to demonstrate non-caseating granulomas. The measurement of angiotensin converting enzyme activity in tears has been recommended as a non-invasive test to support the diagnosis of ocular sarcoidosis and for monitoring its course (*see Figure 9.2*)[8-11].

References

1. LONGCOPE, W.T. and FREIMAN, D.G. (1952) A study of sarcoidosis. *Medicine*, **31**, 1.
2. JAMES, D.G., ANDERSON, R., LANGLEY, D. and AINSLIE, D. (1964) Ocular sarcoidosis. *Br. J. Ophthalmol.*, **48**, 461.
3. SCADDING, J.G. (1967) *Sarcoidosis*. (London: Eyre and Spottiswoode)
4. CRICK, R., HOYLE, C. and SMELLIE, H. (1961) The eyes in sarcoidosis. *Br. J. Ophthalmol.*, **45**, 461.
5. BORNSTEIN, J.S., FRANK, M.I. and RADNER, D.B. (1962) Conjunctival biopsy in the diagnosis of sarcoidosis. *N. Engl. J. Med.*, **267**, 60.
6. CRICK, R., HOYLE, C. and MATHER, G. (1955) Conjunctival biopsy in sarcoidosis. *Br. Med. J.*, **ii**, 1180.
7. MELMON, K.L. and GOLDBERG, J.S. (1962) Sarcoidosis with bilateral exophthalmos as the presenting symptom. *Am. J. Med.*, **33**, 158.
8. SHARMA, O.P. and VITA JOAO BRASIL (1983) Determination of angiotensin-converting enzyme activity in tears: A non-invasive test for evaluation of ocular sarcoidosis. *Arch. Ophthalmol.*, **101**, 559.
9. KHAN, F., WESSELY, Z., et al. (1977) Conjunctival biopsy in sarcoidosis: A simple, safe, and specific diagnostic procedure. *Ann. Ophthalmol.*, **9**, 671.
10. WEINREB, R.N., YAVITZ, E.Q. and O'CONNOR, G.R. (1981) Lacrimal gland uptake of gallium citrate Ga[67]. *Am. J. Ophthalmol.*, **92**, 16.
11. KARMA, A. (1979) Ophthalmic changes in sarcoidosis. *Acta Ophthalmol. (Suppl.)*, **141**.

Chapter 10
The reticuloendothelial system in sarcoidosis

Peripheral lymphadenopathy

Superficial lymph-node enlargement is a frequent manifestation of sarcoidosis. Although the incidence varies from series to series, peripheral lymphadenopathy occurs in about three-quarters of all patients. The most frequently involved nodes are cervical, axillary, epitrochlear and inguinal. In the neck, the posterior triangle nodes are more commonly affected as compared with nodes in the anterior triangle. Mesenteric and retroperitoneal lymph-node enlargement can be detected by gallium-67 scanning. Enlarged glands are discrete, shotty, moveable, non-tender, painless and free of surrounding structure.

Unlike tuberculous and fungal lymph nodes, the sarcoid nodes do not ulcerate to form draining skin sinuses. Occasionally, sarcoid nodes may be confused with those of Hodgkin's disease. In the latter, lymph-node enlargement is more often unilateral, and constitutional symptoms are prominent. In sarcoidosis, lymphadenopathy tends to be bilateral and patients are more often asymptomatic. Alcohol-induced pain associated with lymphadenopathy, a well-recognized feature of Hodgkin's disease, occurred in one of our patients with sarcoidosis[1].

Case report—A 29-year-old man came to us with a 1-year history of progressive dyspnoea. During the last 6 months he developed generalized lymphadenopathy and lost 20 lb (9 kg) in weight. Physical examination disclosed firm, non-tender, moveable cervical, axillary, epitrochlear and inguinal lymph nodes. Eyes were normal. There were many reddish flat, non-tender nodules over the back, arms and legs (*see Figure 10.1*). Crackles were heard over both lower lung fields. The liver was enlarged. The chest radiograph showed diffuse infiltration and pleural thickening (*see Figure 10.2*). A dry pleural biopsy showed non-caseating granulomas. Significant eosinophilia and hypercalcaemia were present (*see Figure 10.3*). Serum angiotensin converting enzyme level was 24 IU (normal range 10–36 IU). Serum immunoglobulins: IgG, 3420 mg.(100 ml)$^{-1}$ (342 g.ℓ^{-1}) (normal range, 600–2000 mg.(100 ml)$^{-1}$; 60–200 g.ℓ^{-1}); IgA, 812 mg.(100 ml)$^{-1}$ (81.2 g.ℓ^{-1}) (50–400 mg.(100 ml)$^{-1}$; 5–40 g.ℓ^{-1}); IgM, 361 mg.(100 ml)$^{-1}$ (36.1 g.ℓ^{-1}) (40–250 mg.(100 ml)$^{-1}$; 4–25 g.ℓ^{-1}). Initially, the patient was treated with intravenous saline, magnesium and potassium. Prednisone 40 mg once daily was added after the diagnosis of sarcoidosis was established. After 4 weeks lymphadenopathy subsided and the patient became normocalcaemic. Prednisone was gradually reduced to a maintenance dose of 10 mg daily. At present he has no skin lesions and no lymphadenopathy. His serum calcium level is normal but eosinophilia persists.

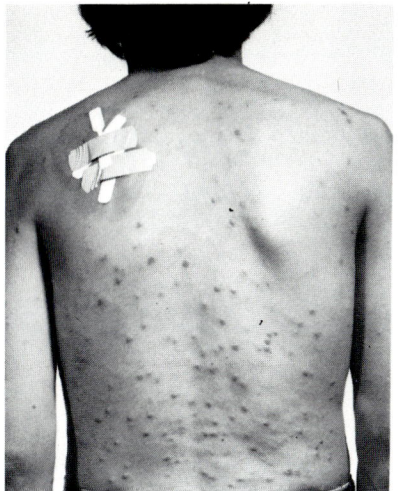 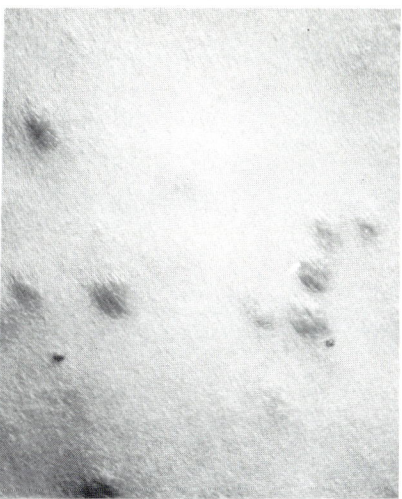

Figure 10.1 Reddish, flat non-tender nodular plaques. Skin biopsy specimens showed non-caseating granulomas.

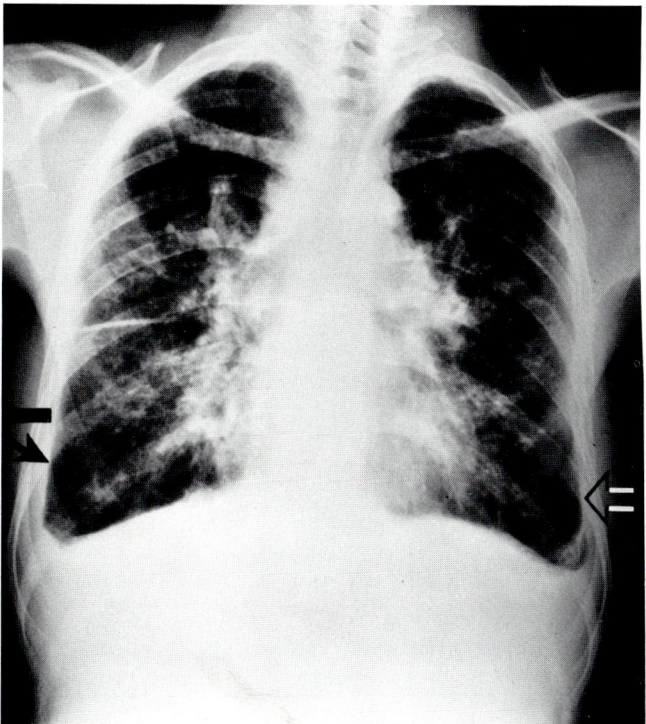

Figure 10.2 Diffuse parenchymal infiltration associated with marked pleural thickening (arrows). A dry pleural biopsy showed non-caseating granulomas.

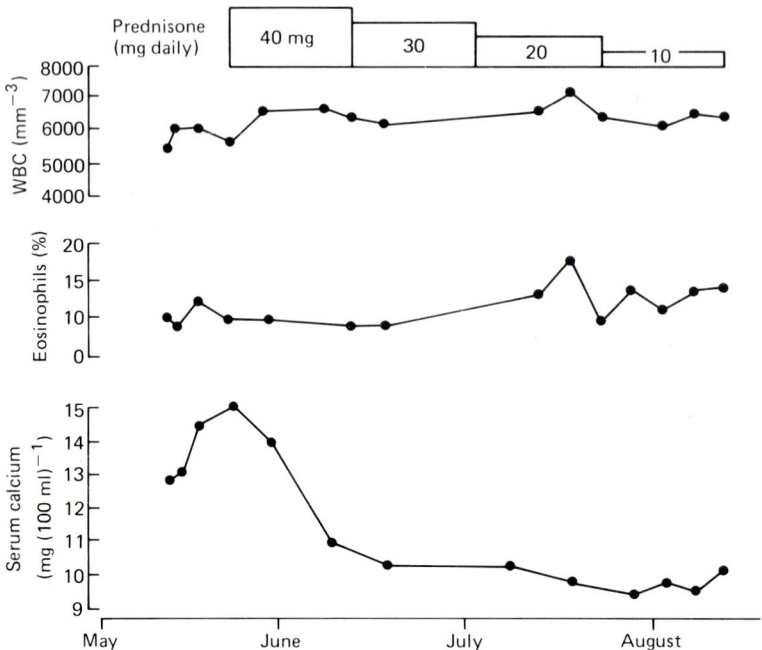

Figure 10.3 Serum calcium, eosinophils and white blood cell count (WBC) in a 29-year-old-man treated with prednisone. The hypercalcaemia responded to prednisone therapy but the peripheral eosinophilia persisted. There was no clinical or laboratory evidence of any parasitic infestation. Conversion factor: serum calcium, $1\,\text{mg}\,.(100\,\text{ml})^{-1} = 0.25\,\text{mmol}.\ell^{-1}$.

Splenic involvement

The incidence of clinically palpable spleen in sarcoidosis varies from 1 to 42%[2]. Using the fine needle aspiration technique, Selroos and Koivunen demonstrated splenic granulomas in 184 (59%) out of 312 patients[3]. Turiaf, Battesti and Helenon performed coeliac arteriography in 28 sarcoidosis patients; in 15 (53%) the spleen was enlarged[4]. Splenomegaly is noticed much more frequently at autopsy. I have been able to palpate the spleen in only 15% of my patients with sarcoidosis.

Splenic enlargement is usually silent but it may cause symptoms due to pressure on adjacent organs. Anaemia, leukopenia, thrombocytopenia and pancytopenia are most likely to occur if the spleen size, on palpation, is larger than 4 cm in the midclavicular line. The primary therapy for symptomatic sarcoid splenomegaly is corticosteroids. The spleen was no longer palpable in 12 of 15 patients with a spleen size less than 4 cm who were treated with corticosteroids for reasons other than the splenic involvement[5]. Splenectomy is indicated in those patients who fail to respond to medical therapy. Young and Mooney reviewed five cases of giant splenomegaly treated by splenectomy[6]. Surgical removal of the spleen is recommended for patients with long-standing massive splenomegaly to prevent splenic rupture, to relieve pressure symptoms and to prevent haemotological abnormalities due to hypersplenism. Guyton and Zumwalt have reported a case of fatal pneumococcaemia in a patient with clinically unsuspected sarcoidosis with a spleen completely infiltrated with granulomatous tissues[7].

Case 1—A 24-year-old woman was admitted for evaluation of severe anaemia and splenomegaly. Physical examination showed cervical, epitrochlear, axillary and inguinal lymphadenopathy. The liver was palpable 2 cm below the right costal margin, and the spleen was enlarged. Laboratory investigations: haemoglobin, 8.1 g.(100 ml)$^{-1}$ (1.26 mmol.ℓ^{-1}); WBC, 4000 mm^{-3} ($4 \times 10^9.\ell^{-1}$) with a normal differential; reticulocytes 2%; thrombocytes, 90 000 ($90 \times 10^9.\ell^{-1}$). A chest radiograph showed minimal hilar adenopathy, and the abdominal film showed splenomegaly (*see Figure 10.4*). The diagnosis was established by a lymph-node biopsy. The patient was given prednisone which improved her blood picture, but every lapse of treatment resulted in a fall in haemoglobin, white blood cell count and platelet values (*see Figure 10.5*).

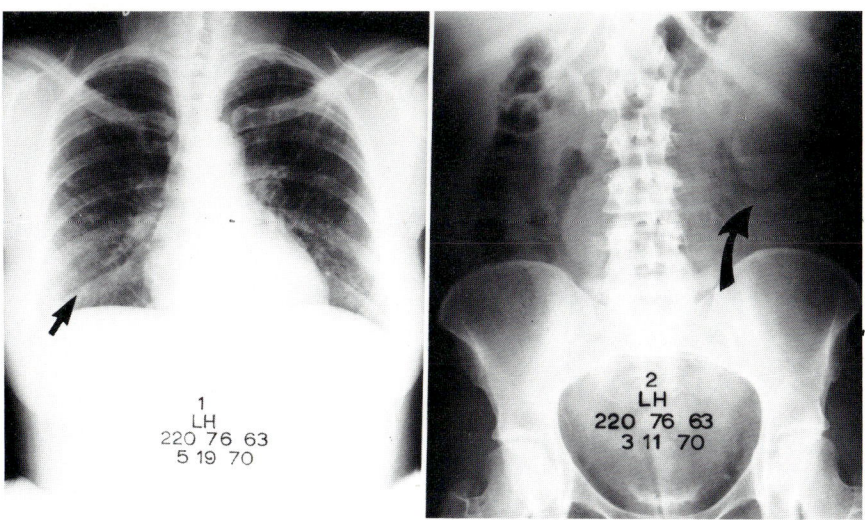

Figure 10.4 A chest radiograph (left) showing bilateral hilar adenopathy and minimal parenchymal infiltration (arrow). An abdominal film (right) shows hepatosplenomegaly (arrow).

Case 2—In 1981 a 31-year-old Negro woman developed a dry, persistent cough. A chest radiograph showed diffuse interstitial infiltrate. She was given prednisone which she discontinued later because of the side-effects. In 1983 the patient was readmitted with an abdominal pain, and a diagnosis of acute cholecystitis was made. Physical examination showed cervical lymphadenopathy, hepatosplenomegaly (8 cm below the left intercostal margin) and skin lesions. Laboratory haemoglobin, 10.3 g.(100 ml)$^{-1}$ (1.6 mmol.ℓ^{-1}); WBC, 6400 mm^{-3} ($6.4 \times 10^9.\ell^{-1}$) with mild eosinophilia (8%). Platelet levels were normal. Angiotensin converting enzyme activity was 56 IU (normal range 10–30 IU). The patient's spleen was huge but she did not complain of any pressure symptoms or show evidence of hypersplenism (*see Figure 10.6*).

Bone marrow

Sarcoidosis of the bone marrow is seldom recognized clinically, but in a carefully conducted autopsy study, Longcope and Freiman demonstrated the presence of non-caseating granulomas in bone marrow in 17% of all patients with sarcoidosis[8]. Browne, Sharma and Salkin described five patients whose bone marrow showed sarcoid granulomas but whose chest radiographs were normal[9]. The authors were careful to exclude infections by using appropriate bacteriological, fungal and

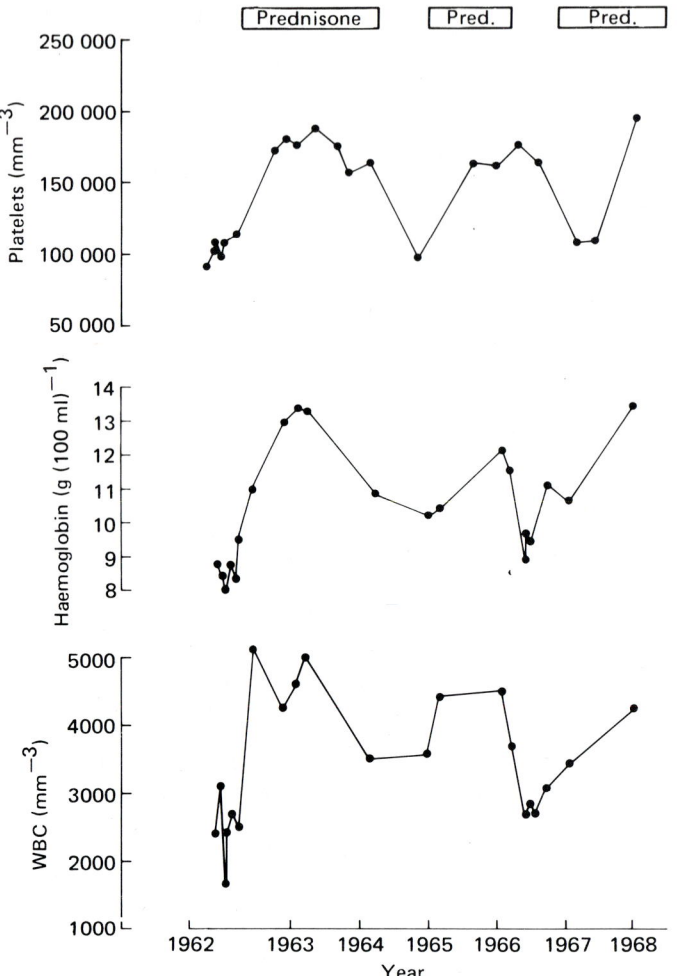

Figure 10.5 Effect of corticosteroid therapy (prednisone) on the thrombocytopenia, anaemia and leucopenia secondary to hypersplenism in a 24-year-old woman with splenic enlargement. Conversion factor: haemoglobin, $1 \text{ g} \cdot (100 \text{ ml})^{-1} = 0.155 \text{ mmol} \cdot \ell^{-1}$.

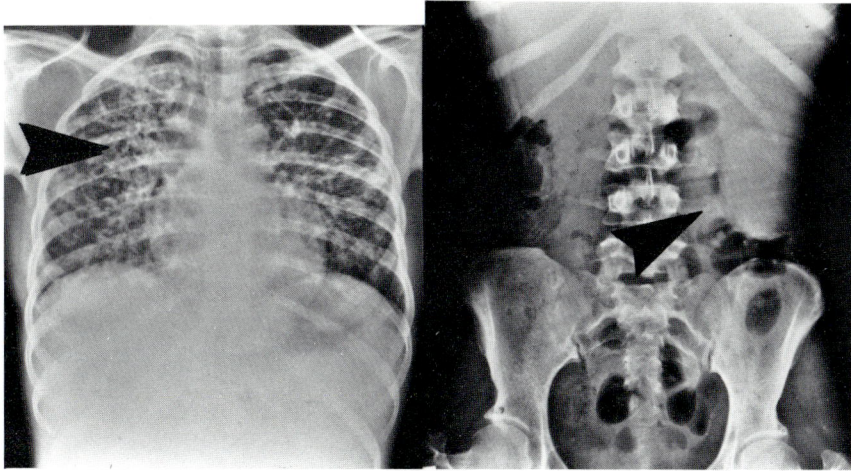

Figure 10.6 Diffuse interstitial fibrosis (left, arrow) and massive splenomegaly (right, arrow) in a 31-year-old woman. The patient showed no evidence of hypersplenism.

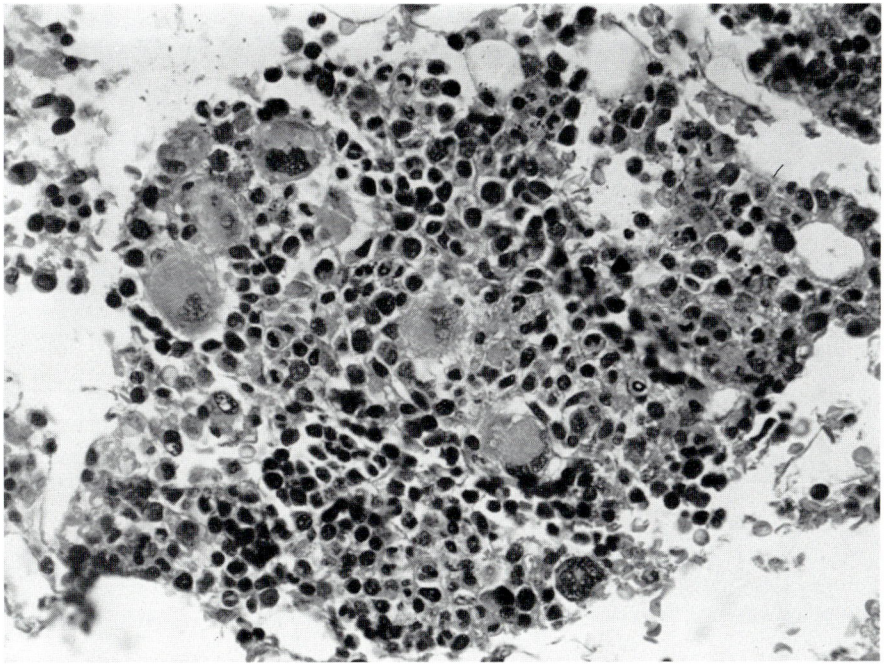

Figure 10.7 Bone-marrow biopsy showing non-caseating granuloma. (Haematoxylin and eosin. × 375.)

TABLE 10.1. Five sarcoidosis patients with bone-marrow involvement*

Patient	Age (years)	Sex	Clinical features	Haematocrit (%)	WBC (mm^{-3})	Differential WBC (%)						Platelet count	Angiotensin converting enzyme (units; normal, 30 units)	Bone marrow Aspiration	Biopsy	Other biopsy specimens showing granuloma
						P	BC	L	E	M	B					
1	51	F	Weakness, malaise, hepatomegaly, skin plaques	34	3900	27	9	58	13	2	0	Decreased	75	Normal	Non-caseating granuloma	Skin
2	25	F	Fever, malaise, hepatosplenomegaly, peripheral lymphadenopathy	19	2600	52	2	28	7	4	0	Normal	50	Normal	Non-caseating granuloma	Liver
3	70	F	Fever, chills, hepatosplenomegaly	31	3300	50	0	29	4	8	0	Decreased	160	Normal	Non-caseating granuloma	Liver
4	40	M	Malaise, abdominal pain	39	5700	40	0	48	7	3	2	Normal	41	Normal	Non-caseating granuloma	None
5	43	M	Fever, chills, splenomegaly	35	7500	60	0	28	7	3	2	Normal	65	Non-caseating granuloma	Not done	None

* Modified from reference 9.
B = Basophils; BC = band cells; E = erythrocytes; L = leucocytes; M = monocytes; P = platelets.

serological studies. Serum angiotensin converting enzyme levels were high in all the patients at the time of diagnosis (*see Table 10.1*).

Thus the presence of non-caseating granuloma in the bone marrow should alert the physician to the possibility of sarcoidosis along with the other common infections (tuberculosis, brucellosis, histoplasmosis) and reticuloendothelial malignancies.

Case report—In 1952, a 46-year-old woman sought medical advice for diffuse maculopapular rash and arthritis of the ankle and wrist joints. Her chest radiograph was normal. She was anaemic and leucopenic. A biopsy specimen of the skin showed non-caseating granulomas. She was given prednisone. Over the following years she remained symptomatic. Further studies included the liver and bone-marrow biopsies; both showed non-caseating granulomas (*see Figure 10.7*). Radiographs of the hands showed bone lesions. The patient is now 72 years old. She has chronic sarcoidosis of low activity. The long-term follow-up, stretching over a 30-year period, showed persistent anaemia, leucopenia and relative lymphocytosis. The patient had no serious infections during this period (*see Figure 10.8*).

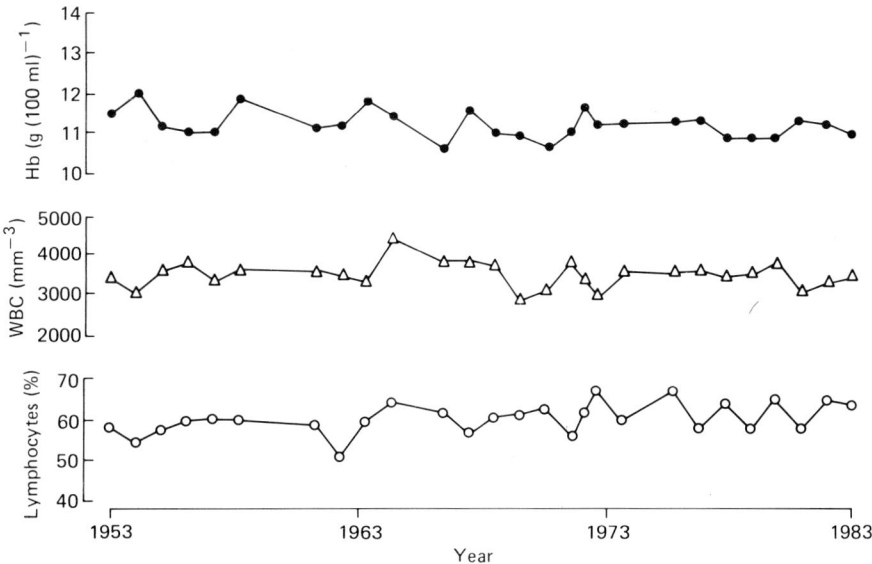

Figure 10.8 30-year follow-up in a patient with bone-marrow involvement, showing anaemia, leucopenia and lymphocytosis. Conversion factor: haemogloblin (Hb), $1 \text{ g.}(100 \text{ ml})^{-1} = 0.155 \text{ mmol.} \ell^{-1}$.

References

1. SHARMA, O.P. and BALCHUM, O.J. (1972) Alcohol-induced pain in sarcoidosis. *Am. Rev. Resp. Dis.*, **106**, 763.
2. SILTZBACH, L.E., JAMES, D.G., NEVILLE, E., *et al.* (1974) Course and prognosis of sarcoidosis around the world. *Am. J. Med.*, **57**, 847.
3. SELROOS, Q. and KOIVUNEN, E. (1983) Usefulness of fine needle aspiration biopsy of spleen in diagnosis of sarcoidosis. *Chest*, **83**, 193.
4. TURIAF, J., BATTESTI, J.P. and HELENON, C. (1976) Selective arteriography of the coeliac artery in patients with thoracic sarcoidosis. *Ann. N.Y. Acad. Sci.*, **278**, 433.
5. KATARIA, Y.P. and WHITCOMB, M.E. (1980) Splenomegaly in sarcoidosis. *Arch. Intern. Med.*, **140**, 35.
6. YOUNG, H.B. and MOONEY, R.A.H. (1968) Giant splenomegaly in sarcoidosis. *Br. J. Surg.*, **55**, 554.
7. GUYTON, J.R. and ZUMWALT, R.E. (1975) Pneumococcemia with sarcoid infiltrated spleen. *Ann. Intern. Med.*, **82**, 847.

8. LONGCOPE, W.T. and FREIMAN, D.G. (1952) A study of sarcoidosis based on a combined investigation of 160 cases including 30 autopsies. *Medicine*, **31**, 1.
9. BROWNE, P.M., SHARMA, O.P. and SALKIN, D. (1978) Bone marrow sarcoidosis. *J. Am. Med. Assoc.*, **240**, 2654.

Chapter 11
Sarcoidosis of the liver

The liver is palpable in only about 20% of patients with sarcoidosis, but granulomas are found in 63-87% depending on the stage and activity of the disease. Klatskin has reported an even higher incidence of 94%[1]. Scadding performed liver biopsies in 73 patients with sarcoidosis and found granulomas in 48 (66%)[2]; when the chest radiograph showed hilar lymph-node enlargement only (stage I), 87% were positive; when there was bilateral hilar adenopathy and infiltration (stage II), 67% were positive; and when the chest X-ray showed pulmonary infiltration (stage III), 59% were positive. Thus liver biopsy is more frequently positive in early, active disease; whereas in chronic sarcoidosis the frequency of hepatic involvement is low. Liver involvement in sarcoidosis may therefore be summarized as follows:

1. Clinically palpable liver in 20% of patients.
2. Raised alkaline phosphatase activity in 30-40% of patients.
3. Positive liver biopsy in 60-80% of patients.

Liver granuloma

Liver granuloma is a well-demarcated cluster of epithelioid cells and occasional multinucleated giant cells. A thin peripheral rim of lymphocytes is present. Small areas of central necrosis are usually seen, but caseation is absent (*see Figure 11.1*). Granulomas predominantly involve the portal zones. It should be realized that the aetiology of hepatic granuloma can seldom be established on histological grounds without clinical, radiological and laboratory evidence. The differential diagnosis of hepatic granuloma particularly in the absence of any evidence of multisystem sarcoidosis requires an extensive search for acid-fast organisms, other bacteria and fungi. Non-caseating granulomas resembling sarcoidosis can be seen in tuberculosis, brucellosis, berylliosis, coccidioidomycosis, histoplasmosis, acquired cytomegalovirus infection, schistosomiasis and neoplastic disorders[3]. Hepatic granulomas are frequently found in primary biliary cirrhosis[4].

90 Sarcoidosis of the liver

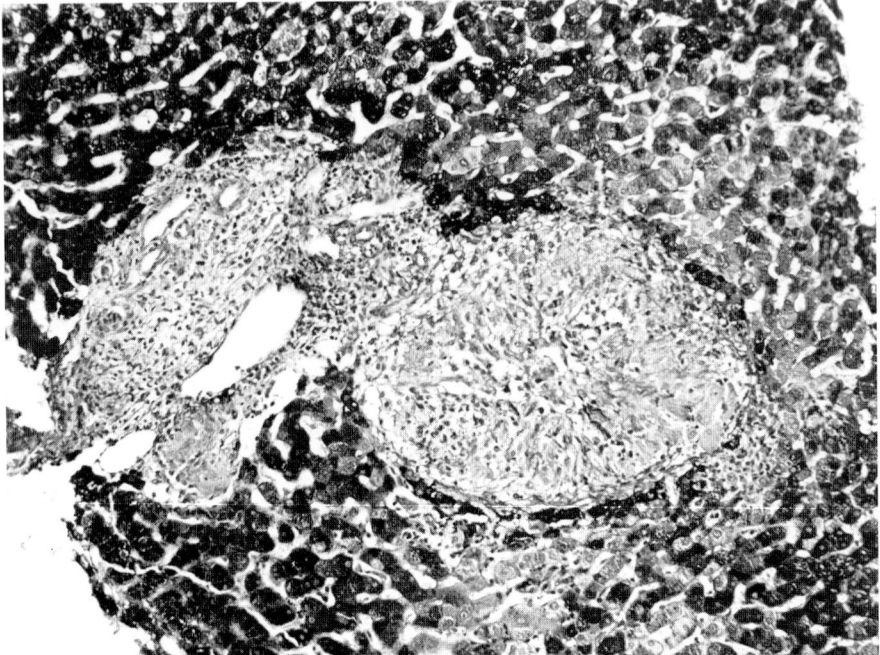

Figure 11.1 Noncaseating granuloma in liver. (Haematoxylin and eosin. × 125.)

Liver function tests

Liver involvement may be extensive without apparent clinical or laboratory evidence of hepatic dysfunction. The granulomas are scattered and often heal with little or no fibrosis. Severe jaundice is uncommon. Maddrey *et al.* described 20 patients, five had severe liver function abnormality and jaundice[4]. Mild elevations of alkaline phosphatase and serum bilirubin are common and may occur in as many as 80% of the patients (*see* Figure 11.2).

Portal hypertension and hepatic failure

Portal hypertension is rare in sarcoidosis. Mistillis, Green and Schiff proposed a presinusoidal mechanism of portal hypertension[5]. Maddrey *et al.*[4] found no evidence of presinusoidal obstruction and concluded that obliteration of the hepatic venous bed by granulomas and fibrosis is the likely mechanism. Chronic intrahepatic cholestasis may occasionally occur and produce jaundice, pruritus and hepatosplenomegaly[6, 7]. Gastrointestinal haemorrhage secondary to oesophageal varices has been reported. Corticosteroids are of no benefit in established portal hyptertension; portosystemic shunt is the treatment of choice.

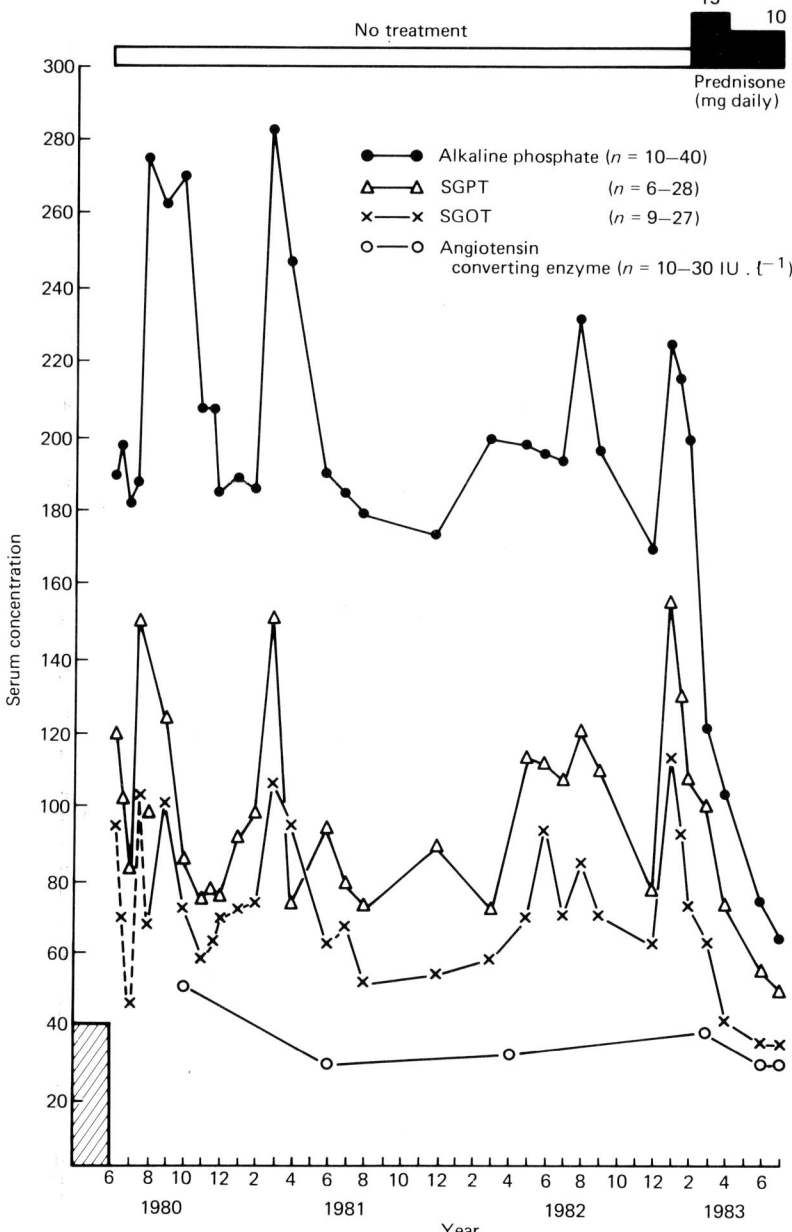

Figure 11.2 Liver function test in a 53-year-old woman with asymptomatic granulomatous hepatitis. Note the fluctuating course and the dramatic effect of a small dosage of prednisone. The patient had no signs and symptoms and worked full time as a secretary. SGOT = serum glutamic–oxaloacetic transaminase; SGPT = serum glutamic–pyruvic transaminase.

References

1. KLATSIN, G. (1977) Hepatic granulomata: Problems in interpretation. *Mt. Sinai J. Med.*, **44,** 798.
2. SCADDING, J.G. (1967) *Sarcoidosis.* (London: Eyre and Spottiswoode)
3. SIMON, H.B. and WOLFF, S.M. (1973) Granulomatous hepatitis and prolonged fever of unknown origin. A study of 13 patients. *Medicine*, **52,** 1.
4. MADDREY, W.C., JOHNS, C.J., BOITNOTT, J.K. and IBER, F.L. (1970) Sarcoidosis and chronic hepatic disease: A clinical and pathological study of 20 cases. *Medicine*, **49,** 375.
5. MISTILLIS, S.P., GREEN, J.R. and SCHIFF, L. (1964) Hepatic sarcoidosis with portal hypertension. *Am. J. Med.*, **36,** 470.
6. BASS, N.M., BURROUGHS, A.K., SCHEUER, P.J., *et al.* (1982) Chronic intrahepatic cholestasis due to sarcoidosis. *Gut*, **23,** 417.
7. TACHIBANA, T. (1976) Peritoneoscopy of sarcoid hepatosplenomegaly. *Ann. N.Y. Acad. Sci.*, **278,** 520.

Chapter 12
The kidneys in sarcoidosis

The kidneys can be affected by sarcoidosis in the following ways:
1. Hypercalcaemia.
2. Hypercalciuria.
3. Granulomatous infiltration of the renal parenchyma.
4. Glomerular disease.
5. Granulomatous renal arteritis.

Hypercalcaemia

This occurs in about 13% of the patients with sarcoidosis and may have a direct depressant action on the renal concentrating ability[1]. In addition, it may lead to impaired renal acid excretion and a decrease in glomerular filtration rate. Blood urea nitrogen levels are high; improvement follows if serum calcium levels are reduced. Adequate hydration and corticosteroid therapy quickly reverses the abnormal calcium metabolism. In this group of patients there is no physical damage to renal parenchyma.

Hypercalciuria

Hypercalciuria leads to nephrocalcinosis and nephrolithiasis—which may or may not be visible radiographically—with obstructive lesions in collecting tubules and finally to renal failure.

Granulomatous infiltration of the renal parenchyma

The incidence of renal granulomas varies from 4 to 40%. Longcope and Freiman recorded renal granulomas in four out of 30 autopsies[2]. In a review of the literature Branson and Park recorded that the kidneys were affected in only eight (7%) of 117 patients[3]. Lebacq reported that epithelioid granulomas are present in 40% of sarcoidosis kidneys[4]. The granulomatous lesion usually consists of a few scattered tubercles in the renal cortex and medulla; massive infiltration is rare. Mild albuminuria and an abnormal urinary sediment (red and white blood cells, granular casts) are frequent[5].

Alterations of tubular functions including impaired concentrating ability, depressed tubular function, water reabsorption and abnormal renal acidification have been reported[6]. In patients with extensive granulomas severe impairment of renal function is present. Interstitial infiltration by mononuclear cells is another pathological feature which occurs in about 32% of the patients. The lesion has been considered to be a forerunner of true granuloma formation[7]. Corticosteroids improve filtration rate, urinalysis, acid excretion and concentrating ability. Follow-up renal biopsies in a few patients have demonstrated the disappearance of granulomas and improvement of interstitial infiltration.

Glomerular disease

Recently, both membranous and proliferative glomerular abnormalities have been described in sarcoidosis. Proliferative glomerulonephritis seems to be less frequent than membranous nephropathy. Immunofluorescent studies may show immune-complex deposits (IgG and complement) along the glomerular basement membrane. Most of the patients have either proteinuria or clinical nephrotic syndrome[8-10]. The latter may be the expression of membranous glomerulonephritis and focal glomerulosclerosis[11]. Hypertension occurs frequently but is rarely a serious problem. Corticosteroids have not been successful in the treatment of membranous nephropathy.

Granulomatous renal arteritis

Although hyaline deposits in arterial walls occur frequently in sarcoidosis, true obliterative granulomatous endarteritis of the renal arterioles is uncommon[12]. When it occurs, it is usually associated with severe hypertension and carries a poor prognosis.

Case report:—In October 1980, a 42-year-old man was admitted for the treatment of haematuria, diffuse skin lesions, arthritis, pain and redness of the eyes, and bouts of depression. Although the diagnosis of sarcoidosis had been made 12 years earlier, he had received corticosteroid treatment only for 1 year, 1975. In the past he had had nephrostomies on both kidneys. Physical examination: blood pressure, 120/85 mmHg; pulse, 80 beats per minute, regular; respiration, 18 per minute. Eye examination reveleaed an atonic pupil on the right side. Intraocular tension was normal. Slit-lamp examination showed a trace of posterior subcapsular haziness in the right eye.

A maculopapular rash was present on the back, forearms and legs. Laboratory results: Haemoglobin, $16.8\,g.(100\,ml)^{-1}$ $(2.6\,mmol.\ell^{-1})$; WBC, $5\,300\,mm^{-3}$ $(5.3\times10^9.\ell^{-1})$ with a normal differential. Urine showed 40–50 white blood cells and 15–20 red blood cells per high power field. Serum electrolytes, calcium and liver function tests were normal. Twenty-four hour urine calcium results on three consecutive days were 129.0, 135.0 and 148 mg (normal range, 100–300 mg. (24 hour)$^{-1}$). Immunoglobulin analysis: IgG, $752\,mg.(100\,ml)^{-1}$ $(7.52\,g.\ell^{-1})$ (normal range, $560\text{--}1512\,mg.(100\,ml)^{-1}$; $5.6\text{--}15.12\,g.\ell^{-1}$); IgM, $95.0\,mg.(100\,ml)^{-1}$ $(0.95\,g.\ell^{-1})$ (normal range, $43\text{--}323\,mg.(100\,ml)^{-1}$; $0.43\text{--}3.23\,g.\ell^{-1}$); and IgA, $75.0\,mg.(100\,ml)^{-1}$ $(0.75\,g.\ell^{-1})$ (normal range, $104\text{--}448\,mg.(100\,ml)^{-1}$; $1.04\text{--}4.48\,g.\ell^{-1}$). Serum angiotensin converting enzyme activity was 55 units (normal range 12–36 units).

A skin biopsy specimen showed non-caseating granulomas. Special stains for acid-fast bacilli and fungi were negative. A chest radiograph showed diffuse, disseminated small rounded and irregular opacities with prominence of the main pulmonary artery segment. An intravenous pyelogram displayed large calcifications in the region of the left kidney with hydronephrosis. The right kidney demonstrated only some blunting of the minor calyces and a few small calculi (*see Figure 12.1*). A gallium-67 scan showed slight diffuse uptake in both lungs and in parotid and lacrimal glands (*see Figure 12.2*).

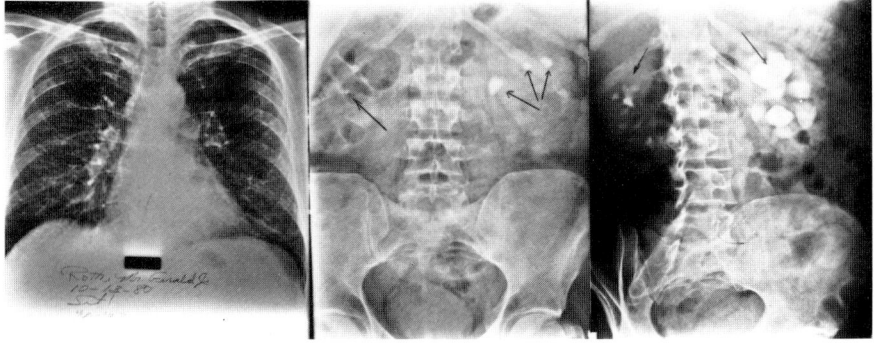

Figure 12.1 Renal stones and hydronephrosis (arrows) in a 42-year-old man.

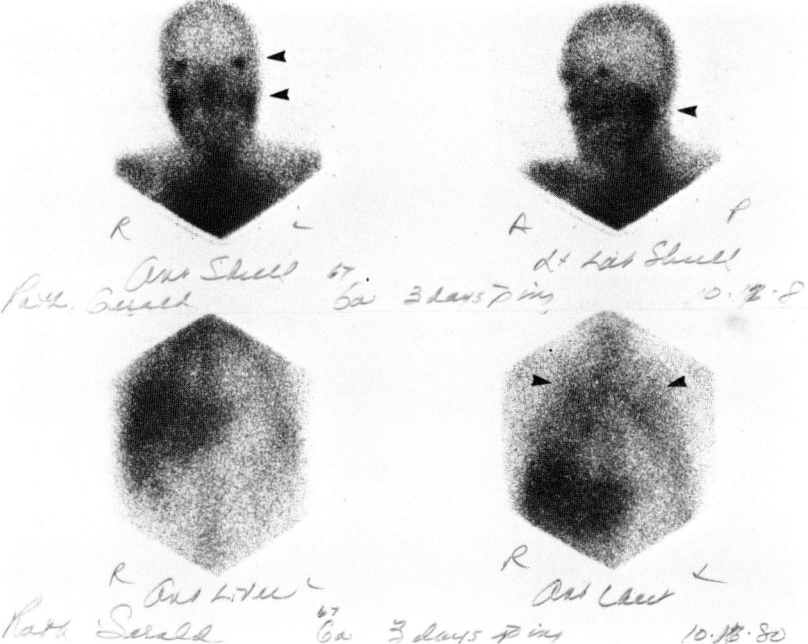

Figure 12.2 Gallium-67 uptake by lacrimal and parotid glands. Mild diffuse pulmonary uptake is also noted.

Comment — In this patient, uncontrolled hypercalcaemia and hypercalciuria were responsible for nephrocalcinosis and obstructive uropathy. On the present examination his serum and urine calcium results were normal because he was taking Dyazide (triamterine and hydrochlorothiazide). I treated him with hydrochlorothiazide 50 mg twice daily and prednisone 30 mg daily, which was gradually reduced to 20 mg daily. He was advised to avoid milk, cheese, nuts and other high-calcium foods and to spend as little time as possible in direct sunlight. His low serum IgA level was probably an incidental finding.

References

1. EPSTEIN, F.H., RIVERA, M.J. and CARONE, F.A. (1958) Effect of hypercalcemia induced by calciferal upon renal concentrating ability. *J. Clin. Invest.*, **37,** 1702.
2. LONGCOPE, W.T. and FREIMAN, D.G. (1952) A study of sarcoidosis. *Medicine*, **31,** 1.
3. BRANSON, J.H. and PARK, J.H. (1954) Sarcoidosis-hepatic involvement: Presentations of cases with fatal liver involvement, including autopsy findings and review of evidence for sarcoid involvement of liver as found in literature. *Ann. Intern. Med.*, **40,** 111.
4. LEBACQ, E.G. (1970) Renal involvement in sarcoidosis. *Postgrad. Med. J.*, **46,** 526.
5. LOFGREN, S., SNELLMAN, B. and LINDGREN, A.G.H. (1957) Renal complications in sarcoidosis: Functional and biopsy studies. *Acta Med. Scand.*, **159,** 295.
6. MORRIS, R.C., JOHNSON, L.B. and FUDENBERG, H. (1965) Impairment of renal acidification in hyperglobulinemia patients. *Clin. Res.*, **13,** 115.
7. ROMER, F.K. (1980) Renal manifestations and abnormal calcium metabolism in sarcoidosis. *Q. J. Med.*, **49,** 233.
8. MCCOY, R.C. and TISHER, C.C. (1972) Glomerulonephritis associated with sarcoidosis. *Am. J. Pathol.*, **68,** 339.
9. MACSEARRAIGH, D., DOYLE, C.T., TWOMEY, M., *et al.* (1978) Sarcoidosis with renal involvement. *Postgrad. Med. J.*, **54,** 528.
10. RICHMOND, J.M., CHAMBERS, B., D'APICE, A.J.F., *et al.* (1981) Renal disease in sarcoidosis. *Med. J. Aust.*, **ii,** 36.
11. TAYLOR, T.K., SENEKJIAN, H.O., KNIGHT, T.F., *et al.* (1979) Membranous nephropathy with epithelial crescent in a patient with pulmonary sarcoidosis. *Arch. Intern. Med.*, **139,** 1183.
12. NUTHER, R.S., MCCARRON, D.A. and BENNETT, W.M. (1981) Renal manifestations of sarcoidosis. *Arch. Intern. Med.*, **141,** 643.

Chapter 13
Myocardial sarcoidosis

Although clinically recognizable involvement of the heart occurs in about 5% of patients with sarcoidosis, at autopsy myocardial granulomas are found in as many as 27%[1-4]. No portion of the heart is immune to sarcoidosis. The granulomas most commonly involve the free wall of the left ventricle, followed by the ventricular septum, the right ventricle and lastly the atrial wall (see Figure 13.1). Aorta, pulmonary arteries, superior vena cava and pulmonary veins are infrequently affected. The granulomatous invasion of the pericardium and the valves is rare[5].

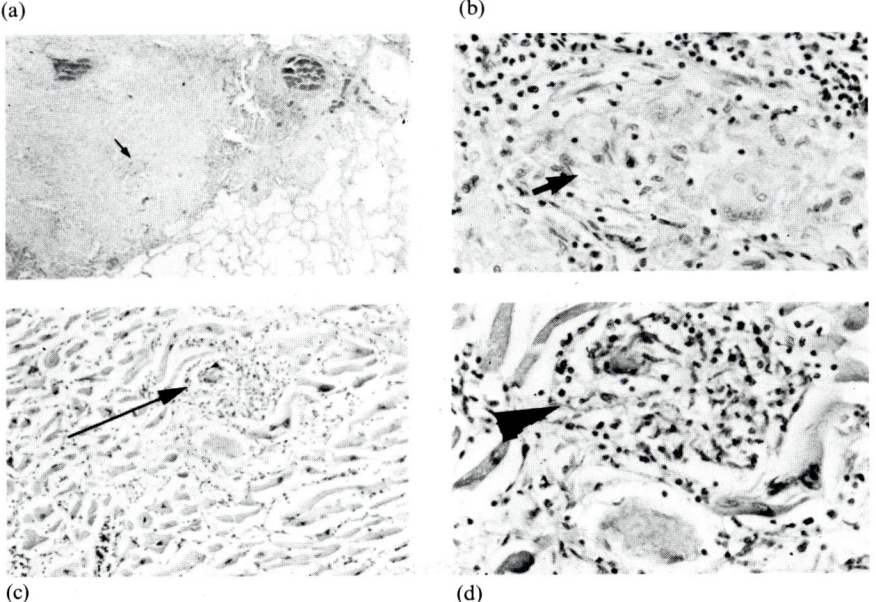

Figure 13.1 Myocardial granulomas (arrows) in a young healthy man who died suddenly. (a) × 75, (b) × 50; (c) × 100; (d) × 150.

Diagnosis

The diagnosis of myocardial sarcoidosis is often difficult because in most cases the cardiac lesion is minimal, patchy and asymptomatic. Signs and symptoms of the disease depend on the number and location of the granulomas and the presence or absence of the myocardial scarring. The clinical evidence of myocardial disease may precede other manifestations of sarcoidosis by many years[6]. Cardiac sarcoidosis may present clinically in the following ways.

Alterations of rhythm

Conduction disturbances

Conduction disturbances are the most frequent clinical evidence of myocardial sarcoidosis. The disturbances occur in the form of partial heart block including intraventricular conduction defects and complete heart block. Complete heart block was a feature in 44 (22%) and partial block (including right bundle-branch block) in 70 (35%) of 200 patients studied by Fleming[7]. Nineteen (54%) out of 35 patients reported by Bashour et al. showed varying degrees of conduction disturbances[8]. Miyaji et al., in a review of 12 patients, discovered seven with atrioventricular block[9]. Complete heart block occurred in five and partial heart block in two out of 11 patients described by Gozo and his colleagues[10]. The high incidence of conduction disturbances in the disease is not surprising because granulomas involved the ventricular septum in 19 (73%) of 26 patients with cardiac dysfunction due to sarcoidosis; the left ventricular wall was infiltrated in 25 (96%) and the right ventricular wall in 12 (46%) patients[5]. Of the 70 cases reviewed by Gozo et al. granulomas were found in the ventricular septum in 30 (43%) and right or left ventricular walls in 57 patients (81%)[10].

Cardiac arrhythmias

Disturbances of rhythm are the second most common presenting features of myocardial sarcoidosis. Of the 200 cases studied by Fleming, 77 (38.5%) suffered ventricular arrhythmia, and 46 (23%) had supraventricular arrhythmias[7]. Multiple ventricular premature contractions occur occasionally. Atrial arrhythmias are rare[11, 12]. Rhythm disturbances may produce palpitation, dizziness, syncope and rarely, psychiatric manifestations[13].

Sudden death

Sudden death is common and is frequently the first manifestation of myocardial sarcoidosis. It occurred in 49 (24.5%) of 200 patients reported by Fleming[7]. Autopsy studies on the patients who died showed extensive infiltration of the myocardium by granulomas and fibrosis[6].

Congestive heart failure

Congestive heart failure (CHF) may result either from severe rhythm disturbances or from extensive granulomatous infiltration causing impaired cardiac contractility[5]. In Porter's series, CHF occurred in one-third of the patients[14]. Fourteen out of 16 patients studied by Bashour et al. had evidence of heart failure[8]. Of the six patients described by Ghosh et al., three were in heart failure[15]. Autopsy studies in the patients dying of heart failure usually reveal extensive myocardial damage. In the early stages when the damage is limited to minimal mitochondrial damage the granulomatous process might be reversible[16].

Myocardial infarction-like picture

About 7% of the patients with cardiac sarcoidosis develop chest pain resembling angina pectoris or myocardial infarction. The electrocardiographic changes suggestive of transmural myocardial infarction may occur if there is a full-thickness replacement of the myocardium by sarcoid granulomas[17-19].

Valvular involvement

Valvular involvement is rare. Six (3%) of 200 patients in Fleming's series were noted to have aortic diastolic murmurs. In one patient a congenitally stenotic aortic valve was replaced which showed non-caseating granulomas[7,15].

Mitral valve involvement is more frequent. The mitral systolic murmurs which are usually transient or recurrent may often become permanent and are probably produced due to papillary muscle involvement. An echocardiographic examination should always be performed in a patient with sarcoidosis who develops a mitral systolic murmur. Raftery, Oakley and Goodwin have described a sarcoid patient who had developed mitral incompetence due to papillary muscle dysfunction. The mitral valve was replaced. Histology of the papillary muscle showed granulomas[20]. Sarcoid involvement of the tricuspid valve has also been reported[21].

Ventricular aneurysm

Ventricular aneurysm may occur in patients with cardiac sacoidosis. The aneurysm may be small, occupying a relatively limited area of the ventricular wall; or it may be diffuse, encompassing a large portion of the cardiac wall. Roberts et al. suggested that the aneurysmal dilation in a sarcoid patient may be related in part to the administration of corticosteroids[5]. Excision of a left ventricular aneurysm may be beneficial[22].

Pericardial involvement

Shiff, Blatt and Colp reported the first case of clinically significant pericardial effusion with histological evidence of granulomas in the pericardium[23]. Roberts et al. have described three deaths to pericardial effusion. All three patients had epicardial sarcoid granulomas[5]. Recurrent pericardial effusion is rare, although the use of echocardiography, in one study, has disclosed small pericardial effusion in 19% of 48 cases[24].

Electrocardiographic abnormalities

Siltzbach noted abnormal electrocardiographic changes in 40 (50%) of 80 patients with histologically confirmed sarcoidosis but without complaints. The abnormalities included conduction or rhythm disturbances, ST deviations or T-wave changes[25,26]. Similar findings were recorded by Mikhail et al. from London in 14 (10%) of their 147 patients[27]. Numao et al. studied electrocardiograms of 963 patients with sarcoidosis and compared with 946 sex-age-matched healthy controls; 22.1% of patients had ECG abnormalities including premature ventricular contraction, right bundle-branch block, premature atrial contraction and ST-T wave changes[28].

Endomyocardial biopsy

Endomyocardial biopsy is of limited value because of the patchy distribution of the disease. Sekiguchi *et al.* performed simulated myocardial biopsies on the seven hearts involved in fatal sarcoidosis. They biopsied 10 different sites in both the right and the left ventricle. Even in those heavily infiltrated hearts, there was a high rate of false-negative biopsies—37% in the right ventricle and 53% in the left ventricle[29].

Thallium-201 imaging

Thallium-201 is routinely used to study myocardial perfusion. Bulkley *et al.* noted focal abnormalities in a small number of sarcoid patients[30]. Kinney detected focal defects in 30% of the patients with sarcoidosis[31]. Haywood *et al.*[32] found focal left ventricular defects in four (13%) out of 30 patients. All the defects decreased in size during thallium stress imaging, a finding opposite of that usually seen in myocardial ischaemia. Nine patients had abnormal right ventricular visualization at rest. Thus, 11 (37%) out of 30 patients had abnormal myocardial scans at rest. Two-dimensional echocardiograms in these patients failed to demonstrate segmental ventricular contraction abnormalities[32].

Diagnosis, evaluation and importance

The diagnosis of primary myocardial sarcoidosis is usually made on the basis of one or more of the cardiac abnormalities (described above) occurring in a patient with histologically proved multisystem sarcoidosis. When the diagnosis has been established, a 24-hour Holter monitoring with exercise testing may be needed to exclude significant arrhythmia. Echocardiography should be used, particularly in the presence of a murmur, to exclude any abnormality of the mitral value, ventricular septum, the left ventricular wall and the pericardium. Thallium-201 scanning may be of value in detecting myocardial lesions and monitoring the effect of therapy on the size of the focal defect. The role of endomyocardial biopsy remains to be established. Because of a high incidence of sudden death, all patients with myocardial sarcoidosis should be aggressively treated and closely monitored. Fleming believes that no one with sarcoidosis should fly single-handedly and this prohibition should be life-long because the myocardial involvement may occur many years after other manifestations of the disease have appeared[6]. This certainly is a wise prophylactic step which needs further evaluation.

References

1. SILVERMAN, K.J., HUTCHINS, G.M. and BUCKLEY, B.H. (1978) Cardiac sarcoid: A clinicopathologic study of 84 unselected patients with systemic sarcoidosis. *Circulation*, **58**, 1204.

2. MAYOCK, R.L., BERTRAND, P., MORRISON, C.E., et al. (1963) Manifestations of sarcoidosis: Analysis of 145 patients with a review of nine series. *Am. J. Med.*, **35**, 67.
3. LONGCOPE, W.T. and FREIMAN, D.G. (1952) A study of sarcoidosis. *Medicine*, **31**, 1.
4. RIKER, W. and CLARK, M. (1949) Sarcoidosis. *Am. J. Clin. Pathol.*, **19**, 725.
5. ROBERTS, W.C., MCALLISTER, H.A. and FERRANS, V.J. (1977) Sarcoidosis of the heart: A clinicopathologic study of 35 necropsy patients (group I) and review of 78 previously described necropsy patients (group II). *Am. J. Med.*, **63**, 86.
6. FLEMING, H.A. and BAILEY, S.M. (1981) Sarcoid heart disease. Report of 197 United Kingdom cases with necropsy confirmation in 62. *J. R. Coll. Phys.*, **15**, 245.
7. FLEMING, H.A. (1981) Review of sarcoid heart disease 1981. In *Sarcoidosis* (eds Chretien, J., Marsac, J. and Saltiel, J.C.), p. 312. (Paris: Pergamon Press)
8. BASHOUR, F.A., MCCONNELL, T., SKINNER, W., et al. (1968) Myocardial sarcoidosis. *Dis. Chest*, **53**, 413.
9. MIYAJI, T., OHARA, M., FUNAKI, M., et al. (1967) A case of myocardial sarcoidosis with Adams–Stokes syndrome. *J. Jap. Soc. Intern. Med.*, **56**, 360.
10. GOZO, E.G., Jr., COSNEW, I., COHEN, H.G., et al. (1971) The heart in sarcoidosis. *Chest*, **60**, 379.
11. PASCOE, H.R. (1964) Myocardial sarcoidosis. *Arch. Pathol.*, **77**, 299.
12. NISSEN, A.W. and BERTE, J.B. (1964) Cardiac arrhythmias in sarcoidosis. *Arch. Intern. Med.*, **113**, 275.
13. RAJASENON, V. and COOPER, F.S. (1969) Myocardial sarcoidosis, bouts of ventricular tachycardia, psychiatric manifestations and sudden death. *J. Natl. Med. Assoc.*, **61**, 306.
14. PORTER, G.H. (1960) Sarcoid heart disease. *N. Engl. J. Med.*, **263**, 1350.
15. GHOSH, P., FLEMING, H.A., GRESHAM, G.A., et al. (1972) Myocardial sarcoidosis. *Br. Heart J.*, **34**, 769.
16. FERRANS, V.J., HIBBS, R.G., BLACK, W.C., et al. (1965) Myocardial degeneration in sarcoidosis. Histochemical and electron microscopic studies. *Am. Heart J.*, **69**, 159.
17. GOLD, J.A. and CANTOR, P.J. (1959) Sarcoid heart disease. A case with an unusual electrocardiogram. *Arch. Intern. Med.*, **104**, 101.
18. HINES, H.D. and SANCETTA, S.M. (1963) Myocardial sarcoidosis simulating healed myocardial infarction. *Ohio State Med. J.*, **59**, 689.
19. CHISOLM, J.C., Jr. (1966) Sarcoid cardiomyopathy. *J. Natl. Med. Assoc.*, **58**, 265.
20. RAFTERY, E.B., OAKLEY, G. and GOODWIN, J.F. (1966) Acute subvalvular mitral incompetence. *Lancet*, **ii**, 360.
21. STEIN, M.H., GROSS, J.M. and SHULMAN, H. (1962) A case of cardiac sarcoidosis manifested by uncontrollable ventricular tachycardia. Review of cardiac manifestations in sixteen cases of sarcoidosis. *Am. J. Cardiol.*, **10**, 864.
22. LULL, R.J., DUNN, B.E., GREGORATOS, G., et al. (1972) Ventricular aneurysm due to cardiac sarcoidosis with surgical cure of refractory ventricular tachycardia. *Am. J. Cardiol.*, **30**, 282.
23. SHIFF, A.D., BLATT, C.J. and COLP, C. (1969) Recurrent pericardial effusion secondary to sarcoidosis of the pericardium. A biopsy-proved case. *N. Engl. J. Med.*, **281**, 141.
24. KINNEY, E., MURTHY, R., ASCUNLE, J., et al. (1979) Effusions in sarcoidosis. *Chest*, **76**, 476.
25. DENEBERG, M. (1965) sarcoidosis of the myocardium and aorta. *Am. J. Clin. Pathol.*, **44**, 445.
26. STEIN, E., JOCKLEV, I., STIMMEL, B., et al. (1973) Asymptomatic electrocardiographic alterations in sarcoidosis. *Am. Heart. J.*, **86**, 474.
27. MIKHAIL, J.R., MITCHELL, D.N. and BALL, K.R. (1974) Abnormal electrocardiographic findings in sarcoidosis. In *Proceedings of the International Conference on Sarcoidosis* (eds Iwai, K. and Hosoda, Y), p. 365. (Tokyo: University of Tokyo Press)
28. NUMAO, Y., SEKIGUCHI, M., FRUIE, T., et al. (1980) Study of cardiac involvement in 963 cases of sarcoidosis by ECG and endomyocardial biopsy. In *Sarcoidosis and Other Granulomatous Diseases* (eds Williams, W.J. and Davies, B.H.), p. 607. (Cardiff: Alpha Omega Publishing)
29. SEKIGUCHI, M., NUMAO, Y., IMAI, M., et al. (1980) Clinical and histopathological profile of sarcoidosis of the heart and acute idiopathic myocarditis. Concepts through a study employing endomyocardial biopsy. I Sarcoidosis. *Jap. Circ. J.*, **44**, 249.
30. BULKLEY, B.H., ROULEAU, R., WHITTAKER, J.Q., et al. (1977) The use of thallium-201 for myocardial imaging in sarcoid heart disease. *Chest*, **72**, 27.
31. KINNEY, E.L., JACKSON, G.L., REEVES, W.C., et al. (1980) Thallium scan myocardial defects and echocardiographic abnormalities in patients with sarcoidosis without clinical cardiac dysfunction. *Am. J. Med.*, **68**, 497.
32. HAYWOOD, L.J., SHARMA, O.P., SIEGEL, M.E., et al. (1982) Detection of myocardial sarcoidosis by thallium-201 imaging. *J. Natl. Med. Assoc.*, **74**, 959.

Chapter 14
Neurosarcoidosis

Sarcoidosis may involve the nervous system in 1–29% of cases with an average of about 5%[1, 2].

Clinical diagnosis of neurosarcoidosis depends on the finding of neurological involvement in a patient with the multisystem disease. When the neural lesions occur in the absence of other tissue involvement, the diagnosis is open to misinterpretation and requires histological confirmation. Cranial nerves, meninges, hypothalamus and pituitary gland are the most frequently involved sites in the central nervous sytem.

Cranial nerve involvement

Facial nerve

Of the cranial nerves, the facial nerve is most frequently affected. Facial nerve palsy is also the most common neurological manifestation of sarcoidosis[3]. Colover found facial paralysis in 58 (50%) of 118 cases reviewed from the literature[4]. This was unilateral in 65% and bilateral in 35% of these patients. Facial nerve was affected in 12 (67%) of 18 cases studied by Silverstein, Feurer and Sitzbach[5]. The palsy was right-sided in eight, left-sided in two and two more patients had bilateral involvement. Seventh-nerve palsy occurred in 25 patients studied by James and Sharma. The lesion was right-sided in nine, left-sided in seven, and seven were bilateral. In most cases, the palsy is sudden, transient, and of lower motor neurone type. If the lesion is above the level of chorda tympani, loss of taste may occur.

The pathogenesis is unclear. Initially, it was suggested that pressure due to an inflamed, swollen parotid gland was responsible for the lesion. Parotid gland enlargement, however, accompanied the facial palsy in only two out of 12 cases reported by Silverstein, and four out of 25 cases reported by James and Sharma. Also, the nerve compression in the region of mastoid foramen does not explain the occurrence of loss of taste sometimes associated with facial palsy.

Furthermore, facial paralysis may follow parotitis by days or weeks, or precede it[2]. Wells postulated that apart from direct invasion, the sarcoid may have some distant effects on neural and glial tissues. He pointed out that areas of increased vascularity such as hypothalamus, optic nerve head and the sites of spinal fluid secretions are frequently affected by sarcoidosis. A small increase in serum concentration of any granulomagenic toxin would have a maximum effect at these places. Facial palsy and the parotid gland swelling might also be due to an exposure to such a hypothetical toxin[6].

Optic nerve

The optic nerve is the second most commonly involved cranial nerve. Visual symptoms—including blurred vision, field defects, and pupillary abnormalities—occur due to the granulomatous infiltration of the nerves, chiasma, or tracts.

Glossopharyngeal and vagus nerves

Involvement of the pharynx, soft palate and vocal cords is the third most frequent cranial nerve syndrome.

Auditory

Colover[4] noted deafness in eight out of 118 patients. Delaney[2] studied three patients with the eighth nerve involvement. Fluctuating deafness and vertigo were the main symptoms. Other cranial nerves may be involved, in the following order of decreasing frequency: oculomotor, trigeminal, hypoglossal, olfactory, abducens, accessory and trochlear. Matthews[7] and Delaney[2] have, independently, reported the occurrence of multiple cranial nerve palsies.

Papilloedema

Papilloedema was observed in seven out of 38 patients reported by James and Sharma[3]. They advised that in patients with papilloedema, the diagnosis of neurosarcoidosis should be entertained when it develops rapidly in young adults, particularly women of childbearing age and especially if there is facial weakness or other cranial nerve palsies. About 5% of the patients have demonstrable changes in the optic papilla.

Intracranial involvement

Hypothalamus and pituitary gland

The most common intracranial sites of sarcoid involvement are the hypothalamus, the third ventricle, and the pituitary gland. Pennell reported symptoms of diabetes insipidus in 35% of patients with neurosarcoidosis[8]. Other manifestations of the hypothalamus pituitary axis disturbances include obesity, lethargy, sleep disturbances, hypogonadism and amenorrhoea. Enlargement of sella turcica may cause bitemporal hemianopia.

Space-occupying lesions

Localized granulomatous mass lesions have been found in practically every part of the central nervous system, including the floor of the third ventricle; lateral ventricle; occipital, frontal and temporal lobes; optic chiasma; basal ganglia; cerebellum and the spinal cord[9].

Localized lesions show a certain predilection for the base of the brain. The clinical features are similar to any space-occupying mass and include headaches, lethargy, seizures, diminution of visual acuity, papilloedema and optic atrophy[10]. The cerebrospinal fluid usually shows high protein levels. Skull radiographs are usually normal, but CAT scans have been found useful in defining the mass-occupying lesions[11].

Meningitis

Meningitis in sarcoidosis is usually of chronic nature. Naumann, however, has described a 3-month-old infant who presented with fever, neck rigidity and spinal fluid pleocytosis associated with cutaneous manifestations of sarcoidosis. The child died, and an autopsy revealed granulomas in the subdural layer of the falx, tentorium and under the sutures of the skull[12]. Meningitis was clinically suspected in nine (64%) of the 14 patients. Subsequent autopsies revealed granulomatous involvement of the meninges in all of the 14 cases. The CSF findings include pleocytosis (predominantly lymphocytes) and elevated protein in about 70% of the patients. One in every five patients shows low CSF glucose.

Seizures

Seizures occur in 5-22% of the patients with neurosarcoidosis. Grand mal, focal, Jacksonian, psychomotor and myoclonic seizures have been described. The presence of seizures indicates chronicity and poor prognosis.

Peripheral neuropathy

Peripheral nerve involvement may occur either alone or in association with other cranial nerve palsies which is infrequent. The overall frequency of peripheral neuropathy is 15%. Manifestations of sarcoid neuropathy include paraesthesia, root pains, weakness and wasting of muscles, and absence or depression of tendon reflexes[13]. Neuralgia, symmetrical or asymmetrical, is a frequent symptom. Matthews described three cases of sarcoidosis with evidence of peripheral nerve involvement which consisted of hyperaesthesia and weakness in the leg in one and sensory changes in the left hand in another. Cranial nerves were involved in all three. Two of the four patients described by Silverstein et al.[5] had exclusively motor manifestations and in the other two both motor and sensory disturbances were noted. Three of the four patients had cranial neuropathy. In 14 out of 21 published reports on peripheral neuritis reviewed by Colover,[4] cranial as well as peripheral nerves were involved.

A Landry-Guillain-Barré syndrome has been described. The pathogenesis of peripheral neuropathy is uncertain. The cause may be a toxin, but granulomatous infiltration of the nerve and segmental demyelination have been demonstrated[3,4].

Electromyographic studies in the patients with neuropathy may show increased insertional activity, spontaneous electrical activity consisting of fibrillation potentials and positive waves from the muscles at rest. Conduction velocities may be prolonged[5].

Psychiatric manifestations

Occasionally, the granulomatous infiltration of the central nervous system may produce a wide variety of mental symptoms. In one of the five patients with psychiatric manifestations described by Hook, symptoms were so profound that the patient had to be committed to a mental institution[14]. The symptoms of apathy, lack of judgement and memory loss were thought to be due to an obstructing lesion in the inferior horn of the right ventricle. Other manifestations include agitation, hallucination, irritability, memory loss, lethargy, persecution ideas and confused states[15].

Spinal-cord involvement

Involvement of the spinal cord is rare[13]. Less than 20 cases have been reported. Delaney described two patients who presented with signs of spinal-cord dysfunction including paraparesis, back and leg pains and incontinence. The CSF showed increased protein and pleocytosis. X-rays of the spinal cord are usually normal. Myelograms may reveal a partial block or arachnoiditis (*see* case report below).

Cerebrospinal fluid

Hook observed a marked pleocytosis and raised protein levels in two (22%) of his nine patients[14]. Pernell, in a review of the cerebrospinal changes in sarcoidosis, noted that at least 50% of the patients had a moderate pleocytosis and moderate to marked increase in serum protein values. Colover reported that serum protein values were raised in about 80% of cases with an average value of $275 \text{ mg} . (100 \text{ ml})^{-1}$ ($2.75 \text{g} . \ell^{-1}$). Protein content is usually high in patients with spinal-cord lesion or peripheral neuropathy. A significant lowering of the blood glucose level to the range of $10-40 \text{ mg} . (100 \text{ ml})^{-1}$ ($0.55-2.2 \text{ mmol} . \ell^{-1}$) has been reported. Cerebrospinal fluid is usually normal in patients with a localized brain lesion. The CSF examination could be of diagnostic value in patients suspected of having neurosarcoidosis.

Miscellaneous studies

Electroencephalograms (EEG) show abnormal features in 80% of patients with central nervous system lesions. In the patients with peripheral neuropathy, electromyograms reveal increased insertional as well as spontaneous electrical activity[16]. Cranial computed axial tomography (CAT) is the most informative study. The non-caseating granulomas show as slightly attenuating, homogeneously enhancing mass lesions, with little surrounding low attenuation[17]. Hydrocephalus is best diagnosed by CAT and enhancement of the basal meninges may indicate the presence of active granulomas.

Case report—A 39-year-old man developed fatigue and left-sided pain extending from the midline anteriorly to the back and from the nipple line to upper border of the pelvis. Despite the symptomatic therapy, the pain persisted. Gradually, the pain became severe and localized in his mid-back between the scapulae. It did not radiate down to the arms, neck or the anterior chest wall. He denied any numbness or weakness. His son had sarcoidosis.

Physical examination showed a large area of hyperaesthesia over the region supplied by the lower thoracic nerve roots on the left. The rest of the examination was normal. Laboratory results: the serum protein electrophoresis showed mildly elevated gamma globulin levels. CSF: glucose, $61 \text{ mg.}(100 \text{ ml})^{-1}$ ($3.4 \text{ mmol} . \ell^{-1}$); chloride, $116 \text{ mEq (mmol)} . \ell^{-1}$ proteins, $168 \text{ mg}. (100 \text{ ml})^{-1}$ ($1.68 \text{ g.})^{-1}$). Radiographs of the chest, cervical spine and thoracic spine were normal. A myelogram showed a filling defect from T1 to T8 which was felt to be consistent with malignant tumour.

Because of the significant elevations in serum glutamic–pyruvic transaminase (SGPT), serum glutamic–

oxaloacetic transaminase (SGOT), lactate dehydrogenase (LDU) and liver alkaline phosphatase (LAP) activities, a liver biopsy sample was obtained, which showed non-caseating granulomas. The spinal-cord tumour mass was explored. It also revealed non-caseating granulomas. The patient was given prednisone and an aggressive physical therapy. After the operation the back pain subsided but the left-sided pain continued.

Comment—This patient suffered from initial paraesthesia associated with severe intractable back pain due to intramedullary tumour which responded to corticosteroids.

References

1. SHARMA, O.P. (1975) *Sarcoidosis: A Clinical Approach*, p. 97. (Springfield, Il.. Charles C. Thomas)
2. DELANEY, P. (1977) Neurologic manifestations in sarcoidosis: Review of the literature, with a report of 23 cases. *Ann. Intern. Med.*, **87,** 336.
3. JAMES, D.G. and SHARMA, O.P. (1967) Neurosarcoidosis. *Proc. R. Soc. Med.*, **60,** 1169.
4. COLOVER, J. (1948) Sarcoidosis with involvement of nervous system. *Brain*, **71,** 451.
5. SILVERSTEIN, A., FEUER, M.M. and SLITZBACH, L.E. (1965) Neurologic sarcoidosis. *Arch. Neurol.*, **12,** 1.
6. WELLS, C.E.C. (1967) The natural history of neurosarcoidosis. *Proc. R. Soc. Med.*, **60,** 1172.
7. MATTHEWS, W.B. (1959) Sarcoidosis of the nervous system. *Br. Med. J.*, **i,** 267.
8. PENNELL, W.H. (1951) Boeck's sarcoid with involvement of the central nervous system. *Arch. Neurol. Psychiatr.*, **66,** 728.
9. WHELAN, M.A. and STERN, J. (1981) Sarcoidosis presenting as a posterior fossa mass. *Surg. Neurol.*, **15,** 455.
10. KARNIK, A. (1982) Nodular cerebral sarcoidosis stimulating metastatic carcinoma. *Arch. Intern. Med.*, **142,** 385.
11. KENDALL, B.E. and TATLER, G.L.V. (1978) Radiologic findings in neurosarcoidosis. *Br. J. Radiol.*, **51,** 81.
12. NAUMANN, O. (1938) Kasuistischer Bertrag zur Kenntnis de Schaumannschen benignen 'granulomatose' (Morbus Besnier–Boeck–Schaumann). *Z. Klinderheilkd*, **60,** 1.
13. NATHAN, M.P.R., CHASE, P.H., ELGUENZABEL, H., *et al.* (1976) Spinal cord sarcoidosis. *N. Y. State J. Med.*, **76,** 748.
14. HOOK, O. (1954) Sarcoidosis with involvement of the nervous system. *Arch. Neurol. Psychiatr.*, **71,** 554.
15. MATTHEWS, W.B. (1965) Sarcoidosis of the nervous system. *J. Neurol. Neurosurg. Psychiatr.*, **23,** 28.
16. WANMAN, J.S. and SHER, J.H. (1979) The spectrum of CNS sarcoidosis: A clinical and pathologic study. *Mt. Sinai J. Med.*, **46,** 309.
17. ROSENBLOOM, M.A. and UPHOFF, D.E. (1983) The association of progressive multifocal leukoencephalopathy and sarcoidosis. *Chest*, **83,** 572.

Chapter 15
The musculoskeletal system

Bones

Karl Kreibich of Prague was the first to demonstrate bone lesions in sarcoidosis. In 1904, he described a 26-year-old man with chronic skin lesions involving the nose, cheek and right ear associated with swellings of both hands and feet. A radiograph disclosed radiolucencies in the phalanges of both hands[1].

The incidence of bone involvement, like other manifestations, varies from 1-4 to 34% depending on the primary interest of the author and whether a radiological evaluation of the bones was performed[2]. Bone lesions are more common in patients with persistent disease, particularly in those with lupus pernio and other chronic skin lesions[3]. Negro patients with extensive and progressive disease frequently have bone changes. Bone lesions are rare in early disease at the stage of bilateral hilar adenopathy and erythema nodosum. James noted that among the 200 patients with sarcoidosis in his series, bone involvement occurred only once in the absence of skin lesions[4].

Jungling[5] described three types of bone lesions. Type 1 comprised diffusely expanded bone with cysts of various sizes (*see Figure 15.1a*). Type 2 comprised round, well-defined, punched-out areas (*see Figure 15.1b*). Type 3 comprised a uniform lattice-like appearance (*see Figure 15.1c*). Jungling considered that type 1 was the early active lesion and type 2 was the stage of healing[5].

The bones of hands and feet are most often involved; the nasal bones—particularly in patients with lupus pernio—skull, vertebrae, pelvis, ribs, sternum and the distal ends of long bones may also be affected. The bone lesions are often asymptomatic but, in many cases, the affected part may be tender and painful. The association of the bone and skin lesions indicates a poor prognosis.

Joints

Although Jonathan Hutchinson was the first to recognize the existence of sarcoid arthritis, the articular involvement in sarcoidosis became established through the studies of Burman and Mayer[6], Gendel, Young and Greiner[7], Myers *et al.*[8], Sokoloff and Bunim[9], Spilberg, Siltzbach and McEwen[10] and Grigor and Hughes[11].

The incidence of joint involvement varies from 25 to 39% in various series. Onset of articular symptoms have ranged from 4 months to 59 years of age. The joint disease

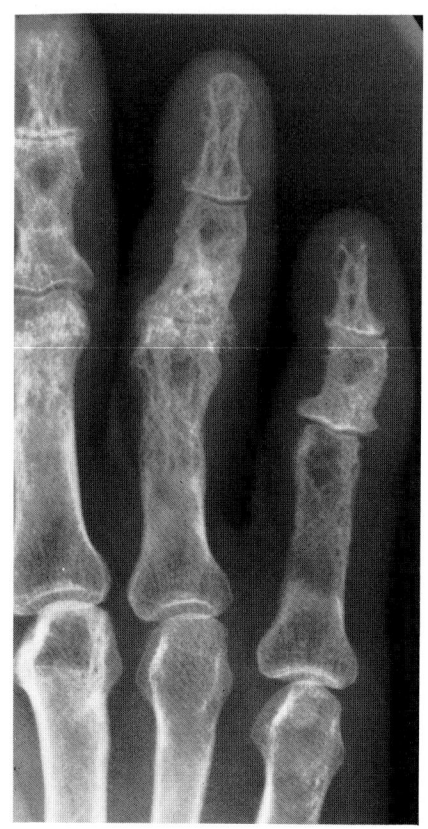 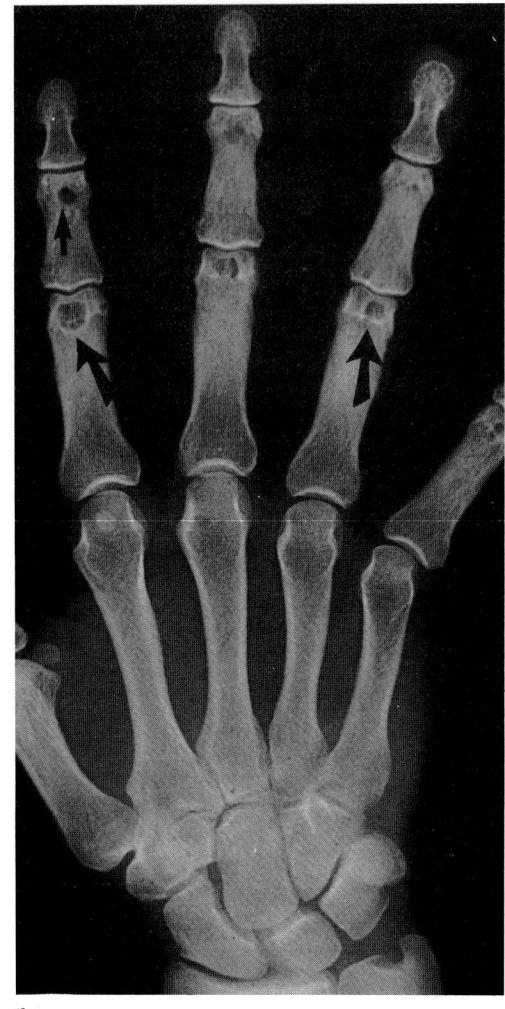

(a) (b)

Figure 15.1(*a*) Various sizes of bone cysts. (*b*) Rounded punched-out cysts (arrows).

was an initial manifestation of sarcoidosis in 74 (90%) of 83 patients reviewed by Kaplan[12]. In some cases, the joint involvement preceded the other manifestations of sarcoidosis by many years. In one of the 10 patients described by Patterson, Israel and Smukler, acute arthritis preceded the established diagnosis by 16 years[13].

The joints most commonly affected by sarcoidosis are the knees, ankles, elbows, wrists and small joints of hands (*see Figure 15.2*). The joint lesions are usually swollen, warm, tender and painful; effusions are common, particularly in patients with chronic recurrent exacerbations. Sarcoid arthritis may be indistinguishable from that observed in rheumatic fever or rheumatoid disease. The articular involvement in sarcoidosis may be divided as follows.

Transitory, migrating arthralgias—There is no evidence of arthritis. It may sometimes be associated with erythema nodosum. Sokoloff considers this to be a non-

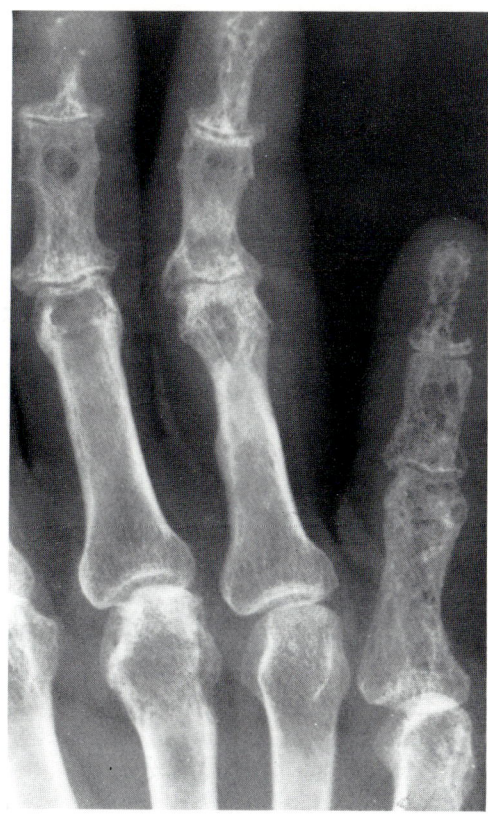

(c)

Figure 15.1 (c) Lattice-like bone lesions.

specific reaction which may also be observed in other systematic diseases including primary tuberculosis, fungal and viral infections.

Migratory polyarthritis associated with fever, erythema nodosum and bilateral hilar adenopathy—This type of joint involvement commonly affects the larger joints such as the ankles, knees, wrists and elbows. Extreme pain and tenderness of the joints, especially the proximal ends of the long bones and phalanges, are often out of proportion to the objective evidence of the arthritis. Radiographic examination of the bones is normal, but a synovial biopsy specimen may show non-caseating granulomas. It is a self-limiting lesion which subsides within 1–2 months, leaving no sequelae; recurrence is rare. Clinical and radiological recovery is a rule. Analgesics are indicated for symptomatic relief.

Acute relapsing mono or polyarticular arthritis—The picture is similar to the one seen in type 2, but with multiple episodes. Joint deformity is likely to occur. Relapsing monoarticular arthritis of the great toe, simulating gout, has been reported.

Chronic persistent polyarthritis or, rarely, monoarticular arthritis—This type of joint abnormality usually occurs in patients with advanced systemic disease, particularly of the lungs and of the skin. Joint deformities are common; occasionally, destruction of the affected joint may occur. Eight out of 28 patients studied by Spilberg *et al.*[10]

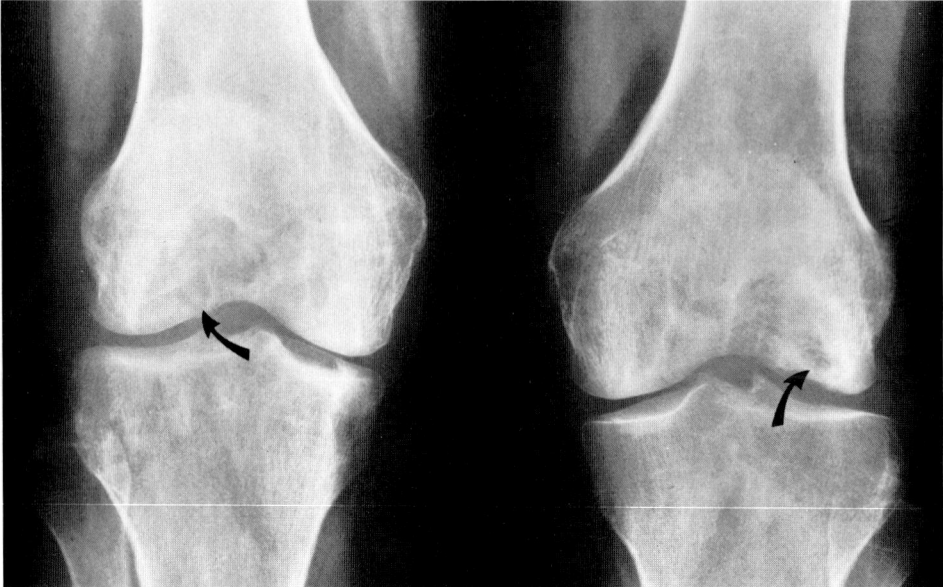

Figure 15.2 Sarcoid lesions (arrows) of the medial aspects of both lateral femoral condyles and both distal femoral epiphyses. (Reproduced from *J. Bone Joint Surg.* (1973), **55A,** 618, by courtesy of publishers.)

experienced recurrences ranging from three to seven in number, and in four patients the articular lesions become chronic. Synovial thickening and effusions were present in all. None of the patients with persistent arthritis had erythema nodosum which is a feature of acute benign sarcoidosis.

Differential diagnosis of sarcoid arthritis

Sarcoidosis should be included in the differential diagnosis in a patient with arthritis. The diagnosis can be established on the basis of a typical chest radiographic finding and by demonstrating non-caseating granulomas in a synovial-membrane, lymph-node, skin or lung biopsy sample. Serum angiotensin converting enzyme activity may be high. At times, the distribution between 'gouty' arthritis and monoarticular sarcoid arthritis may be difficult. This is particularly so if the patient also has elevated uric acid levels. Hyperuricaemia occurs in about 20% of sarcoid patients. In acute stages, sarcoidosis may be confused with rheumatic fever or rheumatoid arthritis. However, the characteristic pulmonary lesions, normal ASO titres and negative serological tests for rheumatoid arthritis and the demonstration of non-caseating granulomas by organ biopsy confirm the diagnosis of sarcoidosis. Tuberculosis—typical and atypical—can produce a destructive arthritis. The isolation of organism from culture and the presence of draining skin sinuses indicate mycobacteriosis or fungal infections rather than sarcoidosis.

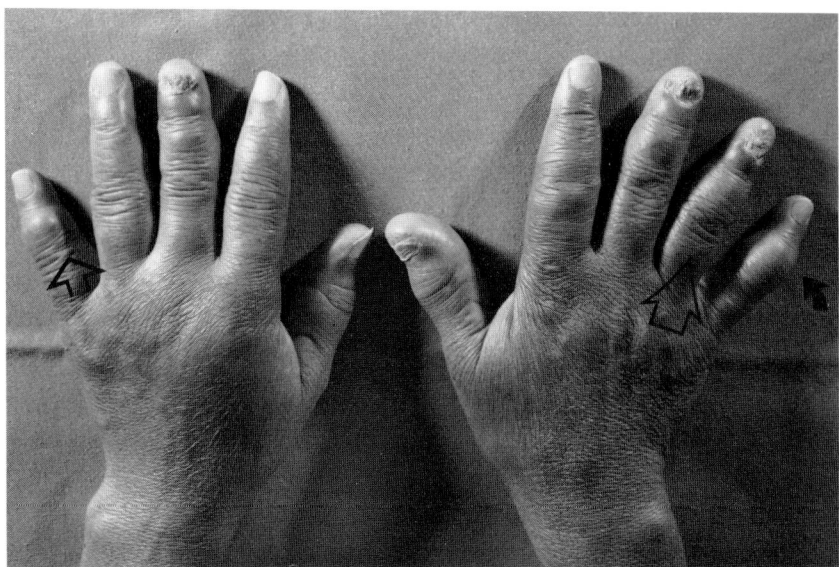

Figure 15.3 Sausage-shaped swellings (arrows) of small joints of hands.

Muscles

Sarcoidosis of muscle may manifest in the following ways.

Asymptomatic granulomatous muscle involvement

In the early stages of sarcoidosis, asymptomatic granulomatous muscle involvement is common. The prevalence rate, based on the presence of non-caseating granulomas in random muscle biopsies, have ranged from 50 to 80%. Silverstein and Siltzbach obtained non-caseating granulomas by random biopsy in eight patients, none of whom had musculoskeletal or neurological symptoms[14]. In three out of four patients with early active sarcoidosis reported by Myers et al.[15] a biopsy of the gastrocnemius muscle detected non-caseating granuloma. None of these patients had any symptoms suggesting muscle involvement. Wallace et al. found non-caseating granulomas in 23 out of 42 patients with histologically confirmed sarcoidosis[16]. They also stressed the importance of making serial sections; the yield of granulomas is directly proportional to the number of sections studied.

The symptomless muscle granulomas occur frequently in active disease, especially in patients with erythema nodosum. Muscle biopsy may be a useful source for obtaining the histological evidence of sarcoidosis. The finding of non-caseating granuloma in muscle without any overlying skin lesion is fairly characteristic of sarcoidosis and rarely ever due to tuberculosis and fungal infections.

Palpable muscle nodules

Licharew[17] was the first to recognize the multiple nodules in muscles of a 17-year-old girl with extensive sarcoidosis[18]. This type of muscle lesion is rare and was discovered only once in a series of 800 patients with histologically confirmed disease. Microscopic examination of muscle nodules reveals non-caseating granulomas.

Polymyositis

This form of symptomatic muscular sarcoidosis is seen more often in women than in men and is characterized by fever, severe muscle pain and tenderness involving principally the proximal shoulder and pelvic girdle muscles. This acute syndrome may be the initial manifestation of sarcoidosis. Electromyographic findings resemble non-granulomatous polymyositis. Response to corticosteroid therapy is good.

Chronic myopathy

Muscle wasting and weakness indicate chronic myopathy and are associated with chronic multisystem disease[19]. This type of sarcoid myopathy has an insidious onset and affects mainly women in the fourth and fifth decades of their lives. Electromyography shows non-specific changes. Corticosteroids may be beneficial in a few cases. Muscle hypertrophy and contractures have been reported.

Isolated sarcoid myopathy

This type of myopathy is extremely rare[20]. In patients who appear to have isolated sarcoid myopathy a careful examination will often reveal clinical, radiological or histological evidence of multisystem sarcoidosis.

References

1. KREIBICH, K. (1904) Uber Lupus Pernio. *Arch. Dermatol. Syph.*, **71**, 3.
2. SHARMA, O.P. (1975) *Sarcoidosis: A Clinical Approach*, p. 103. (Springfield, Il.: Charles C. Thomas)
3. NEVILLE, E., CARSTAIRS, L.S. and JAMES, D.G. (1977) Sarcoidosis of bone. *Q. J. Med.*, **46**, 215.
4. JAMES, D.G. (1959) Dermatological aspects of sarcoidosis. *Q. J. Med.*, **28**, 109.
5. JUNGLING, D. (1928) Uber Ostitis Multiplex cystoides, zugleich ein Beitrag zur Lehre von der Tuberkuliden des knochesn. *Beitr. Klin. Chirurg.*, **143**, 401.
6. BURMAN, M.S. and MAYER, L. (1936) Arthroscopic examination of the knee joint. Report of cases observed in the course of arthroscopic examination, including instances of sarcoid and multiple polypoid fibromatosis. *Arch. Surg.*, **32**, 846.
7. GENDEL, B.R., YOUNG, J.M. and GREINER, D.J. (1952) Sarcoidosis: review with 24 additional cases. *Am. J. Med.*, **12**, 205.
8. MYERS, G.B., GOTTLIEB, A.M., MATTMAN, P.E., et al. (1952) Joint and skeletal manifestations in sarcoidosis. *Am J. Med.*, **12**, 161.
9. SOKOLOFF, L. and BUNIM, J.J. (1959) Clinical and pathological studies of joint involvement in sarcoidosis. *N. Engl. J. Med.*, **260**, 841.
10. SPILBERG, I., SILTZBACH, L.E. and MCEWEN, C. (1969) The arthritis of sarcoidosis. *Arthr. Rheum.*, **12**, 126.
11. GRIGOR, R.R. and HUGHES, G.R. (1976) Chronic sarcoid arthritis. *Br. Med. J.*, **ii**, 1044.
12. KAPLAN, H. (1963) Sarcoid arthritis: a review. *Arch. Intern. Med.*, **112**, 924.
13. PATTERSON, J.R., ISRAEL, H.L. and SMUKLER, N. (1971) The musculoskeletal manifestations of sarcoidosis. In *Proceedings of the Fifth International Conference on Sarcoidosis* (eds Levinsky, L. and Macholda, F.), p. 590. (Prague: Charles University)

14. SILVERSTEIN, A. and SILTZBACH, L.E. (1969) Muscle involvement in sarcoidosis. *Arch. Neurol.*, **21,** 235.
15. MYERS, G.B., GOTTLIEB, A.M., MATTMAN, P.E., *et al.* (1952) Joint and skeletal manifestations in sarcoidosis. *Am. J. Med.*, **12,** 161.
16. WALLACE, S.L., LATTES, R., MALIA, J.P., *et al.* (1958) Muscle involvement in Boeck's sarcoid. *Ann. Intern. Med.*, **48,** 497.
17. LICHAREW, W. (1908) Moskauer, Venereologische and dermatologische. *Gesellschaft Derm. Zbl.*, **11,** 258.
18. BRUN, A. (1961) Chronic polymyositis on the basis of sarcoidosis. *Acta Psychiat. Neurol. Scand.*, **36,** 515.
19. WARBURG, M. (1955) A case of symmetrical muscular contractures due to sarcoidosis. *J. Neuropathol. Exp. Neurol.*, **14,** 313.
20. MUCHA, V. and ORZECHOWSKI, K. (1919) Ein Fall von tuberculoser Dermatomyositis. *Wiener Klin. Wochenschr.*, **32,** 35.

Chapter 16
Endocrine involvement

Pituitary

Among the endocrine glands, the pituitary and hypothalamus are the most commonly affected by sarcoidosis. Hypothalamic involvement is more common than the pituitary dysfunction.

Diabetes insipidus

Heerfordt was the first to postulate the relationship between diabetes insipidus and uveoparotid fever[1]. Later, Tillgren provided the histological evidence of granulomatous infiltration in a patient with clinical pituitary involvement[2]. Winnacker, Becker and Katz surveyed the literature and uncovered 60 cases of diabetes insipidus caused by sarcoidosis[3]. Most sarcoidosis patients with diabetes insipidus have other features of the disease, including parotid enlargement, uveitis, facial palsy and pulmonary involvement. However, it is difficult to establish the diagnosis if polyuria and polydipsia are the initial and only features of sarcoidosis. Occasionally, diabetes insipidus has been associated with other manifestations of hypothalamic–pituitary dysfunction, e.g. somnolence and obesity, hypothermia, impotence, amenorrhoea, sleep disturbances, hypogonadism, alveolar hypoventilation and hypothyroidism[4–11]. Rarely, neighbouring parts of the base of the brain may also be involved, resulting in optic atrophy, bitemporal hemianopia, deafness and vertigo and anosmia[12,13].

The diagnosis of diabetes insipidus due to sarcoidosis is based on the occurrence of polydipsia and polyuria in a patient with a clinical or radiological picture of the disease and histological evidence of non-caseating granulomas; it must be differentiated from the renal disease which causes a large output of low-specific-gravity urine. Eosinophilic granuloma can closely mimic sarcoidosis; both diseases may produce pulmonary infiltration and diabetes insipidus. In such cases, a lung biopsy specimen is needed to establish the diagnosis.

Stuart, Neelen and Leboritz have demonstrated that the hypothalamus is the predominant site of functional impairment in patients with neuroendocrine sarcoidosis. In their study of 10 patients with sarcoidosis and hypopituitarism, a disturbance of water metabolism was present in seven. However, dysfunction of thirst regulation and normal ADH reserve were more common than true diabetes insipidus. It is suspected that excessive thirst with normal ADH might be due to the overactivity of angiotensin II in the hypothalamus[9].

Hypopituitarism

Sarcoidosis may also involve the anterior pituitary gland[10]. Winnacker et al.[3] reviewed 19 randomly selected sarcoid patients and found 17 who showed deficiency of one or more anterior pituitary hormones. Stuart et al. studied 10 patients with sarcoidosis and hypopituitarism and observed a deficiency of at least two anterior pituitary hormones in all 10 cases[9]. Other reported manifestations of hypopituitarism have included hypoglycaemia, dwarfism, Fröhlich's syndrome and infantilism. The occurrence of anterior hypopituitarism without associated diabetes insipidus is rare.

Brun, Revol and Perrin-Fayolle[14] studied the metyrapone response in 14 patients with sarcoidosis. Eleven showed an abnormal increase in basal urinary 17-hydroxycorticosteroids and compound-S. The response was higher and pronounced in patients with active sarcoidosis; whereas, in chronic disease the metyrapone response was normal. The authors suggested that pituitary hyperactivity might be due to granulomas in the pituitary or hypothalamus.

Turkington and MacIndoe reported that 32% of patients with disseminated sarcoidosis had elevated prolactin levels. The authors suggested that hyperprolactinaemia was a sensitive marker of hypothalamic sarcoidosis[15]. Caro, Glennon and Israel[16] found five patients with galactorrhoea amongst 300 women with sarcoidosis. Prolactin levels were elevated in three out of five patients. Prolactin responses to L-dopa and thyrotrophin releasing hormone (TRH) were normal but not to chlorpromazine, suggesting a hypothalamic disturbance.

Nakao et al. found elevated prolactin levels in 12 out of 80 patients with sarcoidosis and in 10 patients these levels returned to normal after corticosteroid therapy[17]. However, Munt, Marshall and Underwood could find hyperprolactinaemia in only two out of 61 patients and it was not present in nine patients with neurosarcoidosis[18]. Thus, the value of serum prolactin as an indicator of hypothalamic involvements needs further investigation.

Thyroid

Spencer and Warren gave us the first description of sarcoid involvement of the thyroid gland[19]. The association, however, remained obscure for more than 25 years until Mayock et al. in their study of 145 patients mentioned in passing that two (1.4%) had clinical evidence of thyroiditis[20]. Karlish and MacGregor described four (1.3%) patients with clinical features of thyroiditis amongst their 300 sarcoidosis patients[21]. Clinically recognizable thyroid involvement occurs in less than 1% of sarcoidosis patients. Autopsy reports, however, indicate that thyroid may be affected in about 5% of the patients[22].

Hypothyroidism

Brun described a patient with sarcoidosis and myxoedema. Although the gland was not palpable, a surgical biopsy revealed granulomatous infiltration and fibrosis of the gland[23]. The patient reported by Buckle had a diffusely enlarged thyroid gland which on biopsy showed non-caseating granulomas[24]. Richards studied a patient with prolonged tendon reflexes, but showed no evidence of hypothyroidism[25].

Hyperthyroidism

Sarcoid granulomas have been observed in the thyroid gland removed at surgery on the patients with sarcoidosis and hyperthyroidism[26,27]. Hancock reported on five patients with thyrotoxicosis and sarcoidosis. He reviewed the literature and uncovered the 20 previously reported and concluded that such an association could result from an autoimmune disturbance resulting from loss of T-cell control[28]. Proptosis without associated hyperthyroidism has been reported[29].

Parathyroids

Sarcoidosis rarely involves the parathyroid glands. The coexistence of sarcoidosis and primary hyperthyroidism has been reported only 24 times[30]. Functional hypoparathyroidism is frequently observed in sarcoidosis. Increased intestinal absorption of calcium reduces PTH secretion[31,32]. Rarely, sarcoid granulomas are found within a parathyroid adenoma[33]. From the practical point of view, hypercalcaemia resistant to corticosteroid therapy should suggest the possibility of primary hyperparathyroidism or malignancy rather than sarcoidosis[34].

Adrenals

Unlike tuberculosis, sarcoidosis rarely affects the adrenal glands. Sarcoidosis has been reported with Addison's disease only eight times. Mayock *et al.* described a patient who died suddenly in Addisonian crisis. At autopsy, granulomas were found in the lungs, liver, spleen and bone marrow; the adrenals, however, showed dense fibrosis[35]. TASS syndrome—an unusual association of thyroiditis, Addison's disease, Sjögren's syndrome and sarcoidosis—has been described[36].

References

1. HEERFORDT, C.F. (1909) Uber eine 'Febris uveoparotidea subchronica.' *Albrecht e. Graefes Arch. Ophthalmol.*, **70**, 254.
2. TILLGREN, J. (1935) Diabetes insipidus as a symptom of Schaumann's disease. *Br. J. Dermatol.*, **47**, 223.
3. WINNACKER, J.L., BECKER, E.L. and KATZ, S. (1968) Endocrine aspects of sarcoidosis. *N. Engl. J. Med.*, **278**, 483.
4. POSNER, I. (1952) Sarcoidosis: Case report. *J. Pediatr.*, **20**, 486.
5. BLEISCH, V.R. and ROBBINS, S.L. (1952) Sarcoid-like granulomata of pituitary gland: Cause of pituitary insufficiency. *Arch. Intern. Med.*, **89**, 877.
6. SPILLANE, J.D. (1952) Four cases of diabetes insipidus and pulmonary disease. *Thorax*, **7**, 134.
7. SHEALY, C.N., KAHANA, L., ENGEL, F.L., *et al.* (1961) Hypothalamic–pituitary sarcoidosis: Report on four patients, one with prolonged remission of diabetes insipidus following steroid therapy. *Am. J. Med.*, **30**, 46.
8. CAMPBELL, I.W., SNORT, A.T.K. and DOUGLAS, A. (1980) Hypothalamic manifestations of sarcoidosis—with particular reference to hypothalamic hypothyroidism. In *Sarcoidosis and Other Granulomatous Disease* (eds Williams, W.J. and Davies, B.H.), p. 579. (Cardiff: Alpha Omega Publications)
9. STUART, G.A., NEELEN, F.A. and LEBOVITZ, H.F. (1978) Hypothalamic insufficiency: The cause of hypopituitarism in sarcoidosis. *Ann. Intern. Med.*, **88**, 589.

10. VESELEY, D.L., MALDONODO, A. and LEVY, G.S. (1977) Partial hypopituitarism and possible hypothalamic involvement in sarcoidosis. Report of a case and review of the literature. *Am. J. Med.*, **62**, 425.
11. DAWN, J.J., KANTER, H.G. and KATZ, S. (1965) Central nervous system sarcoidosis with alveolar hypoventilation. *Am. J. Med.*, **38**, 893.
12. WALSH, F.B. (1959) Ocular importance of sarcoid: Its relation to uveo-parotid fever. *Arch. Ophthalmol.*, **21**, 421.
13. LEVIN, P.N. (1935) The neurological aspects of uveo-parotid fever. *J. Nerv. Ment. Dis.*, **81**, 176.
14. BRUN, J., REVOL, A. and PERRIN-FAYOLLE, M. (1965) Metyrapone ditartrate (Metopirone) test during ganglio-pulmonary sarcoidosis of Besnier–Boeck–Schaumann: Diagnostic and etiopathogenic value. *Dis. Chest*, **48**, 337.
15. TURKINGTON, R.W. and MACINDOE, J.H. (1972) Hyperprolactinaemia in sarcoidosis. *Ann. Intern. Med.*, **76**, 545.
16. CARO, J.F., GLENNON, A. and ISRAEL, H. (1980) Neuroendocrine studies in sarcoidosis. In *Sarcoidosis and Other Granulomatous Diseases* (eds Williams, W.J. and Davies, B.H.), p. 587. (Cardiff: Alpha Omega Publishers)
17. NAKAO, K., NOMA, K., SATO, B., *et al.* (1978) Serum prolactin levels in eighty patients with sarcoidosis. *Eur. J. Clin. Invest.*, **8**, 37.
18. MUNT, P.W., MARSHALL, R.N. and UNDERWOOD, L.E. (1975) Hyperprolactinaemia in sarcoidosis. *Am. Rev. Respir. Dis.*, **112**, 269.
19. SPENCER, J. and WARREN, S. (1938) Boeck's sarcoid: report of a case with clinical diagnosis confirmed at autopsy. *Arch. Intern. Med.*, **62**, 285.
20. MAYOCK, R.L., BERTRAND, P., MORRISON, C.E., *et al.* (1963) Manifestations of sarcoidosis: Analysis of 145 patients with a review of nine series selected from literature. *Am. J. Med.*, **35**, 67.
21. KARLISH, A.J. and MACGREGOR, G.A. (1970) Sarcoidosis, thyroiditis and Addison's disease. *Lancet*, **ii**, 330.
22. VOGT, H. (1949) Morbus Besnier–Boeck–Schaumann: Klinsche und pathologische anatomische Studie. *Helv. Med. Acta (Suppl.)*, **25**, 1.
23. BRUN, J., MOURIGUAND, C., COMBEY, P., *et al.* (1959) Thyroidite sclereuse d'origine sarcoidosique avec myxodema et fibrose pulmonaire diffuse. *Lyon Med.*, **91**, 179.
24. BUCKLE, R.M. (1963) Sarcoid goitre. *Proc. R. Soc. Med.*, **56**, 611.
25. RICHARDS, A.G. (1962) 'Myxodema reflex' as presenting sign in sarcoidosis. *Can. Med. Assoc. J.*, **96**, 32.
26. COWDELL, R.H. (1954) Sarcoidosis with special reference to diagnosis and prognosis. *Q.J. Med.*, **23**, 29.
27. CUMMINS, S.D., CLARK, D.H. and GANDY, T.H. (1951) Boeck's sarcoid of thyroid gland. *Arch. Pathol.*, **51**, 68.
28. HANCOCK, B.W. and MILLARD, L.G. (1976) Sarcoidosis and thyrotoxicosis: A study of five patients. *Br. J. Dis. Chest*, **70**, 129.
29. MELMON, K.L. and GOLDBERG, J.S. (1962) Sarcoidosis and exophthalmos as initial symptom. *Am. J. Med.*, **33**, 158.
30. LEBACQ, L.E. (1983) An update of biochemical findings and diagnostic procedures in sarcoidosis. In *Sarcoidosis* (eds Chretien, J., Marsac, J. and Saltiel, J.), p. 263. (Paris: Pergamon Press)
31. CUSHARD, W.G., SIMON, A.B., CANTERBURY, J.M., *et al.* (1972) Parathyroid function in sarcoidosis. *N. Engl. J. Med.*, **286**, 395.
32. REINER, M., SIGURDSSON, G., NUNZIATA, V., *et al.* (1976) Abnormal calcium metabolism in normocalcaemic sarcoidosis. *Br. Med. J.*, **ii**, 1473.
33. ROBINSON, R.G., KERWIN, D.M. and TSOU, E. (1980) Parathyroid adenoma with coexistent sarcoid granuloma. *Arch. Intern. Med.*, **140**, 1547.
34. ABERG, H., JOHANSSON, H., WERNER, I., *et al.* (1972) Sarcoidosis, hypercalcemia, and hyperparathyroidism. *Scand. J. Respir. Dis.*, **53**, 259.
35. MAYOCK, R.L., BERTRAND, P., MORRISON, C.E., *et al.* (1963) Manifestations of sarcoidosis: Analysis of 145 patients with a review of nine series selected from literature. *Am. J. Med.*, **35**, 67.
36. SEINFELD, E.D. and SHARMA, O.P. (1983) The TASS syndrome: An unusual association of thyroiditis, Addison's disease, Sjögren's syndrome and sarcoidosis. *Proc. R. Soc. Med.*, **76**, 883.

Chapter 17
The parotid glands

Waldenstrom was the first to recognize the parotid enlargement as one of the manifestations of sarcoidosis[1]. The frequency of the parotid gland involvement varies. Although the gland was palpable only in 6% out of 388 patients reported by Greenberg et al.[2], the subclinical involvement is more common and may be detected by technetium-99m concentration and by measuring salivary volume and amylase[2-4]. Granulomas in minor salivary glands may be demonstrated in as many as 50% of the patients with mediastinal sarcoidosis. Gallium-67 uptake by the parotid glands occurred in as many as 75% of the patients with acute symptomatic sarcoidosis[5,6].

Sarcoid parotitis may be asymptomatic or symptomatic (dryness of the mouth); enlarged bilaterally (usually) or unilaterally (rarely); and transient or persistent. The gland is usually firm, non-tender and smooth. Occasionally, the surface of the gland may be nodular. Associated enlargement of the lacrimal glands is similar to that found in Mikulicz syndrome. Enlargement of the lacrimal glands and keratoconjunctivitis sicca resemble that found in Sjögren's syndrome. In about 40% of the patients the parotid enlargement is transient and self-limiting. No therapy is needed for asymptomatic parotitis, but persistently enlarged glands with dry mouth call for corticosteroids.

Case report—This 32-year-old woman developed painless enlargement of the parotid and lacrimal glands associated with fever, dry cough, and dyspnoea on exertion. The patient had lost about 10 lb (4.5 kg) in weight. Physical examination revealed bilateral, non-tender swellings of the parotids and the lacrimal glands (*see Figures 17.1 and 17.2*). A chest radiograph showed bilateral hilar adenopathy and parenchymal infiltration. Gallium-67 scans showed a bilateral increase in activity in the parotids, lacrimal and hilar glands (*see Figure 17.3*). Non-caseating granulomas were seen in biopsy specimens of the right lacrimal and the right parotid gland (*see Figures 17.4 and 17.5*). The patient responded to prednisone 20 mg daily, and in about 8 weeks the swelling of the lacrimal and parotid glands subsided.

References

1. WALDENSTROM, J. (1937) Some observations on uveoparotitis and allied conditions with special reference to the symptoms from the nervous system. *Acta Med. Scand.*, **91**, 53.
2. GREENBERG, G., ANDERSON, R., SHARPSTONE, P. and JAMES, D.G. (1964) Enlargement of parotid glands due to sarcoidosis. *Br. Med. J.*, **ii**, 861.
3. BHOOLA, K.D., MCNICOL, N.W., OLIVER, S. and FORAN, J. (1969) Changes in salivary enzymes in patients with sarcoidosis. *N. Engl. J. Med.*, **281**, 877.
4. TURIAF, J. and BATTESTI, P. (1976) Gougerot–Sjögren syndrome and sarcoidosis. *Ann. N.Y. Acad. Sci.*, **278**, 401.

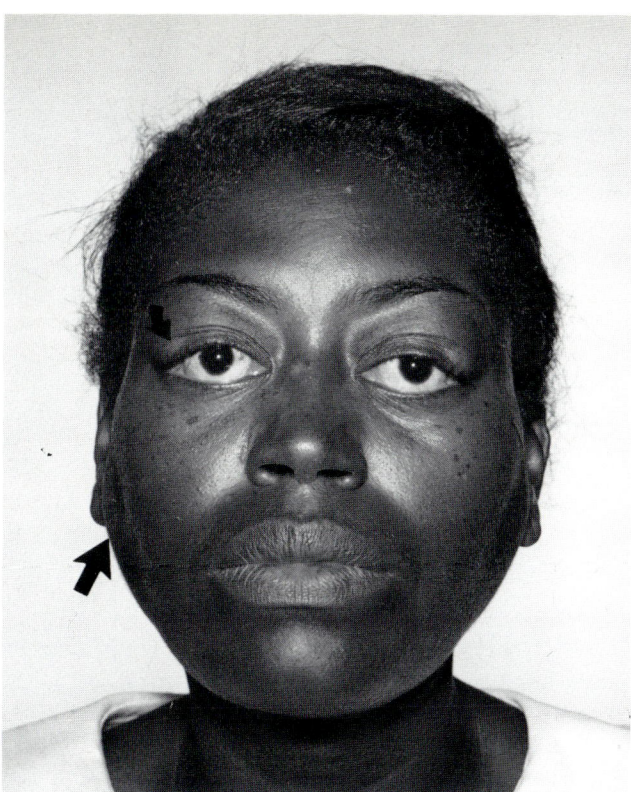

Figure 17.1 A 32-year-old woman with bilateral parotid and lacrimal gland enlargement (arrow).

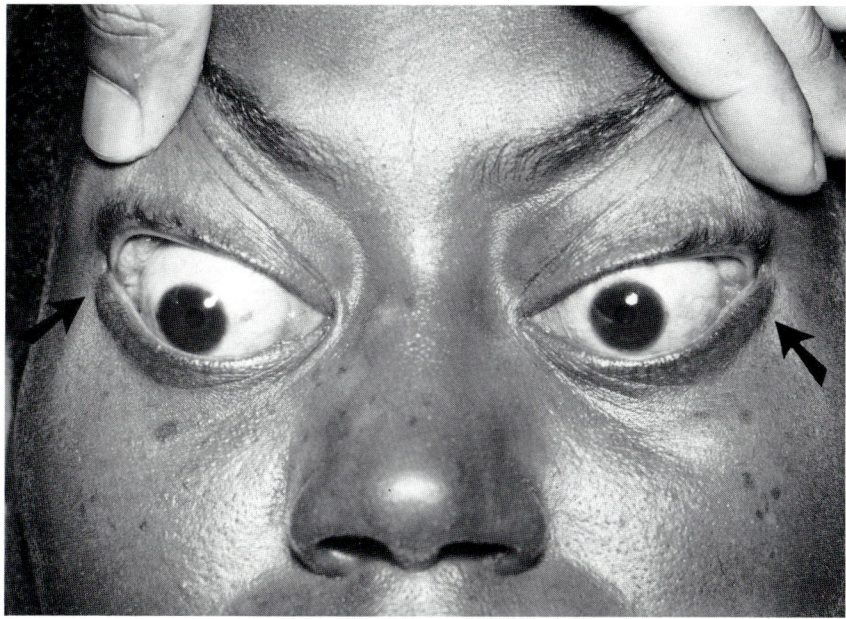

Figure 17.2 Lacrimal glands showing greyish-white sarcoid tubercles (arrows).

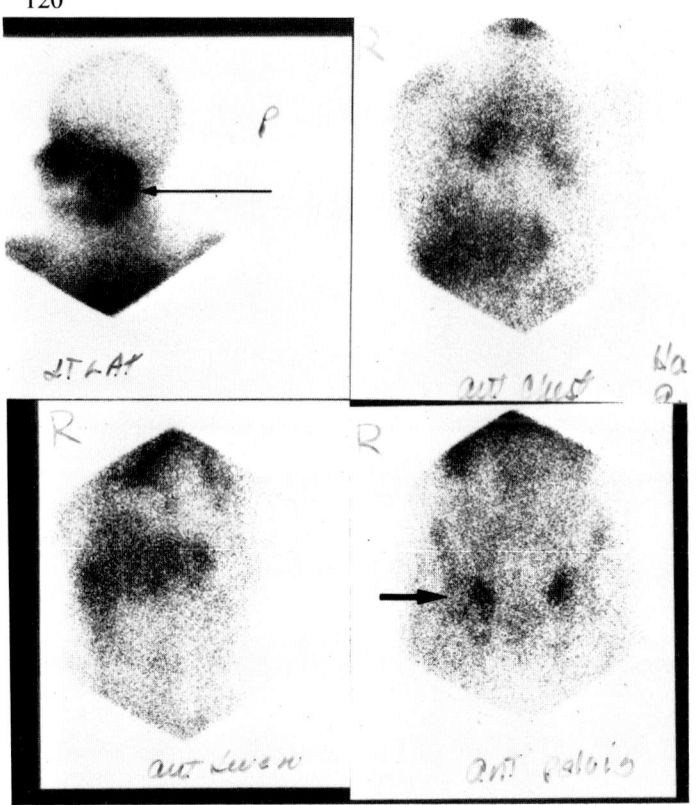

Figure 17.3 Gallium-67 scan showing increased activity in the parotids, hilar and inguinal glands (arrows).

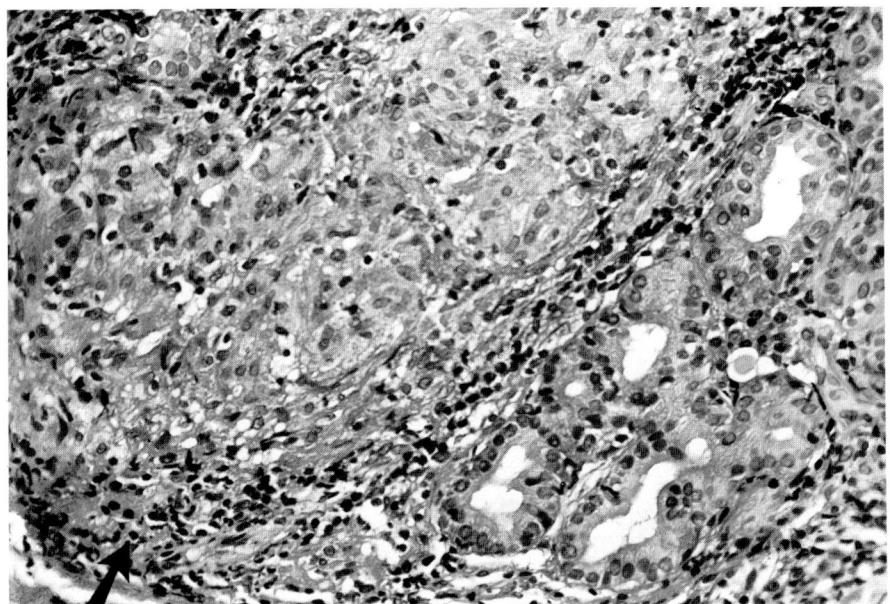

Figure 17.4 Non-caseating sarcoid granuloma in a lacrimal gland biopsy specimen. (Haematoxylin and eosin. × 250.)

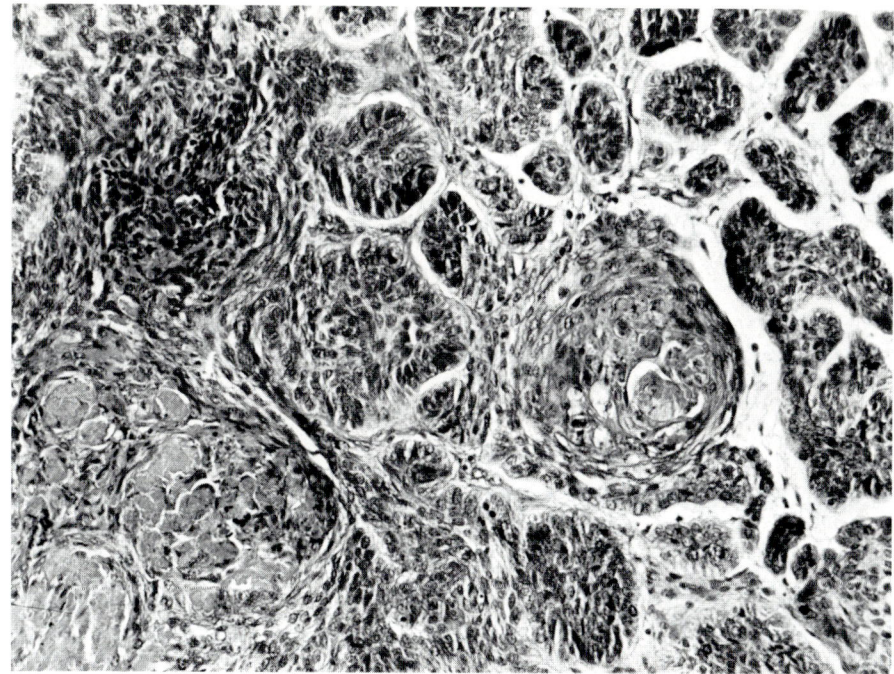

Figure 17.5 Parotid salivary gland showing sarcoid granulomas. (Haematoxylin and eosin. × 150.)

5. WIENER, S.N. and PATEL, B.P. (1979) ^{67}Ga-citrate uptake by the parotid glands in sarcoidosis. *Radiology*, **130**, 753.
6. NESSAN, V.J. and JACOWAY, J.R. (1979) Biopsy of minor salivary glands in the diagnosis of sarcoidosis. *N. Engl. J. Med.*, **301**, 922.

Chapter 18
Gastrointestinal tract

Unlike tuberculosis, sarcoidosis rarely affects the gastrointestinal system.

Oesophagus

Of all the organs of the digestive tract, the oesophagus is least frequently involved in sarcoidosis. Polacheck and Matre described a 65-year-old man with weight loss, abdominal pain, hepatosplenomegaly and pulmonary infiltration. An upper gastrointestinal barium meal study revealed an irregularity of the oesophagus. Biopsy specimens of the liver, lung, lymph node and the oesophagus showed non-caseating granulomas[1].

Stomach

Less that 50 cases of gastric sarcoidosis have been reported in the literature[2-7]. Sarcoidosis of the stomach may be divided into the following three categories.

Symptomless granulomatous involvement of the gastric mucosa

Studies by Palmer[8] suggest that symptomless involvement of the stomach may be more frequent than is generally realized. Six (10%) of 60 patients with sarcoidosis who had no gastrointestinal symptoms and had normal gastroscopic appearance showed granulomas in the gastric mucosal biopsy specimens.

Gastric ulcer/ulcers

Granulomatous lesion of the gastric musosa may result in single or multiple ulcerations[2]. The patient may complain of nausea, epigastric pain and vomiting. Haematemesis may occur[9-11]. In a case described by Ona, serial gastroscopic studies showed resolution of the sarcoid ulcer within 5 months on antacid therapy[7]. Corticosteroid therapy can avert the surgical intervention if the diagnosis is established early.

Granulomatous infiltration

Granulomatous infiltration of the gastric mucosa may be localized or generalized.

Local sarcoid infiltration—Sarcoidosis has a predilection for the antrum and the pylorus. The lesion may produce a 'funnel-shaped' distortion of the stomach[12,13]. In some patients gastric immobility may be demonstrated by barium studies[14]. Korsager described a 76-year-old woman with diffuse pulmonary infiltration who developed abdominal discomfort and explosive vomiting. Fibreoptic bronchoscopy revealed a segmental, circumscribed, firm lesion producing constriction with a diameter of 1.5 cm. Biopsy specimens from the fundus, antrum, the pyloric canal and the duodenum showed non-caseating granulomas. The patient responded to prednisone treatment[5].

Generalized extensive infiltration or *linitis plastica syndrome*—Intense granulomatous infiltration of the gastric wall may simulate the appearance of linitis plastica due to carcinoma or syphilis. The symptoms at this stage may include epigastric pain, nausea, abdominal cramps and, occasionally, diarrhoea.

Intestines

Histological and immunological similarities between sarcoidosis and Crohn's disease have led some to believe in a common aetiological identity. However, clinical differences between the two conditions are vast. There are only a few documented cases of sarcoidosis involving the small intestine. Dines *et al.*[15] reported on two patients with sarcoidosis and regional ileitis. This most likely represents a fortuitous occurrence. Gould, Handley and Bernado reported the first authentic case of sarcoidosis involving the large bowel[16]. Konda *et al.* described a 31-year-old Negro male with generalized sarcoidosis including involvement of both the stomach and the rectum[6].

Pancreas

Pancreatic sarcoidosis was first reported by Nickerson[17]. Maher, Choi and Dodds reviewed the literature and found only four cases of pancreatic sarcoidosis diagnosed in a living patient. They added one more patient with histological evidence of non-caseating granulomas in the pancreas. The patient also had granulomas in the distal common bile duct[18].

Peritoneum

Becker and Coleman[19] and Wong and Rosen[20] have described three patients with sarcoidosis and associated peritoneal involvement; two developed gross ascites; at laparotomy granulomas were seen in the peritoneum.

References

1. POLACHEK, A.A. and MATRE, W.J. (1964) Gastrointestinal sarcoidosis: Report of a case involving oesophagus. *Am. J. Dig. Dis.*, **9,** 429.
2. MCKUSICK, V.A. (1953) Boeck's sarcoid of the stomach with comments on the etiology of regional enteritis. *Gastroenterology*, **23,** 103.
3. WADINA, G.S. and MELAMED, A. (1966) Gastric granuloma (sarcoidosis?). *Am. J. Gastroenterol.*, **45,** 11.

4. ISRAEL, H. and SONES, M. (1953) Sarcoidosis: clinical observations on one hundred and sixty cases. *Arch. Intern. Med.*, **102**, 766.
5. KORSAGER, S. (1979) Sarcoidosis of the stomach. *Scand. J. Resp. Dis.*, **60**, 24.
6. KONDA, J., RUTH, M., SASSARIS, M., et al. (1980) Sarcoidosis of the stomach and rectum. *Am. J. Gastroenterol.*, **73**, 516.
7. ONA, F.V. (1981) Gastric sarcoid. *Am. J. Gastroenterol.*, **75**, 286.
8. PALMER, E.D. (1968) A note on silent sarcoidosis of the stomach. *J. Lab. Clin. Med.*, **52**, 231.
9. FUNG, W.P., KOO, K.T. and LEE, Y.S. (1975) Gastric sarcoidosis presenting with haematemesis. *Med. J. Austr.*, **ii**, 47.
10. PALMER, E.D. (1970) *Upper Gastrointestinal Haemorrhage*, p. 328. (Springfield, Il.: Charles C. Thomas)
11. BERENS, D.L. and MONTES, M. (1975) Gastric sarcoidosis. *N.Y. St. J. Med.*, **75**, 1290.
12. LEVERE, R.D. (1962) Sarcoidosis with gastric involvement. *Gastroenterology*, **42**, 189.
13. BLACKSTONE, M.O., JEELANI, D.G., MIZUNO, H., et al. (1976) Gastric sarcoidosis presenting as antral scarring. *Gastrointest. Endosc.*, **22**, 211.
14. LIEHR, H. (1962) Sarcoides des Magnes. *Med. Klin.*, **64**, 975.
15. DINES, D., DEPREMEE, R.A. and GREEN, P. (1971) Sarcoidosis associated with regional enteritis (Crohn's disease). *Minn. Med.*, **54**, 617.
16. GOULD, S.R., HANDLEY, A.J. and BERNARDO, D.F. (1973) Rectal and gastric involvement in a case of sarcoidosis. *Gut*, **14**, 971.
17. NICKERSEN, D.A. (1937) Boeck's sarcoid. *Arch. Pathol.*, **24**, 19.
18. MAHER, L., CHOI, H. and DODDS, W.J. (1981) Non-caseating granulomas of the pancreas. *Ann. J. Gastroenterol.*, **75**, 222.
19. BECKER, W.F. and COLEMAN, W.D. (1961) Surgical significance of abdominal sarcoidosis. *Ann. Surg.*, **153**, 987.
20. WONG, M. and ROSEN, S.W. (1962) Ascites in sarcoidosis due to peritoneal involvement. *Ann. Intern. Med.*, **57**, 277.

Chapter 19

Upper respiratory tract

The nose: Nasal mucosa and the septum

The upper respiratory tract involvement occurs in 5-20% of the patients[1-3]. The nasal mucosa is most frequently involved particularly in the patients with lupus pernio. Nasal stuffiness, dryness and crusting are the common symptoms. When obtaining a history of a patient with sarcoidosis, always inquire, 'Do you have any nasal stuffiness or congestion?' If the answer is yes, do not ignore it. It may be the first symptom of sarcoidosis of the upper respiratory tract (SURT). Physical examination at this stage may reveal pale, yellowish, slightly raised, firm tiny nodules. The lesions are small and may be easily overlooked. Later the mucosa becomes erythematous, granular and polypoid. The polypoidal growth may then cause obstruction, stagnation, discharge and rarely epistaxis. Nasal septal perforation may follow[4]. A biopsy specimen of the nasal mucosa, in such cases, almost always shows non-caseating granulomas.

The nasal involvement is an indicator of chronic persistent disease and finding of a nasal granuloma even in the early stage of the disease constitutes an indication for treatment. Systemic steroids are the sheet anchor of therapy. Intralesional corticosteroids may be beneficial for polypoidal growths. Nasal congestion and obstruction, occasionally, responds to beclomethasone diproprionate nasal spray. One should resist the temptation of removing polyps caused by SURT, because nasal septal perforations have been reported to occur after submucosal resections[5].

Case report—Nasal stuffiness and gradually increasing swelling of the third and fourth fingers on the right hand were responsible for a 60-year-old woman's first visit to the hospital. She had no history of any trauma, infections or major illness. She had always been in relatively good health. Physical examination revealed flesh-coloured nodules on the nasal bridge and nasal alae and hypopigmented atrophic macules on the chin. The third and fourth fingers of the right hand were swollen (*see Figure 19.1*). A chest radiograph showed bilateral hilar adenopathy and pulmonary infiltration. Bone lesions were seen (*see Figure 19.2*). Serum angiotensin converting enzyme level was 42 $IU.\ell^{-1}$ (normal range 10-30 $IU.\ell^{-1}$). The skin and transbronchial lung biopsy specimens showed non-caseating granulomas. Serum immunoglobulins: IgG, 2170 mg.$(100\,ml)^{-1}$ (21.7 g.ℓ^{-1}) (normal range, 600-2000 mg.$(100\,ml)^{-1}$; 6-20 g.ℓ^{-1}); IgA, 723 mg.$(100\,ml)^{-1}$ (7.23 g.ℓ^{-1}) (normal range, 50-400 mg.$(100\,ml)^{-1}$; 5-40 g.ℓ^{-1}); IgM, 210 mg.$(100\,ml)^{-1}$ (2.1 g.ℓ^{-1}) (normal range, 40-250 mg.$(100\,ml)^{-1}$; 4-25 g.ℓ^{-1}). She was given prednisone which produced partial amelioration of the nasal stuffiness. The chest radiograph has remained unchanged.

Comment—Nasal stuffiness was one of the early symptoms in this patient, with chronic multisystem involvement.

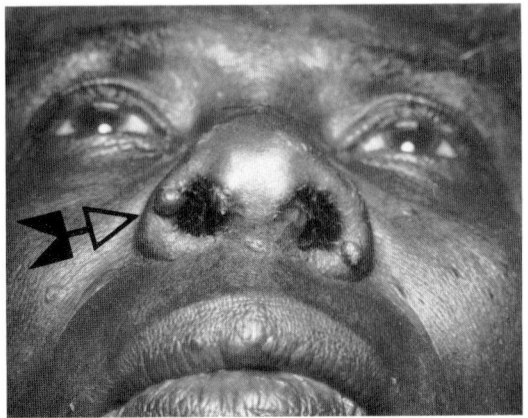

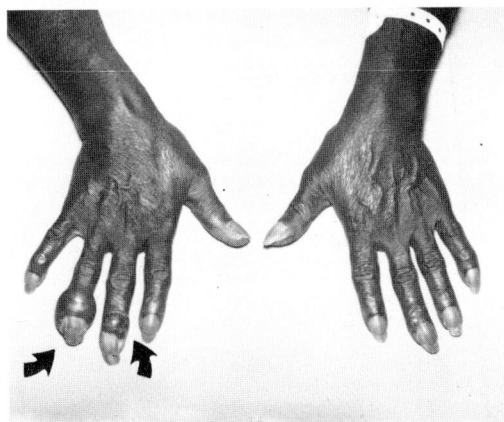

Figure 19.1 Flesh-coloured nodules on the nose and the septum and swellings of the right hand (arrows). Nasal mucosa is dry and crusted.

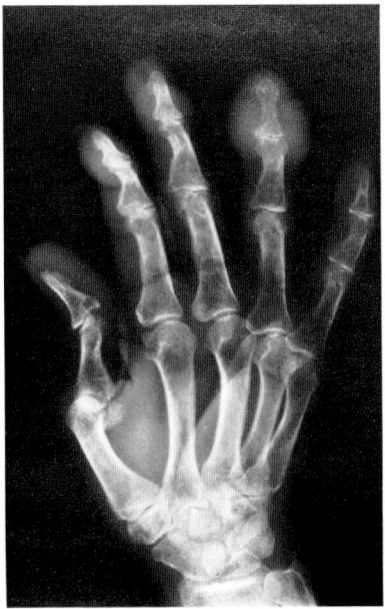
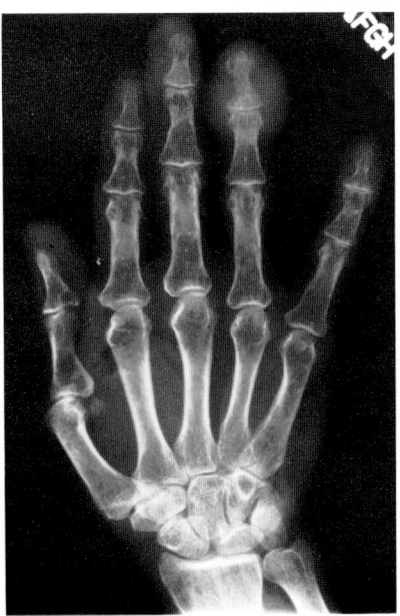

Figure 19.2 Bone and joint involvement: swelling of the distal interphalanges.

Laryngeal sarcoidosis

The larynx is involved in about 5% of the sarcoidosis patients[6]. The granulomatous lesion most commonly affects the epiglottis; the aryepiglottic folds, arytenoids, false cords and subglottic areas are also frequently involved. Sarcoidosis seems to affect the areas of the larynx that are rich in lymphatics and spares the true vocal cords which are relatively devoid of lymphatics. In general, the laryngeal involvement is associated with other manifestations of the disease. Isolated affliction of the larynx may also occur. The lesion may vary in appearance from a localized submucosal induration to a solid polypoid tumour. Ulceration is rare. A large exophytic lesion may produce fatal airway obstruction.

Since the disease has a tendency towards spontaneous remission, patients with mild to moderate airway obstruction can be followed up on a regular basis by flow–volume loops. Treatment of severe airway obstruction consists of the systemic administration of high-dose steroids (prednisone 80 mg daily). Local injection of corticosteroids is beneficial in patients with diffuse infiltrating lesions. Tracheostomy and surgical removal of the lesion is necessary when the obstruction fails to respond to corticosteroids[7,8]. The laryngologist should include laryngeal sarcoidosis in the differential diagnosis in patients with airway obstruction[9,10].

Case report—A 21-year-old secretary noticed a gradual change in her voice. She described her voice as somewhat 'bubbly'. Physical examination and the chest radiograph were normal. Laryngeal examination revealed marked narrowing due to swelling of the epiglottis and the false cords (*see Plate 19.1a*). The

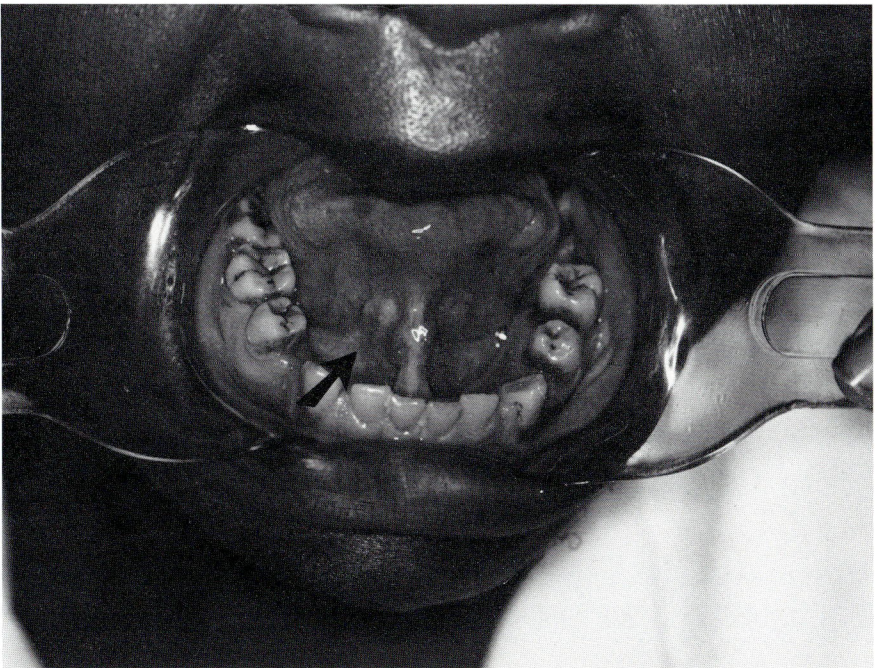

Figure 19.3 Nodular sarcoid lesion on the under-surface of the tongue and frenulum (arrow). Histological investigation showed a non-caseating granuloma. The lesion subsided after treatment with corticosteroids.

true cords were not involved. A biopsy specimen showed a granulomatous reaction (*see Plate 19.1b*). Serum angiotensin converting enzyme activity was only mildly elevated. She was given prednisone 60 mg daily which promptly improved her symptoms.

The tonsils

Involvement of the tonsils varies considerably. Mayock *et al.*[11] found no evidence of tonsillar granulomas in their series, whereas Gravesen[12] and Lightner[13] found 64% and 50% tonsillar involvement, respectively. Weiss found only two positive biopsy samples in 22 patients[14]. Occasionally, tiny nodules or large, pale tubercles may be visible on the tonsillar surface. Markedly enlarged tonsils may cause fullness of the throat and dysphagia. Injection of corticosteroids locally into the tonsils have resulted in regression of markedly hypertrophied tonsils[15]. Rarely palate, tongue and trachea are also affected by sarcoidosis (*see Figure 19.2*).

References

1. NEVILLE, E., MILLS, R.G.S. and JAMES, D.G. (1976) Sarcoidosis of the upper respiratory tract. *Ann. N.Y. Acad. Sci.*, **278**, 416.
2. DIBENEDETTO, R. and LEFRAK, S. (1970) Systemic sarcoidosis with severe involvement of the upper respiratory tract. *Am. Rev. Respir. Dis.*, **102**, 801.
3. SELROOS, O. and NIEMISTO, M. (1977) Sarcoidosis of the nose. *Scand. J. Respir. Dis.*, **58**, 1.
4. ALLEN, B.R. (1978) Sarcoid of nose with collapse of nasal cartilage. *Br. J. Dermatol.*, **99** (Suppl. 16), 54.
5. SHARMA, O.P. (1978) Sarcoidosis of the upper respiratory tract. *Arch. Intern. Med.*, **138**, 1064.
6. DEVINE, K.D. (1965) Sarcoidosis and sarcoidosis of the larynx. *Laryngoscope*, **75**, 533.
7. WEISMAN, R.A., CANALIS, R.F. and POWELL, W.J. (1980) Laryngeal sarcoidosis with airway obstruction. *Ann. Otol. Rhinol. Laryngol.*, **89**, 58.
8. CARASSO, B. (1974) Sarcoidosis of the larynx causing airway obstruction. *Chest*, **65**, 693.
9. NEEL, B.H. and MCDONALD, D.J. (1982) Laryngeal sarcoidosis: Report of 13 patients. *Ann. Otol. Rhinol. Laryngol.*, **91**, 359.
10. BOWER, J.S., BELEN, J.E. and WEG, J.G. (1980) Manifestations and treatment of laryngeal sarcoidosis. *Am. Rev. Resp. Dis.*, **122**, 325.
11. MAYOCK, R.L., BERTRAND, P., MORRISON, C.E. and SCOTT, J.H. (1963) Manifestations of sarcoidosis: Analysis of 145 patients with a review of nine series selected from literature. *Am. J. Med.*, **35**, 67.
12. GRAVESEN, P.B. (1942) *Lymphogranulomatoses Benigna*. (Odense, Denmark. I Kommission hos Andelsbog-trykkeriet).
13. LIGHTNER, S.J. (1949) *Der Morbus Besnier–Boeck–Schaumann*. (Basel: B. Schwabe and Co.)
14. WEISS, J.A. (1960) Sarcoidosis in otolaryngology. *Laryngoscope*, **70**, 1351.
15. MIGLETS, A.W. and BARTON, C.L. (1970) Sarcoid of the tonsils: Response to local steroid injection. *Arch. Otolaryngol.*, **92**, 516.

Chapter 20

The reproductive system

Male

Sarcoidosis may rarely affect any portion of the male reproductive system, but the epididymis and the testis are the most frequently involved structures.

Epididymis

Less than 20 cases of clinically apparent epididymal sarcoidosis have been reported[1]. Commonly, sarcoid epididymitis occurs during the multisystem disease; rarely, it may be the initial manifestation (*see Figure 20.1*)[2,3].

Sarcoid epididymitis is characterized by painless nodular swelling which may be unilateral or bilateral. Unilateral involvement is more common, occurring in about two-thirds of the patients. Acute epididymitis has a good prognosis; it subsides either spontaneously or after a course of corticosteroid therapy. Rarely, epididymal lesions may produce recurrent, painful swellings, ductal obstruction, oligospermia and infertility.

Testis

Wees reviewed the literature and found three cases with testicular disease and added one more, bringing the total to four histologically confirmed cases of sarcoidosis of the testis. All four patients had evidence of generalized sarcoidosis[4,5].

The testicular lesion may remain asymptomatic or may appear as a painless scrotal mass. The latter may mimic a tumour. Testicular granuloma may be unilateral or bilateral. Rarely, Leydig-cell dysfunction may produce changes in secondary sexual characters. Corticosteroids are effective in reducing the swelling and preserving the gonadal dysfunction.

Miscellaneous

Rarely, the scrotum, spermatic cord and penis may be affected by sarcoidosis[6,7]. Asymptomatic involvement of the prostate gland and seminal vesicles may occur[8]. Involvement of the urinary bladder has been reported[9,10].

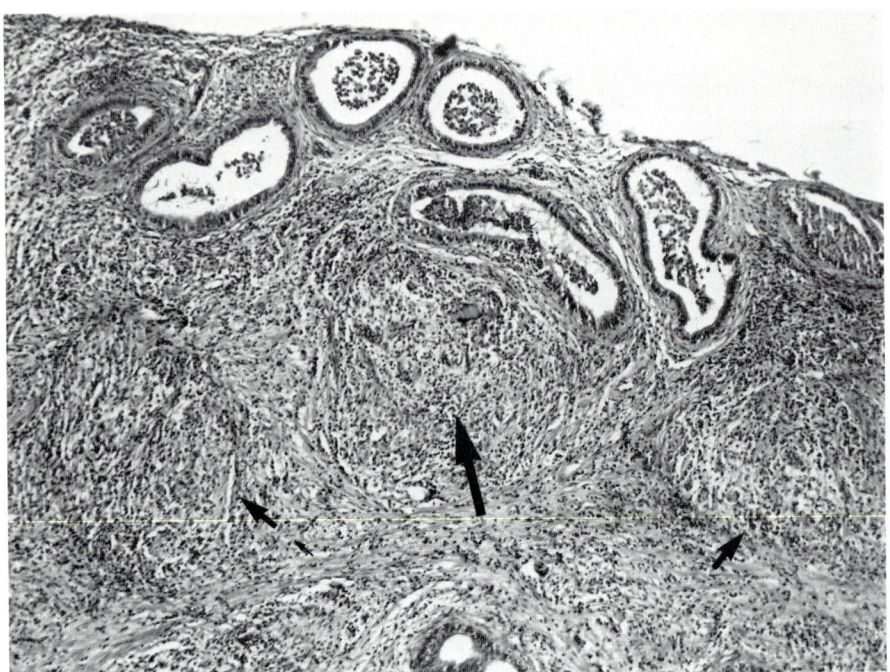

Figure 20.1 Epididymis biopsy: sarcoid granulomas (arrows). (Haematoxylin and eosin. × 125.) This 24-year-old man complained of left testicular swelling, parotid gland enlargement, anorexia and weight loss. A chest radiograph showed bilateral hilar adenopathy and pulmonary infiltration. The patient was given 20 mg prednisone daily. His appetite improved and the testicular and parotid swellings subsided.

Female

Uterus

Although the granulomas have occurred in nearly every part of the female reproductive system, the uterus is the organ most commonly affected by sarcoidosis. Clinical manifestations of uterine sarcoidosis include amenorrhoea, menorrhagia, metrorrhagia and cervical erosion. The diagnosis may be established by a curettage or a cervical biopsy. Mayock *et al.* described a patient with cervical erosion; a biopsy specimen of the lesion showed sarcoid granulomas[11]. Longcope and Freiman studied a woman with endometrial sarcoidosis. The diagnosis was made on curettage for menorrhagia[12]. Altchek, Gains and Siltzbach[13] described a 39-year-old woman who had a hysterectomy 5 years after the diagnosis of sarcoidosis was made. Both endometrium and myometrium were infiltrated with non-caseating granulomas. Taylor studied two patients who showed sarcoid tubercles on endometrial curettages[14].

Fallopian tubes

Cowdell[15] and Castoldi and Guidici[16] described patients with granulomatous lesions of the fallopian tubes. Kay reported on a patient who showed granulomatous infiltration of the bowel, the peritoneum and both fallopian tubes[17].

Breast

Reisner described two patients with sarcoidosis who developed breast nodules which regressed on follow-up. No biopsy was obtained[18]. Scadding reported on a 48-year-old woman with pulmonary infiltration and a breast nodule which showed non-caseating granulomas[19]. Scott[20] and Dalmark[21] have also reported sarcoid lesions of the breast.

References

1. OPAL, S.M., PITTMAN, D.L. and HOFELDT, F.D. (1979) Testicular sarcoidosis. *Am. J. Med.*, **67**, 147.
2. KRAUS, L. (1958) Genital sarcoidosis: A case report and review of the literature. *J. Urol.*, **80**, 367.
3. GERTESENBACHER, B.J., GREEN, R. and SACHS, F.L. (1977) Epididymal sarcoidosis: A report of two cases and review of the literature. *Yale J. Biol. Med.*, **50**, 669.
4. WEES, S.J. (1981) Testicular sarcoidosis. *S. Med. J.*, **24**, 255.
5. WINNACKER, J.L., BECKER, K.L., KATZ, S., et al. (1967) Recurrent epididymitis in sarcoidosis: Report of patients treated with corticosteroids. *Ann. Intern. Med.*, **66**, 743.
6. HANSFELD, K.F. (1961) Primary sarcoidosis of scrotum: Case report. *J. Urol.*, **86**, 269.
7. CARLI, G. (1955) Sarcoide di Boeck-Schaumann del solco balano prepuziale. *Minnerva Dermatol.*, **30**, 178.
8. HARDEBECK, H. (1953) Boeschsches Sarkoid der Prostata. *Ztschr. Urol.*, **46**, 202.
9. RADEWILL, F.H. (1943) Malakoplakia of the urinary bladder and generalized sarcoidosis. *J. Urol.*, **49**, 401.
10. FRENCH, A.J. and MASON, J.T. (1951) Malakoplakia of urinary bladder and sarcoidosis. *J. Urol.*, **66**, 229.
11. MAYOCK, R.L., BERTRAND, P., MORRISON, C.E., et al. (1963) Manifestations of sarcoidosis. Analysis of 145 patients with a review of nine series selected from the literature. *Am. J. Med.*, **35**, 67.
12. LONGCOPE, W.T. and FREIMAN, D.G. (1952) A study of sarcoidosis. *Medicine*, **31**, 1.
13. ALTCHEK, A., GAINES, J.A. and SILTZBACH, L.E. (1955) Sarcoidosis of the uterus. *Am. J. Obstet. Gynecol.*, **70**, 540.
14. TAYLOR, A.B. (1960) Sarcoidosis of the uterus. *J. Obstet. Gynecol. Br. Emp.*, **67**, 32.
15. COWDELL, R.H. (1954) Sarcoidosis with special reference to diagnosis and prognosis. *Q.J. Med.*, **23**, 29.
16. CASTOLDI, P. and GUIDICI, E. (1955) Granuloma di Besnier-Boeck-Schaumann con localizzazioni alle salpingi. *Minerva Ginaecol.*, **7**, 627.
17. KAY, S. (1956) Sarcoidosis of the fallopian tubes. Report of a case. *J. Obstet. Gynaecol. Br. Emp.*, **63**, 871.
18. REISNER, D. (1944) Boeck's sarcoid and systemic sarcoidosis. A study of thirty-five cases. *Am. Rev. Tuberc.*, **49**, 289.
19. SCADDING, J.G. (1967) *Sarcoidosis*. (London: Eyre and Spottiswoode)
20. SCOTT, R.B. (1938) The sarcoidosis of Boeck. *Br. Med. J.*, **ii**, 777.
21. DALMARK, G. (1942) Lymphogranulomatose benigne: Un cas avec des alterations mannaires comme seul symptome. *Acta Chir. Scand.*, **86**, 108.

Chapter 21

The immunology of sarcoidosis

The immunological functions in the body are carried out by two distinct populations of immunocompetent lymphoid cells: thymus-dependent or T cells and bursa-dependent or B cells.

Thymus-dependent or T cells are mediators of cellular immunity. The T lymphocytes, for their maturation, require direct contact with thymic epithelial cells and exposure to thymic hormones. The T lymphocytes carry antigen-receptor sites on their surface, retain long-lasting immunological memory and are responsible for delayed-type hypersensitivity reactions. Mature T cells seed the thymic-dependent zone or paracortical areas of peripheral lymphoid tissue. Post-thymic lymphocytes can be divided into:

1. Suppressor–cytotoxic cells.
2. Helper–inducer cells.
3. Null cells.
4. Delayed-hypersensitivity cells.

All peripheral T cells can be identified by the monoclonal antibody OKT-3. Suppressor–cytotoxic cells are identified by OKT-5, OKT-8 or Leu-2 monoclonal antibodies. Helper–inducer T-cell subsets are identified by OKT-4 or Leu-3 monoclonal antibodies.

Bursa-dependent or B cells produce and secrete immunoglobulins or circulating (humoral) antibodies responsible for resistance to most of the bacterial infections. B cells do not have antigen receptors on their surface. These cells are abundant in the lymph nodes, spleen, appendix and Peyer's patches. In the peripheral blood B cells represent 10–20% of the total circulating lymphocytes. The majority of patients with sarcoidosis display depression of delayed-type hypersensitivity. The immune reactions mediated by circulating antibodies remain unimpaired.

Cutaneous anergy

Tuberculin test

Cutaneous anergy has long been established as a cardinal immunological feature of sarcoidosis. Of the skin tests commonly used, the testing of existing hypersensitivity with intracutaneous tuberculin is the most widely used. Approximately two-thirds of the patients with sarcoidosis do not respond to tuberculin test in all conventional strengths between 1 and 250 TU[1]. Scadding observed that 61% of 260 patients gave no reaction to 100 TU. He further noted that patients with acute disease (stage I, BHL) had a lower incidence of negative reactors, for 50% of the patients with erythema nodosum and 54% of those with asymptomatic hilar adenopathy were non-reactors to 100 TU[2]. Lofgren and Lundback made similar observations[3]. However, Wurm demonstrated that the percentage of non-reactors increased with increasing chronicity of sarcoidosis; 68.2% of his stage I patients were anergic as opposed to 85.9% at stage III disease[4]. Of the 150 patients in my series, 128 (85%) failed to react to intermediate PPD (5 TU)[5]. The behaviour of tuberculin sensitivity, however, did not correlate with activity of the disease although a majority of the patients in the series had long-standing sarcoidosis.

Recovery from sarcoidosis and cutaneous anergy

It was generally accepted that patients with sarcoidosis regained tuberculin sensitivity on recovery[6-8]. However, Israel and Sones performed serial tuberculin tests in 170 patients over an interval of at least 2 years with a mean interval of 6 years[9]. At the end of the period, they found that tuberculin test was not influenced by the activity of the disease; the 65 patients with active disease, the 45 patients with inactive disease and the 60 patients who had recovered displayed inability to regain tuberculin sensitivity. Chusid, Shah and Siltzbach observed essentially similar results in a study of 69 patients with clinically recovered sarcoidosis[10]. Seventy-two per cent of patients with clinically and radiographically improved sarcoidosis, studied by Sharma and Beresford, demonstrated tuberculin anergy[11].

Effect of cortisone on tuberculin sensitivity

Citron and Scadding demonstrated that 50% of the patients with sarcoidosis who were anergic to tuberculin became tuberculin responsive if cortisone was added directly to the tuberculin test solution[12]. This effect of corticosteroids in uncovering or bringing out delayed hypersensitivity skin response to an antigen is called paradoxical response. Gross observed that paradoxical response to tuberculin and Candida antigens occurred in about one-third of all patients with sarcoidosis, and in more than one-half of those anergic to tuberculin[13]. It has been suggested that paradoxical responders have a defect in their ability to express delayed-type response, in addition to the known lymphocyte defect.

Thus, in sarcoidosis about two-thirds of patients have tuberculin anergy; the immunological defect persists despite clinical and radiological recovery in most of the patients; and the paradoxical response occurs in approximately one-third of all patients with sarcoidosis.

Effect of superimposed tuberculosis and BCG vaccination on tuberculin skin test in patients with sarcoidosis

Patients with sarcoidosis who develop active tuberculosis react strongly to tuberculin test at the time tuberculosis is diagnosed. Most of these patients, however, become anergic again after the recovery from tuberculosis. Similarly, when vaccinated with BCG vaccine, patients with sarcoidosis may acquire and retain, albeit temporarily, the sensitivity of tuberculin antigen. Thus, the relative depression of delayed-type hypersensitivity in sarcoidosis can be overcome by a strong antigenic challenge by tuberculous infection; but the cellular deficiency reappears when the infection is no longer active.

If a patient with sarcoidosis, particularly the one treated with corticosteroids, develops a positive tuberculin test *think of active tuberculosis.*

Other bacterial and fungal skin tests

In patients with sarcoidosis, cutaneous anergy can also be demonstrated by using other bacterial, fungal and viral antigen skin tests. Friou, using *Candida albicans* (oidiomycin), noted positive reaction in 95% of controls and 53% of sarcoidosis patients[14]. Citron utilized the same antigen and observed reactions in 90% of controls and in 40% of 30 patients with sarcoidosis[15]. Sones and Israel tested the patients with pertussis and histoplasmin antigens and recorded similar results[16]. Six of the seven patients studied by Quinn, Bunch and Yagle produced no cutaneous response to intradermal injection of mumps antigen despite the development of complement-fixing antibodies[17].

Chemical sensitization

As described above, sarcoid patients often show anergy to a few or all recall skin test antigens including tuberculin, mumps, Candida and Trichophyton. Most of these patients also fail to develop skin sensitivity after active sensitization with synthetic chemical sensitizer such as 2,4 dinitro-1-chlorobenzene (DNCB). Epstein and Mayock were able to demonstrate DNCB sensitivity in 96 (68%) of 141 controls and in only eight (35%) of 23 patients with sarcoidosis[18]. We reported anergy to DNCB in 55% of our sarcoidosis patients[5]. Like tuberculin anergy, defective response to DNCB seems to persist after clinical recovery from the disease.

Keyhole limpet (*Megathura crenulata*)

Haemocyanin (KLH) is a potent antigen which elicits both humoral and delayed-type responses in man. The KLH skin test correlates well with the tuberculin sensitivity in predicting the delayed-type hypersensitivity in sarcoidosis[19,20].

In vitro: Alterations in delayed hypersensitivity

Lymphopenia

Lymphopenia is a frequent finding in active sarcoidosis which seems to correlate with skin anergy. The lymphopenia represents an absolute reduction in the number of T cells[21]. Monoclonal antibody techniques have enabled us to assess the helper and suppressor functions of human T cells[22]. In normal subjects the ratio of helper to suppressor cells in the peripheral blood is approximately 1.8:1. The ratio is somewhat lower in low-activity sarcoidosis (1.4:1) but is significantly lower in high-intensity alveolitis (0.8:1). This relatively high number of suppressor cells in the peripheral blood may partly explain the cutaneous and *in-vitro* anergy observed in sarcoidosis[23].

The situation is, however, different in pulmonary and other tissue granulomas, where the helper:suppressor ratio is significantly higher (10.5:1). The cells bearing the suppressor–cytotoxic antigen are located in mantle surrounding the granuloma while the helper–inducer cells are distributed throughout the granuloma among the aggregated epithelioid cells (*see Plate 5.1 i, j*)[24].

Activated T cells

Siltzbach observed that the peripheral blood lymphocytes in sarcoidosis have an unusual potential for a long-term survival and spontaneous proliferation in culture[25]. In about half of the patients with active sarcoidosis atypical lymphocytes are found. There is also a significant increase in the number of lymphocytes that form stable E rosettes at 37°C culture when stimulated by mitogens or allogenic antigens[26,27]. The blood T cells from patients with active disease release a variety of lymphokines and possess minimal capacity to polyclonally activate B cells to secrete immunoglobulins.

Lymphocyte transformation

Phytohaemagglutinin (PHA) and concanavalin A stimulate normal human lymphocytes *in vitro* to undergo mitoses and blast transformation. This phenomenon of lymphocyte transformation has been used to evaluate the immunological competence of T cells[28]. Failure of cultured lymphocytes to respond to PHA is most marked in the active stage as compared with the inactive or recovered sarcoidosis[29]. Sharma, James and Fox observed that a close relationship exists between the *in-vitro* cellular hyperactivity and the *in-vivo* anergy to skin tests. The twin defect was a feature in two-thirds of patients with sarcoidosis[30].

Peripheral blood monocyte function

Goodwin *et al.*[31] have demonstrated that peripheral blood monocytes from patients with active sarcoidosis fail to respond to phytohaemagglutinin (PHA). However, these mononuclear cells manifest almost a normal response after the addition of indomethacin or the removal of glass-adherent cells. The patients with active sarcoidosis also have an increased percentage of monocytes in peripheral blood mononuclear preparations. The authors suggested that an increased suppression by the prostaglandin-producing suppressor cells and an increased percentage of monocytes contribute to the depressed PHA response noted in sarcoidosis.

Homograft survival

The relative depression of delayed-type sensitivity does not appear to delay the rejection of skin homograft[32].

Serum inhibitors

There is some evidence that substances that inhibit mitogen and recall antigen-induced stimulation of sarcoid lymphocytes exist in the serum of about half of the patients with active sarcoidosis. The nature of these inhibitory factors remains unknown[32].

What causes depression of delayed-type hypersensitivity in sarcoidosis?

The information reviewed above shows that cutaneous anergy in sarcoidosis is due to unavailability of the immune effector lymphocytes[13]. Lymphopenia is a prominent feature of the disease. There is a reduction of helper:suppressor ratio in the peripheral blood and an increase in the ratio at the site of granulomatous inflammation. Thus, immunoreactive cells are fighting the inflammation leaving inadequate number in the peripheral blood to elicit a cutaneous reaction[14].

It has been suggested that suppressor cells and serum factors may also contribute to depression of delayed-type hypersensitivity. However, the significance of these observations has not yet been established.

Humoral responses

Although the delayed hypersensitivity responses are impaired in sarcoidosis, the immune reactions mediated by circulating antibodies show evidence of hyperactivity.

Abnormalities of serum proteins and immunoglobulins

Salvesen was the first to draw attention to hyperglobulinaemia in sarcoidosis[33]. Hyperglobulinaemia which is mainly due to increase in the gamma- and beta-globulin fractions, occurs in 23-88% of the patients[34,35]. Hyperglobulinaemia is more frequent in Negro patients.

An elevation of serum gammaglobulin value (> 3.5 g.$(100$ ml$)^{-1}$ $(35$ g.$\ell^{-1}))$ occurs in more than half of the patients with sarcoidosis. In an international study involving 3676 patients, hypergammaglobulinaemia was observed in 23-96% of the patients[36]. Serum immunoglobulin G (IgG) elevations occurred in more than half of the patients; a quarter showed high IgA levels; and IgM values were high in less than 15% of the patients[37]. Serum immunoglobulin levels do not accurately reflect the clinical, radiographical or physiological impairment in sarcoidosis[38,39].

Hypogammaglobulinaemia is rare[40,41]. A few cases of selective IgA deficiency have been reported[42,43], but the relationship, if any, between the disease and various types of immunoglobulin deficiency states remains unknown.

Antibody formation

Circulating antibody production is normal in sarcoidosis. Fleming, Runyon and Cummings[44] and later James[45] using the Middlebrook technique, found normal values of tuberculin antibodies. Others have noted normal circulating antibody response to immunization with pertussis, tetanus toxoid and typhoid-paratyphoid vaccines. Quinn, Bunch and Yagle[46] recorded normal levels of mumps complement-fixing antibodies in seven patients with sarcoidosis. The studies by Chapman[47] (who found precipitin antibodies against atypical mycobacteria), of Hirshaut et al.[48] (who noted elevated antibody titres to herpes-like virus), and Horsmanheimo et al.[49] (who observed antibodies against mycoplasma organisms) further indicate that the humoral antibody production in sarcoidosis remains unaffected.

Serum complement activity

Serum complement activity was significantly increased in 10 of 11 patients studied by Buckley, Nagaya and Sieker[50]. The follow-up studies showed no change in the elevated complement activity. The authors suggested that an infectious agent effectively hidden from humoral immune factors and causing persistent inflammation might be responsible for the increased complement activity in sarcoidosis.

Immune complexes

The prevalence of immune complexes in sarcoidosis varies from 23 to 70%[51-54]. Circulating immune complexes are present in about half of the patients with acute disease, particularly in those with erythema nodosum. In chronic disease immune complexes are less frequent. It has been suggested that humoral antibodies may be important in the pathogenesis of the sarcoid granuloma. By a direct immunofluorescence technique Quismorio, Sharma and Chandor[55] found immunoglobulin deposits in cutaneous granulomas of five of the eight patients. These consisted of IgM within the blood-vessel wall (five patients), IgM at the epidermal-dermal junction (two patients) and IgG within and around the granuloma (two patients). The role of immune complexes in the pathogenesis of sarcoid granuloma is not clear. It has been suggested that the immune complexes alter the distribution and function of helper-suppressor cells and macrophages[56]!

Autoimmune phenomenon

This topic will be discussed in Chapter 30. Rheumatoid factor (RF) has been recorded in the sera of 10-47% of patients with sarcoidosis. However, the presence of rheumatoid factor carries little diagnostic or prognostic significance[57]. Favez has demonstrated circulating antibodies against the Kveim antigen in patients with sarcoidosis[58]. Turkington and Buckley reported the occurrence of macroglobulinaemia in a patient with sarcoidosis[59]. Chapman and Clark found cold precipitable antibodies in 76% of 25 patients they studied[60]. Autoantibodies to lymphocytes have been reported by Daniele and Rowlands[61], and Lobo and Suratt[62], in about half of the patients with active disease. Autoantibodies do not bear a consistent relationship to the severity or clinical manifestations of sarcoidosis[63].

B cells

The absolute number of B cells in the peripheral blood may increase, remain normal, or decrease in patients with active sarcoidosis. *In-vitro* studies of B-cell function, using a plaque forming assay, show that these cells from sarcoid patients have a low plaque-forming response after pokeweed stimulation. This impairment can be corrected by removing adherent monocytes from the cell suspension[64].

Kveim test

In patients with active sarcoidosis, the intracutaneous injection of a previously validated saline suspension of human sarcoid spleen or lymph nodes gives rise to a nodule, at the site of injection, in 2-6 weeks. A biopsy sample of the nodule in a positive reaction should demonstrate a characteristic non-caseating granulomatous reaction.

In an extensive trial conducted by Siltzbach[65] involving 750 subjects, 165 of whom had proven sarcoidosis, the Kveim test was positive in 94% of those with stage I and stage II sarcoidosis, and 73% of those with stage III and normal chest radiographs. Hurley and Bartholomeucz reported positive tests in 59% of 510 proven cases of sarcoidosis, and a false-positive rate of 1.7% in 722 individuals not suffering from sarcoidosis[66].

In general, the Kveim test is positive in about three-quarters of the patients with sarcoidosis[67,68]. Although false-positive tests using validated Kveim antigen suspensions are rare, Israel and Goldstein have reported the occurrence of positive Kveim reactions in patients with tuberculous lymphadenitis, lymphoma, non-specific lymphadenitis and regional enteritis[69].

The immunological mechanism of the Kveim test remains unexplained. One can only speculate that this slowly developing nodule represents a specific type of delayed hypersensitivity to some yet unidentified substance in human sarcoidal tissues. The active principle in the Kveim antigen is particulate and located intracellularly[70]. It is resistant to alcohol, chloroform and radiation[71]. The material remains stable at room temperature or in refrigerators for years[68,72].

Although the Kveim test is generally regarded specific for sarcoidosis, there are many drawbacks which prevent it from being widely used. The major disadvantage is the unavailability of the potent validated Kveim antigen. Other problems include: the 4-6 weeks necessary for maturation of the nodule, the need for punch biopsy, the variability of interpretation of the granulomatous reaction and the need to withhold corticosteroid therapy until the completion of the test. Furthermore, the development of newer diagnostic techniques including fibreoptic transbronchial biopsy, serum angiotensin-1-converting enzyme measurement, bronchoalveolar lavage, and gallium scanning, have significantly reduced the need of the Kveim test in the management of sarcoidosis[73].

Bronchoalveolar lavage (BAL)

Technique

Bronchoalveolar lavage is performed by placing a fibreoptic bronchoscope into a distal airway and instilling 150-200 ml normal saline in 20-30 ml aliquots. Following each injection, fluid is aspirated from the lower respiratory tract and is analysed for cells, soluble substances such as immunoglobulins and other inflammatory and immune mediators[74,75].

Normal BAL

In normal non-smokers, the effector cell population of the alveolar structure consists of $93 \pm 3\%$ alveolar macrophages, $7 \pm 1\%$ lymphocytes, and less than 1% of polymorphonuclear leukocytes. In normal smokers, the cell population is the same except the number of polymorphs which increases from 2 to 8%[74]. In various pulmonary disorders the effector cell population and immune mediators, and non-cellular components are abnormal[76].

BAL in sarcoidosis

In patients with active sarcoidosis there is a significant increase in all lymphocyte subtypes, particularly in the number of T lymphocytes. The proportion of T cells increases to $90 \pm 4\%$ of all lymphocytes and $31 \pm 8\%$ of all effector cells (see Plate 5.1 b-d). In contrast to T lymphocytes, the proportion of B cells is reduced. Thus, in a typical patient with active sarcoidosis, T-cell : B-cell ratio in the lung is 18 to 1; whereas the T-cell : B-cell ratio in blood is only about 3 to 1[77,78].

Furthermore, the expansion of T lymphocytes in BAL in active sarcoidosis consists of T-helper cells, a subset of T lymphocytes that enhances immune effector function.

The effect of T-helper cells is balanced by another subset of T cells called T-suppressor cells. In normal lung the T-helper : T-suppressor ratio is about 1.8 to 1, the same as in peripheral blood. In contrast, the lung helper : suppressor ratio in active sarcoidosis is shifted to 10.5 to 1[79].

Besides the shift in helper : suppressor cell ratio, there is an increase in other T-cell sub-types including 'T_{37}-cell', the T_y-cell, and the T_μ cell[75,78,80]. The role of these cells in the pathogenesis of sarcoidosis is not clear. The concentration of immunoglobulin G (IgG) is also elevated in sarcoidosis.

'High' and 'low' intensity alveolitis

Crystal and co-workers have used the percentage of lymphocytes in bronchoalveolar fluid to separate 'high intensity sarcoid alveolitis' from the 'low intensity sarcoid alveolitis'. If the lavage T cells are more than 28% the patient has high-intensity alveolitis, but if the lymphocyte percentage is less than 28 the alveolitis is of 'low intensity'.

Bronchoalveolar lavage is a more sensitive indicator of sarcoid activity than the serum angiotensin converting enzyme. There is some evidence that the patients with 'high intensity alveolitis' are more likely to develop irreversible functional damage and the prompt institution of corticosteroid therapy may prevent progression of the disease[81,82].

References

1. JAMES, D.G., SILTZBACH, L.E., SHARMA, O.P., *et al.* (1969) A tale of two cities: Comparison of sarcoidosis, London and New York. *Arch Intern. Med.*, **123**, 187.
2. SCADDING, J.G. (1967) *Sarcoidosis*. (London: Eyre and Spottiswoode)
3. LOFGREN, S. and LUNDBACK, H. (1952) The bilateral hilar lymphoma syndrome. A study of the relation to age and sex in 212 cases. *Acta Med. Scand.*, **142**, 259.
4. WURM, K. (1963) Untersuchungen uber das Tuberkulin – verhalten bei Sarcoidose. *Beitr. Klin. Tuberk.*, **127**, 195.
5. SHARMA, O.P. (1970) Immunological relationship between sarcoidosis and tuberculosis. *Ind. J. Med. Res.*, **58**, 1551.
6. NITTER, L. (1953) Changes in chest roentgenogram in Boeck's sarcoid of the lungs. *Acta Radiol.*, (Suppl. **105**) 1.
7. HOSODA, Y. and CHIBA, Y. (1964) Relationship of sarcoidosis to tuberculosis. *Acta Med. Scand.*, **176** (Suppl. **425**), 271.
8. SOMMER, E. (1964) Primary and secondary anergy in sarcoidosis. *Acta Med. Scand.*, **176** (Suppl. **425**), 195.
9. ISRAEL, H. and SONES, M. (1965) Immunological defect in patients recovered from sarcoidosis. *N. Engl. J. Med.*, **273**, 1003.
10. CHUSID, E.L., SHAH, R. and SILTZBACH, L.E. (1971) Tuberculin sensitivity in sarcoidosis. In *Proceedings of the Fifth International Conference on Sarcoidosis* (eds Lavinsky, L. and Macholda, F.), p. 171. (Prague: Charles University).
11. SHARMA, O.P. and BERESFORD, O.S. (1971) Immunological studies in patients recovered from sarcoidosis and tuberculosis. *Ind. J. Tuberc.*, **18**, 84.
12. CITRON, K.M. and SCADDING, J.G. (1957) The effect of cortisone upon the reaction of the skin to tuberculin in tuberculosis and sarcoidosis. *Q.J. Med.*, **26**, 377.
13. GROSS, N.J. (1973) The paradoxical skin response in sarcoidosis. *Am. Rev. Resp. Dis.*, **107**, 1973.
14. FRIOU, G.J. (1952) A study of cutaneous reactions to oidiomycin, trichophytin and mumps skin test antigens in patients with sarcoidosis. *Yale J. Biol. Med.*, **24**, 533.
15. CITRON, K.M. (1957) Skin tests in sarcoidosis. *Tubercle*, **38**, 33.
16. SONES, M. and ISRAEL, H. (1954) Altered immunologic reactions in sarcoidosis. *Ann. Intern. Med.*, **40**, 260.
17. QUINN, E.L., BUNCH, D.C. and YAGLE, E.M. (1955) The mumps skin test and complement fixation test as a diagnostic aid in sarcoidosis. *J. Invest. Dermatol.*, **24**, 595.

18. EPSTEIN, W.L. and MAYOCK, R.L. (1957) Induction of allergic contact dermatitis in patients with sarcoidosis. *Proc. Soc. Exp. Biol. Med.*, **96**, 786.
19. WEIGLE, W.O. (1964) Immunochemical properties of hemocyanin. *Immunochemistry*, **1**, 295.
20. SHARMA, O.P. (1975) *Sarcoidosis: A Clinical Approach*, p. 140. (Springfield, Ill.: Charles C. Thomas).
21. HOFFBRAND, B.T. (1968) Occurrence and significance of lymphopenia in sarcoidosis. *Am. Rev. Resp. Dis.*, **98**, 107.
22. REINHERZ, E.L. (1981) Current concepts in immunology, regulation of the immune response, inducer and suppressor subsets in human beings. *N. Engl. J. Med.*, **305**, 308.
23. KATZ, P., HAYNES, B.F. and FAUCI, A.S. (1978) Alteration of T-lymphocyte subpopulations in sarcoidosis. *Clin. Immunol. Immunopathol.*, **10**, 350.
24. MODLIN, R.L., HOFMAN, F.M., SHARMA, O.P., et al. (1983) *In situ* demonstration of T-lymphocyte subsets in granulomatous inflammation: leprosy, rhinoscleroma and sarcoidosis. *Clin. Exp. Immunol.*, **51**, 430.
25. HIRSCHHORN, K., SCHREIBMAN, R.R., BACH, F.H., et al. (1964) *In vitro* studies of lymphocytes from patients with sarcoidosis and lymphoproliferative diseases. *Lancet*, **ii**, 842.
26. HEDFORS, E., HOLM, G. and PETTERSON, D. (1974) Lymphocyte subpopulations in sarcoidosis. *Clin. Exp. Immunol.*, **17**, 219.
27. ROSSMAN, M.D., DAUBER, J.H. and DANIELE, R.P. (1978) Identification of activated T-cells in sarcoidosis. *Am. Rev. Resp. Dis.*, **117**, 713.
28. GREAVES, M., JANOSSY, G. and DOENHOFF, M. (1974) Selective triggering of human T and B lymphocytes *in vitro* by polyclonal antigens. *J. Exp. Med.*, **140**, 1.
29. DANIELE, R.P. and ROWLANDS, D.T., Jr. (1976) Lymphocyte subpopulations in sarcoidosis: Correlation with disease activity and duration. *Ann. Intern. Med.*, **85**, 593.
30. SHARMA, O.P., JAMES, D.G. and FOX, R.A. (1971) A correlation of *in vivo* delayed-type hypersensitivity with *in vitro* lymphocyte transformation in sarcoidosis. *Chest*, **60**, 35.
31. GOODWIN, J.S., DEHORATIUS, R., ISRAEL, H., et al. (1979) Suppressor cell function in sarcoidosis. *Ann. Intern. Med.*, **90**, 169.
32. SNYDER, G.B. (1964) The fate of skin homografts in patients with sarcoidosis. *Bull. Johns Hopkins Hosp.*, **115**, 81.
33. SALVESEN, H.A. (1935) The sarcoid of Boeck, a disease of importance to internal medicine. *Acta Med. Scand.*, **86**, 127.
34. COWDELL, R.H. (1954) Sarcoidosis with special reference to diagnosis and prognosis. *Q.J. Med.*, **23**, 29.
35. CUMMINGS, M.M., DUNNER, E. and WILLIAMS, J.H., Jr. (1959) Epidemiologic and clinical observations in sarcoidosis. *Ann. Intern. Med.*, **50**, 879.
36. JAMES, D.G., NEVILLE, E., SILTZBACH, L.E., et al. (1976) A worldwide review of sarcoidosis. *Ann. N.Y. Acad. Sci.*, **278**, 321.
37. SHARMA, O.P., JAMES, D.G., BIRD, R., et al. (1971) Immunoglobulins in sarcoidosis. In *Proceedings of the Fifth International Conference on Sarcoidosis* (eds Levinsky, L. and Macholda, F.), p. 171. (Prague: Charles University)
38. CELIKOGIU, S., VIEIRA, L.O.B.D. and SILTZBACH, L.E. (1971) Serum immunoglobulin levels in sarcoidosis. In *Proceedings of the Fifth International Conference on Sarcoidosis* (eds Levinsky, L. and Macholda, F.), p. 168. (Prague: Charles University)
39. GOLDSTEIN, R.A., ISRAEL, H.L. and RAWNSLEY, H.M. (1971) Effect of race and stage of disease on the serum immunoglobulins in sarcoidosis. In *Proceedings of the Fifth International Conference on Sarcoidosis* (eds Levinsky, L. and Macholda, F.), p. 178. (Prague: Charles University)
40. BRONSKY, D. and DUNN, Y. (1965) Sarcoidosis with hypogammaglobulinemia. *Am. J. Med. Sci.*, **250**, 11.
41. SHARMA, O.P. and JAMES, D.G. (1971) Hypogammaglobulinemia depression of delayed-type hypersensitivity and granuloma formation. *Am. Rev. Resp. Dis.*, **104**, 228.
42. SHARMA, O.P. and CHANDOR, S.B. (1972) IgA deficiency in sarcoidosis. *Am. Rev. Resp. Dis.*, **106**, 600.
43. SIEGLER, D. (1978) Sarcoidosis and selective IgA deficiency. *Br. J. Chest. Dis.*, **72**, 143.
44. FLEMING, J.W., RUNYON, E.H. and CUMMINGS, M.M. (1951) An evaluation of the haemagglutination test for tuberculosis. *Am. J. Med.*, **10**, 704.
45. JAMES, D.G. (1966) Immunology of sarcoidosis. *Lancet*, **ii**, 633.
46. QUINN, E.L., BUNCH, D.C. and YAGLE, E.M. (1955) The mumps skin test and complement fixation test as a diagnostic aid in sarcoidosis. *J. Invest. Dermatol.*, **24**, 595.
47. CHAPMAN, J. and SPEIGHT, M. (1964) Further studies of mycobacterial antibodies in the sera of sarcoidosis patients. *Acta Med. Scand.*, **176** (Suppl. **425**), 61.
48. HIRSHAUT, Y., GLADE, P., VIERRA, L.O.B.D., et al. (1970) Sarcoidosis, another disease associated with serologic evidence of herpes-like virus infection. *N. Engl. J. Med.*, **283**, 502.
49. HORSMANHEIMO, J., JANSSON, E., HANNNUKSELA, M., et al. (1978) Studies in sarcoidosis: Intradermal mycoplasma test. *Am. Rev. Resp. Dis.*, **117**, 975.

50. BUCKLEY, C.E., NAGAYA, H. and SIEKER, H.O. (1966) Altered immunologic activity in sarcoidosis. *Ann. Intern. Med.*, **64**, 508.
51. HEDFORS, E. and NORBERG, R. (1974) Evidence of circulating immune complexes in sarcoidosis. *Clin. Exp. Immunol.*, **16**, 493.
52. GUPTA, R.C., KUEPPERS, R., DEREMEE, R.A., *et al.* (1977) Pulmonary and extrapulmonary sarcoidosis in relation to circulating immune complexes. *Am. Rev. Resp. Dis.*, **116**, 261.
53. DANIELE, R.P., MCMILLAN, L.J., DAUBER, J.H., *et al.* (1978) Immune complexes in sarcoidosis: A correlation with activity and duration of disease. *Chest*, **74**, 261.
54. MORNEX, J.F., REVILLAR, J.P., VINCENT, C., *et al.* (1979) Elevated serum B_2-microglobulin levels and Clq-binding immune complexes in sarcoidosis. *Biomedicine*, **31**, 210.
55. QUISMORIO, F., SHARMA, O.P. and CHANDOR, S.B. (1977) Immunopathological studies on the cutaneous lesions in sarcoidosis. *Br. J. Dermatol.*, **97**, 635.
56. WILLIAMS, J.D., SMITH, M.D. and DAVIES, B.H. (1982) Interaction of immunocomplexes and T-suppressor cells in sarcoidosis. *Thorax*, **37**, 602.
57. ORESKES, I. and SILTZBACH, L.E. (1968) Changes in rheumatoid factor activity during the course of sarcoidosis. *Am. J. Med.*, **44**, 60.
58. FAVEZ, G. (1971) Circulating antibodies specific to the Kveim antigen demonstrated in sarcoidosis. In *Proceedings of the Fifth International Conference on Sarcoidosis* (eds Levinsky, L. and Macholda, F.), p. 203. (Prague: Charles University)
59. TURKINGTON, R.W. and BUCKLEY, C.E. (1966) Macrocryoglobulinemia and sarcoidosis. *Am. J. Med.*, **40**, 156.
60. CHAPMAN, J. and CLARK, J. (1971) Cold-precipitable proteins of sarcoidosis serum. In *Proceedings of the Fifth International Conference on Sarcoidosis* (eds Levinsky, L. and Macholda, F.), p. 198. (Prague: Charles University)
61. DANIELE, R.P. and ROWLANDS, D.T., Jr. (1976) Antibodies to T-cells in sarcoidosis. *Ann. N.Y. Acad. Sci.*, **278**, 88.
62. LOBO, P.I. and SURATT, P.M. (1979) Studies on the autoantibody to lymphocytes in sarcoidosis. *J. Clin. Lab. Immunol.*, **1**, 283.
63. TURNER-WARWICK, M. (1978) *Immunology of the Lung*, p. 148. (London: Edward Arnold)
64. KATZ, P. and FAUCI, A.S. (1978) Inhibition of polyclonal B-cells activation by suppressor monocytes in patients with sarcoidosis. *Clin. Exp. Immunol.*, **32**, 554.
65. SILTZBACH, L.E. (1969) The Kveim test in sarcoidosis. *J. Am. Med. Assoc.*, **178**, 476.
66. HURLEY, T.H. and BARTHOLOMEUCZ, G. (1967) The Kveim test: Results obtained in sarcoid and non-sarcoid patients with simultaneous use of Australian(CSL) and American(Chase-Siltzbach type I USA) Kveim suspensions. In *Proceedings of the Fourth International Conference on Sarcoidosis* (eds Tumaf, J. and Chabot, J.), p. 194. (Paris: Masson)
67. JAMES, D.G. and SHARMA, O.P. (1967) The Kveim–Siltzbach test: Report of a new British antigen. *Lancet*, **ii**, 1274.
68. KATARIA, Y., SHARMA, O.P., ISRAEL, H.L., *et al.* (1980) Kveim antigen CR-1: Its sensitivity and specificity in sarcoidosis, a comparative study. In *Sarcoidosis and Other Granulomatous Diseases* (eds Williams, W.J. and Davies, B.H.), p. 660. (Cardiff: Alpha Omega)
69. ISRAEL, H.L. and GOLDSTEIN, R.A. (1971) Relation of Kveim antigen test to lymphadenopathy. Study of sarcoidosis and other diseases. *N. Engl. J. Med.*, **284**, 345.
70. MIDDLETON, W.G. and DOUGLAS, A.C. (1980) Further experiences with Edinburgh prepared Kveim-Siltzbach test suspension. In *Sarcoidosis and Other Granulomatous Diseases* (eds Williams, W.J. and Davies, B.H.), p. 655. (Cardiff: Alpha Omega)
71. SILTZBACH, L.E. and TAUB, R.N. (1978) Sarcoidosis. In *Immunologic Diseases* (ed. Samter, M.), 3rd Edn, p. 548. (Boston: Little, Brown & Co.)
72. DOUGLAS, A.C., WALLACE, A., CLARK, J., *et al.* (1976) The Edinburgh spleen: Source of a validated Kveim–Siltzbach test material. *Ann. N.Y. Acad. Sci.*, **278**, 671.
73. ISRAEL, H.L. (1983) Diagnostic value of the Kveim reaction. In *Sarcoidosis and other Granulomatous Diseases of the Lung* (ed. Fanburg, B.L.), p. 273. (New York: Marcel Dekker).
74. HUNNINGHAKE, G.W., GADEK, J.E., KAWANAMI, O., *et al.* (1979) Inflammatory and immune responses in the human lung in health and disease: Evaluation of bronchoalveolar lavage. *Am. J. Pathol.*, **97**, 149.
75. YEAGER, J., WILLIAMS, M.D., BEEKMAN, J.J.F., *et al.* (1977) Sarcoidosis: Analysis of cells obtained by bronchial lavage. *Am. Rev. Resp. Dis.*, **116**, 951.
76. HUNNINGHAKE, G.W., KAWANAMI, O., FERRANS, V.J., *et al.* (1981) Characterization of the inflammatory and immune effector cells in the lung parenchyma of patients with interstitial lung disease. *Am. Rev. Resp. Dis.*, **123**, 407.
77. WEINBERGER, S.E., KELMANN, J.A., NELSON, N.A., *et al.* (1978) Bronchoalveolar lavage in interstitial lung disease. *Ann. Intern. Med.*, **89**, 459.

78. HUNNINGHAKE, G.W., FULMER, J.D., YOUNG, R.C., *et al.* (1979) Localization of the immune response in sarcoidosis. *Am. Rev. Resp. Dis.*, **120**, 49.
79. HUNNINGHAKE, G.W. and CRYSTAL, R.G. (1981) Mechanism of hypergammaglobulinemia in pulmonary sarcoidosis: Site of antibody production and role of T lymphocytes. *J. Clin. Invest.*, **67**, 86.
80. HUNNINGHAKE, G.W., KEOGH, B.A., LINE, B.R., *et al.* (1980) Pulmonary sarcoidosis: Pathogenesis and therapy. In *Basic and Clinical Aspects of Granulomatous Diseases* (eds Boros, D. and Yosshida, T.), p. 275. (New York: Elsevier-North-Holland)
81. CRYSTAL, R.G., ROBERTS, M.C., HUNNINGHAKE, G.W., *et al.* (1981) Pulmonary sarcoidosis: A disease characterized and perpetuated by activated lung T lymphocytes. *Ann. Intern. Med.*, **94**, 73.
82. HUNNINGHAKE, G.W. and CRYSTAL, R.G. (1981) Pulmonary sarcoidosis: A disorder mediated by excess helper T-lymphocyte activity at sites of disease activity. *N. Engl. J. Med.*, **305**, 492.

Chapter 22
Laboratory investigations

Blood

Anaemia

Anaemia (haemoglobin of less than 11 g) was observed in 31 (22%) of 145 patients studied by Mayock et al.; three patients had haemolytic anaemia[1]. Ferguson and Paris[2], and McCort et al.[3], however, reported an incidence of anaemia of only 3.4% and 7.1%, respectively. In my experience, the true incidence of anaemia in sarcoidosis is about 5%. Haemolytic anaemia is rare. The pathogenesis of haemolytic anaemia in sarcoidosis is not completely understood. Liebling, Bell and Stengle studied production, volume and destruction of red blood cells in sarcoidosis and found no abnormality[4]. Hypersplenism has been proposed as a possible cause. Sordillo and Briggs reviewed a total of 18 cases of haemolytic anaemia in sarcoidosis from the world literature; the spleen was enlarged in 13[5]. Only three of the patients were cured by splenectomy; three did not respond to the procedure; and in five other patients relapse occurred within 1 year after removal of the spleen. The unsatisfactory response to splenectomy, a positive Coombs' test, the presence of a false-positive test to syphilis, and the clinical improvement after treatment with corticosteroids suggest that haemolytic anemia in sarcoidosis might be an antigen-antibody reaction. However, Coombs' test was positive in only eight (40%) out of 18 patients with sarcoidosis and haemolytic anaemia. Although corticosteroid therapy is useful in some cases, spontaneous correction of haemolytic anaemia may occur.

Leukopenia and leukaemoid reaction

Leukopenia is a more frequent finding. It occurs in about one-third of the patients[6]. Longcope and Freiman followed up 33 patients for at least 5 years and found that leukopenia could be correlated with the splenic enlargement rather than the activity of the disease[7]. However, leukopenia may occur in absence of splenomegaly and reflect granulomatous infiltration of the bone marrow (Chapter 10, case report). Leukaemoid reaction and polycythaemia are rare. A 55-year-old woman with myeloblastic leukaemoid reaction accompanying sarcoidosis has been described[8].

Eosinophilia

An eosinophil count of 5% or more was found in 34% of patients studied by Mayock et al.[1] The highest incidence (67%) has been reported by McCort et al.[3] and the lowest incidence (10%) occurred in the series of Ferguson and Paris[2]. The mean incidence of eosinophilia is about 24%.

Monocytosis

Monocytosis occurred in about half of the patients reported by Reisner[9]; however, Longcope and Freiman[7] found it in only 10% of their patients who also had leukopenia.

Thrombocytopenia

The association of thrombocytopenia and sarcoidosis has long been recognized. Dickerman, Holbrook and Zinkham[10] reviewed a total of 39 cases of sarcoidosis and thrombocytopenia and divided them into three groups:

1. 10 patients with moderate thrombocytopenia, leukopenia and anaemia, thought to be secondary to a varying degree of portal hypertension.
2. Six patients with moderate to severe thrombocytopenia with moderate chronic bleeding episodes involving the skin, mucous membranes, gingiva and genitourinary tract. These patients had no evidence of portal hypertension.
3. This group of 19 patients presented with acute severe bleeding from many sites including the skin, mucous membranes, genitourinary tract and central nervous system, and severe thrombocytopenia.

There were five deaths, including three patients with central nervous system bleeding. Nine patients who had splenectomy recovered and four of the five patients who received corticosteroids survived.

Since the review by Dickerman et al., there have been seven more cases of severe thrombocytopenia in sarcoidosis[11-13]. Severe thrombocytopenia, while rare in sarcoidosis, may be an initial manifestation or may occur during the course of the disease. Corticosteroids and platelet replacement may produce a therapeutic remission.

What causes thrombocytopenia in sarcoidosis? In many patients thrombocytopenia is associated with an enlarged spleen, but there is some evidence that thrombocytopenia may be an expression of generalized autoimmune reaction. Veien et al. reported elevated serum immunoglobulins, autoantibodies and antibodies to various microorganisms in sarcoidosis patients[14]. Thomas et al.[13], using a direct immunofluorescence technique, demonstrated IgG antibodies on platelets of a patient with sarcoidosis and thrombocytopenia. The platelet antibodies were also present in the serum. This case represents the first serologically proven case of autoimmune thrombocytopenia in sarcoidosis.

Erythrocyte sedimentation rate (ESR)

An elevated ESR was obtained in about two-thirds of the patients with sarcoidosis reviewed by Mayock et al.[1]. Selroos noted an ESR greater than 40 mm.h^{-1} in 25 (18%) out of 140 patients; 19 out of 25 had erythema nodosum[15]. In the Lofgren series of 113 patients with erythema nodosum[16], none had an ESR under 15 mm.h^{-1}. Thus, a high sedimentation rate occurs in acute disease, particularly in association with erythema nodosum. The finding, however, does not carry any diagnostic or prognostic significance.

Urine

Hydroxyproline excretion

Increased breakdown of connective tissue results in increased excretion of hydroxyproline in the urine. Massaro, Handler and Katz[17] found that hydroxyproline excretion is considerably increased in acute sarcoidosis, returning to normal as the chest radiograph clears and the disease becomes inactive. Hydroxyproline excretion is normal in chronic sarcoidosis.

Hypercalciuria

In a study 75 patients with histologically proven sarcoidosis in whom simultaneous estimation of serum and 24-hour urinary calcium levels were carried out, 37 (49%) had hypercalciuria and only 10 (13%) had hypercalcaemia[18]. Lebacq, Verhaegen and Desmet estimated the incidence of hypercalciuria at 62% and renal stones at 13%[19].

Proteinuria

Lebacq et al. have observed significant proteinuria in roughly one-third of their patients and an abnormal urinary sediment in 13%. Haematuria may occur in patients with nephrocalcinosis and nephrolithiasis.

Hypercalcaemia

Incidence

The reported incidence of hypercalcaemia varies from 2 to 63%. The frequency, with a few exceptions, tends to be higher in the North American series. The highest incidence (63%) was reported by McCort et al.[20]. Cummings found calcium levels above 11 mg.$(100 \text{ ml})^{-1}$ (2.75 mmol.ℓ^{-1}) in 35% of his patients[21]. Mayock et al., in their review of 509 patients, recorded a frequency of 17%[22]. Similar results were obtained by Taylor, Lynch and Wynsor in their study of 345 patients with sarcoidosis[23]. Only six of Scadding's 62 patients in London had serum calcium levels of more than 11.0 mg.$(100 \text{ ml})^{-1}$ (2.75 mmol.ℓ^{-1})[24]. Mather reported a still lower prevalence: only four of his 86 untreated patients with sarcoidosis exhibited hypercalcaemia[25]. In Finland, Putkonen, Hannuksela and Halme could find only two patients with hypercalcaemia in a series of 60[26].

What is the cause of such a wide variation in the frequency of hypercalcaemia?

There is no conclusive evidence that race, age, sex, occupation or geographical distribution influence the development of hypercalcaemia. Although hypercalcaemia appears to be a consistent feature, the studies showing excessively high (10-63%) frequency need to be revised. Goldstein et al. in their positive studies with a controlled intake of calcium[27] found that only 2% of their patients had hypercalcaemia. I believe

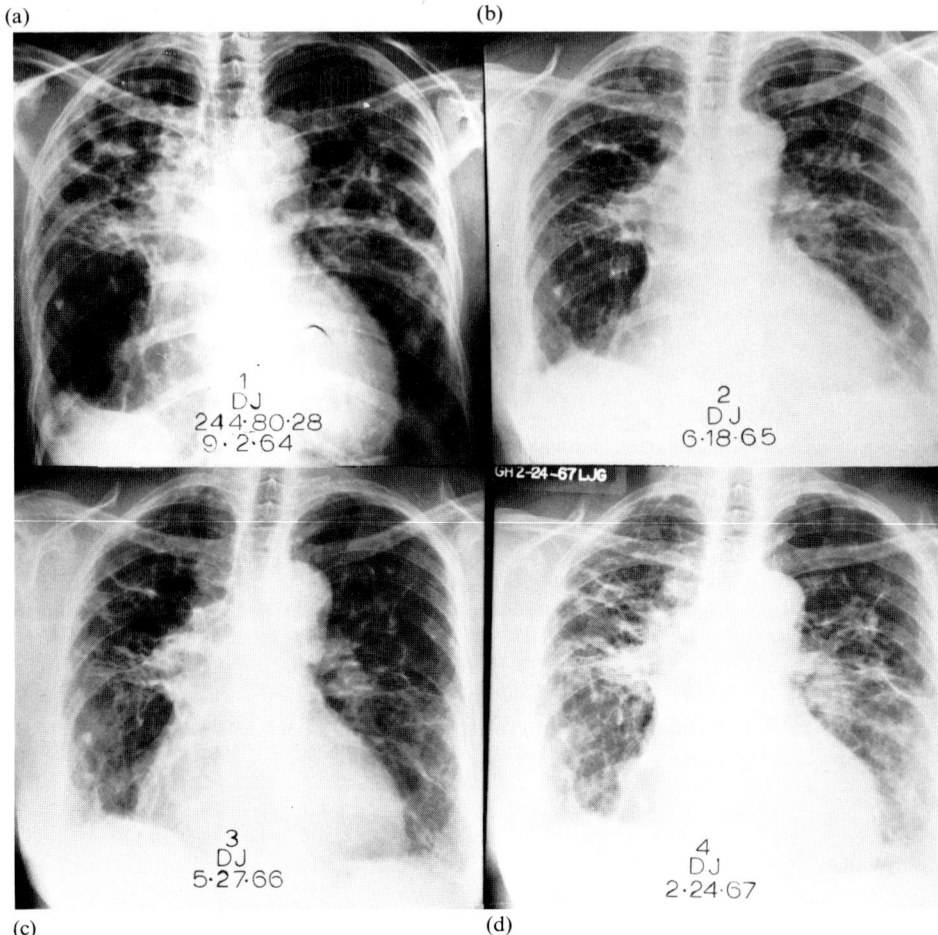

Figure 22.1 (*a–h*) Chest radiographs showing extensive linear reticular infiltrate involving the both lungs. In 1971 the infiltration increased and the patient became more dyspnoeic.

this figure is excessively low and that further studies are needed to establish the frequency of hypercalcaemia. Meanwhile, it seems reasonable to accept the incidence of 11% noted by James *et al*[28] in their world-wide review of 3676 patients with sarcoidosis.

Hypercalcaemia is usually transient in subacute sarcoidosis and may fluctuate in chronic sarcoidosis, depending on the activity of the disease. The following case clearly illustrates that hypercalcaemia may only occur at a certain phase during the long course of chronic sarcoidosis. One is not likely to get a true picture of the calcium abnormality if serum calcium levels are not measured regularly and consistently over a long period of time.

Case report—In 1964, a 49-year-old woman developed dyspnoea and recurrent headaches. She had hypertension for 7 years. Physical examination revealed non-tender hepatosplenomegaly. Laboratory studies showed a reversed serum albumin: globulin ratio. Tuberculin, histoplasmin and coccidioidin skin

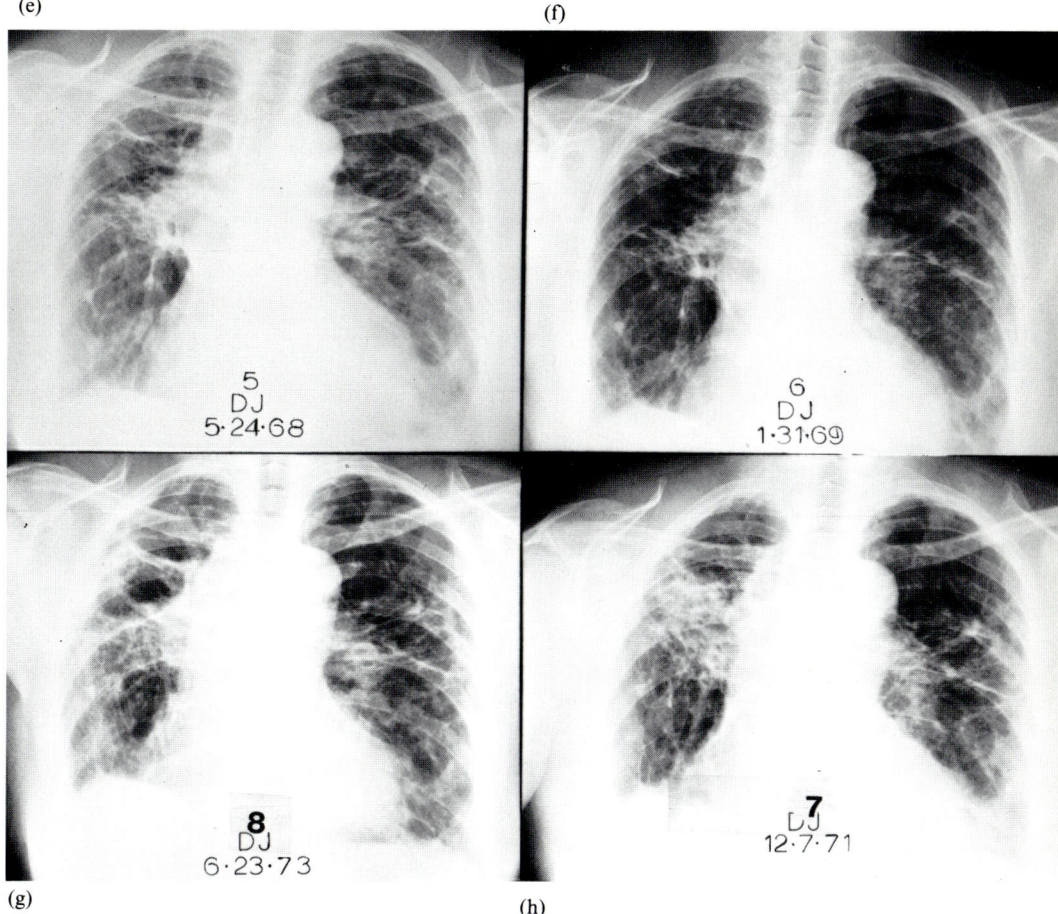

Figure 22.1 (cont.)

tests were negative. The chest radiograph showed fibrocalcific disease in both upper and mid-lung fields (*see Figure 22.1a–d*). A biopsy specimen of the cervical node revealed non-caseating granulomas. The patient was treated with reserpine 0.25 mg twice daily, hydrochlorothiazide 25 mg daily and prednisone 20 mg daily. In 1971, the patient was found to have persistent hypercalcaemia (*see Figure 22.2*). A chest radiograph showed an increase in infiltrate in the right lung field (*see Figures 22.1e–h*). The course was consistent with reactivation of sarcoidosis. No evidence of hyperparathyroidism was found. Prednisone was increased to 40 mg daily. Serum calcium levels eventually returned to normal. Persistently low phosphate values were considered to be due to intrinsic renal disease. Renal biopsy was not performed but an intravenous pyelogram was normal. The patient did well. Serum calcium levels and hypertension remained under control until 1980 when the patient died of a stroke.

Comment—Hypercalcaemia occurred only during one phase of the disease which had lasted more than 16 years.

It has been suggested that hypercalcaemia is more frequent during the summer months when exposure to sun is at its maximum[23]. If this were an important factor then the incidence of hypercalcaemia would be highest in Southern California, the

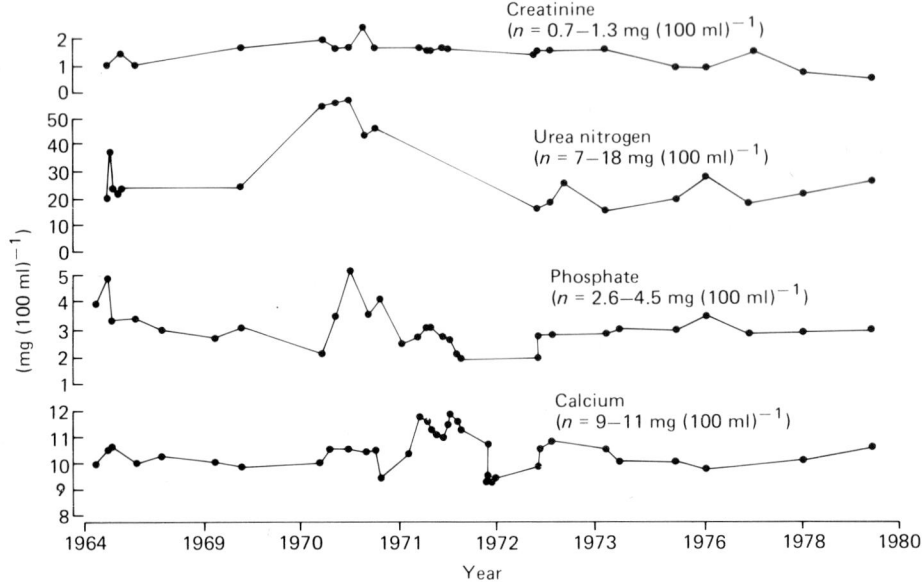

Figure 22.2 Serum calcium, phosphate, urea nitrogen and creatinine levels in a patient with chronic extensive multisystem sarcoidosis. Sixteen-year follow-up shows that hypercalcaemia occurred only during one phase of the disease and would have been easily missed had the serum calcium levels not been so carefully monitored. N = Normal range. *Conversion factors:* serum calcium, 1 mg.(100 ml)$^{-1}$ = 0.25 mmol.ℓ^{-1}; phosphate (inorganic), 1 mg.(100 ml)$^{-1}$ = 0.323 mmol.ℓ^{-1}; urea nitrogen, 1 mg.(100 ml)$^{-1}$ = 0.714 mmol.ℓ^{-1}; creatinine, 1 mg.(100 ml)$^{-1}$ = 88.4 μmol.ℓ^{-1}.

land of sun worshippers. But it is not so! Hypercalcaemia occurs more frequently in sarcoidosis patients in London, Reading (UK), New York and Lisbon[28]. Furthermore, Putkonen et al. found lower values in summer months and slightly higher mean levels in late autumn[26].

What is the cause of hypercalcaemia in sarcoidosis?

Hypercalcaemia occurs in all stages of sarcoidosis. The available evidence indicates that hypercalcaemia is due to increased intestinal absorption. The calcium balance studies of Henneman, Carroll and Dempsey clearly demonstrated the association of hypercalcaemia with increased urinary calcium and decreased faecal calcium excretion. They also observed that hypercalcaemia could not be explained on the basis of an increased release of calcium from bone lesions[29]. Most patients with demonstrable bone lesions have no hypercalcaemia; conversely, increased serum and urine calcium levels occur in young patients without any osseous lesions.

In normal, non-pregnant humans, vitamin D is converted by liver to 25-hydroxy vitamin D which in turn undergoes 1-hydroxylation in the kidney to form 1,25-dihydroxy vitamin D (1-25-(OH)$_2$-D), the most potent metabolite of vitamin D[30, 31]. In sarcoidosis endogenous over-production of 1,25-(OH)$_2$-D is the cause of increased intestinal absorption of calcium[32–34]. Is there an extrarenal site for the manufacture of this active metabolite of vitamin D? The search for an extrarenal site became intense when Barbour et al. reported a patient with sarcoidosis, bilateral nephrectomy and hypercalcaemia[35]. The hypercalcaemia subsided after prednisone therapy. Recently,

Adams, Sharma and Singer[36] demonstrated the production *in vitro* of a (3H) 1,25-$(OH)_2$-D_3 like metabolite of [3H] 25-OH-D_3 by primary cultures of pulmonary alveolar macrophages harvested from patients with active sarcoidosis. Co-elution of the alveolar macrophage-derived metabolite with 1,25-$(OH)_2$-D_3 was obtained on straight-phase high-performance chromatography. Thus, it seems that the alveolar macrophage by metabolizing a sterol hormone precursor 25 OH-D_3 to its active metabolite provides an important extrarenal synthetic site for serum assayable 1,25-$(OH)_2$-D_3 in sarcoidosis. It is probable that the hypercalcaemia in a few reported cases of tuberculosis and berylliosis may also be due to 1,25-$(OH)_2$-D_3 production by active macrophages[37]. Corticosteroids inhibit the peripheral action of 1-25-$(OH)_2$-D and metabolize the compound to an inactive metabolite[12].

What is the role of parathyroids in hypercalcaemia of sarcoidosis?

Roos suggested that increased parathyroid function was responsible for the calcium abnormality[38]. However, normal parathyroids have been found in patients with sarcoidosis and hypercalcaemia. Furthermore, the finding of normal or low parathyroid hormone concentration in serum of these patients indicates the existence of functional hypoparathyroidism in this disease[39].

Primary hyperparathyroidism in association with sarcoidosis has occurred in at least two dozen cases. This coexistence is probably incidental[40].

Serum phosphate

Much less attention has been paid to serum phosphate levels in sarcoidosis. Longcope and Freiman found levels ranging from 2.4 to 4.8 mg.(100 ml)$^{-1}$ (0.78–1.55 mmol.ℓ^{-1}). Putkonen found significantly low serum phosphate levels in eight of his 57 patients; the abnormality was more marked in patients with chronic disease. Twelve of 53 patients investigated by Selroos had phosphate levels under 2.8 mg.(100 ml)$^{-1}$ (0.9 mmol.ℓ^{-1}); six of the twelve patients had stage I disease, four had stage II disease, and the disease was far advanced in two patients. Renal functions were normal in all the patients[41].

Angiotensin converting enzyme

Angiotensin converting enzyme (ACE) catalyses the conversion of angiotensin I to vasoactive angiotensin II and inactivates bradykinin. Although the site of production of ACE in normal individuals is not known, the enzyme is primarily located in endothelial cells of pulmonary capillaries and epithelial cells of proximal renal tubules. It is also present in small amounts in alveolar macrophages. However, alveolar macrophages from smokers synthesize more ACE than those of non-smokers[42].

Increased serum ACE activity in sarcoidosis was first reported by Lieberman[43]. He reported that 83% of patients with active sarcoidosis had abnormally high levels of ACE. Although this observation has been confirmed by others, the reported incidence varies in different centres. Fanburg *et al.*[44] found elevated ACE levels in 27 (48%) out of 56 patients; Abboy, Kanada and Sharma[45] in 48 (54%) out of 89 patients; Silverstein, Friedland and Lyons[46] in 20 (34%) out of 58 patients; Gronhagen-Riska[47] in 34 (60%) out of 57 patients; Khoury *et al.*[48] in 20 (77%) out of 26 patients; Schultz, Miller and Bedrossian[49] in 19 (80%) out of 22 patients; and Lieberman, Nossal and Sclessner in (58%) out of 391 patients with biopsy-proven sarcoidosis[50]. The reason for such differences in sensitivity is not clear.

In a large international study involving 12 centres and 1941 patients, raised ACE activity was present in 1109 (57%) of 1941 patients[51]. Thus, it seems that serum ACE level is raised in about 60% of sarcoidosis patients; the ACE activity is higher in patients with hilar adenopathy and pulmonary infiltration (stage II) than in those with either hilar adenopathy (stage I) or pulmonary infiltrate (stage III)[52]. The test is also positive in patients with extrathoracic sarcoidosis. ACE activity reflects the granuloma load in the body.

Source of ACE in sarcoidosis

The current evidence suggests that ACE is derived from the epithelioid cells of the granulomas in sarcoidosis. ACE was observed to be localized on the cell membrane, particularly on microvillus and pseudopod-like projections of sarcoid epithelioid cells. T lymphocytes modulate ACE synthesis in monotype culture and may do so in a sarcoid granuloma[53].

ACE in diseases other than sarcoidosis

The international experience of 12 centres in six different countries shows that serum angiotensin converting enzyme is elevated in 10% of patients with other granulomatous diseases (*see Table 22.1.*)[51].

TABLE 22.1. Conditions associated with elevated serum angiotensin converting enzyme (ACE) level

Likely to be confused with sarcoidosis	*Unlikely to be confused with sarcoidosis*
Asbestosis[54]	Coccidioidomycosis[59]
Berylliosis[55]	Diabetes mellitus[61]
Granulomatous hepatitis[56]	Gaucher's disease[60]
Hypersensitivity pneumonitis[45, 57]	Idiopathic respiratory disease syndrome[62]
Lymphoma[44]	Inflammatory bowel disease[56]
Miliary tuberculosis[58]	Pulmonary neoplasm[45]
Primary biliary cirrhosis[56]	Leprosy[59]
Silicosis[54]	Liver cirrhosis[63]

ACE and activity of sarcoidosis

The diagnostic value of ACE is limited because the test has a false-negative incidence of 40% and a false-positive incidence of 10%[52]. ACE is most useful in monitoring the clinical course of the disease[52, 64, 65]. Resolution of the active disease or clinical control of sarcoidosis by adequate corticosteroid therapy brings serum ACE level down to the normal range (*see Figure 22.3*). ACE levels occasionally antedate the clinical radiographic and physiological alterations of sarcoidosis. The test is also helpful during pregnancy when repeated radiographs of the chest may not be taken.

Conclusion

Although the importance of ACE as the specific test for the diagnosis of sarcoidosis is limited, it is useful in monitoring the course of the disease.

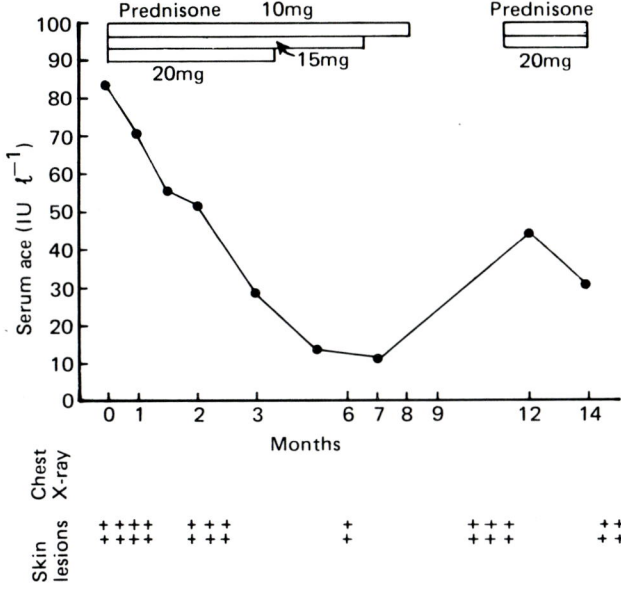

Figure 22.3 Serum angiotensin (ACE) levels in this patient reflect the activity of sarcoidosis and effect of prednisone therapy.

Serum lysozyme

Siltzbach *et al.* observed that serum lysozyme (SLZ) levels above two standard deviation were present in 39 (53%) out of 73 patients with sarcoidosis[66]. SLZ levels were elevated in only 37% of the patients studied by Selroos and Klockars[67]. Simultaneous measurement of serum lysozyme and serum angiotensin converting enzyme might be useful in some patients with active sarcoidosis[68]. The diagnostic value of serum lysozyme determination in sarcoidosis is uncertain. A moderate increase is a non-specific finding and occurs in about 20% of patients with other chest diseases including tuberculosis and silicosis, and a normal value does not exclude sarcoidosis[69, 70].

Transcobalamin II

Measurement of serum unsaturated vitamin B_{12} binding capacity (VBBC) has been proposed to be of value in the diagnosis of sarcoidosis, particularly when combined with ACE and SLZ estimations. In a study of 50 consecutive patients with sarcoidosis, 26 (54%) showed VBBC levels above the normal[71]. Fractionation of VBBC into R binders and transcobalamin (TC) II revealed that elevations of unsaturated B_{12}-binding capacity were attributable primarily to elevations in circulating TC II. However, TC II levels are also elevated in Gaucher's disease, lymphoproliferative disorders, myeloma, Waldenström's macroglobulinaemia and liver disease. The test is of no value in the diagnosis of sarcoidosis.

References

1. MAYOCK, R.L., BERTRAND, P., MORRISON, C.E., et al. (1963) Manifestations of sarcoidosis. Analysis of 145 patients with a review of nine series selected from the literature. *Am. J. Med.*, **35**, 67.
2. FERGUSON, R.H. and PARIS, J. (1958) Sarcoidosis: A study of 29 cases with a review of splenic, hepatic, mucous membrane, retinal and joint manifestations. *Arch. Intern. Med.*, **101**, 1065.
3. MCCORT, J.J., WOOD, R.H., HAMILTON, J.B., et al. (1947) Sarcoidosis: A clinical and roentgenologic study of twenty-eight proved cases. *Arch. Intern. Med.*, **80**, 293.
4. LIEBLING, M.F., BELL, N.H. and STENGLE, J.M. (1961) Studies of the production volume and destruction of erythrocytes in patients with sarcoidosis. *Am. Rev. Resp. Dis.*, **84**, 32.
5. SORDILLO, P.P. and BRIGGS, D.K. (1982) Hemolytic anemia in a patient with sarcoidosis. *N.Y. State J. Med.*, March, 362.
6. ISRAEL, H.L. (1973) Present status of the laboratory diagnosis of sarcoidosis. *Ann. Clin. Lab. Sci.*, **3**, 73.
7. LONGCOPE, WT. and FRIEMAN, D.G. (1952) A study of sarcoidosis. *Medicine*, **31**, 1.
8. BORDELON, J., STONE, M.J. and FRENKEL, E. (1977) Probable myeloblastic reaction with disseminated sarcoidosis. *S. Med. J.*, **70**, 1378.
9. REISNER, D. (1944) Boeck's sarcoid and systemic sarcoidosis: A study of thirty-five cases. *Am. Rev. Tuberc.*, **49**, 289.
10. DICKERMAN, J.D., HOLBROOK, P.R. and ZINKHAM, W.H. (1972) Etiology and therapy of thrombocytopenia associated with sarcoidosis. *J. Pediatr.*, **81**, 758.
11. KNODEL, A.R. and BEEKMAN, J. (1980) Severe thrombocytopenia and sarcoidosis. *J. Am. Med. Assoc.*, **243**, 258.
12. WEILBERG, A.B. and PASSERO, M.A. (1981) Thrombocytopenia and pulmonary hemorrhage in sarcoidosis. *S. Med. J.*, **74**, 254.
13. THOMAS, L.L.M., ALBERTS, C., PEGELS, J.G., et al. (1982) Sarcoidosis associated with autoimmune thrombocytopenia and selective IgA deficiency. *Scand. J. Haematol.*, **28**, 357.
14. VEIEN, M.K., HART, F., BENDIXEN, G., et al. (1976) Immunological studies in sarcoidosis: A comparison of disease activity in various immunological parameters. *Ann. N.Y. Acad. Sci.*, **278**, 47.
15. SELROOS, O. (1969) The frequency, clinical picture and prognosis of pulmonary sarcoidosis in Finland. *Acta Med. Scand.*, **186** (Suppl. **503**) 1.
16. LOFGREN, S. (1953) Primary pulmonary sarcoidosis. *Acta Med. Scand.*, **145**, 424.
17. MASSARO, D., HANDLER, A.E. and KATZ, S. (1966) Excretion of hydroxyproline in patients with sarcoidosis. *Am. Rev. Resp. Dis.*, **93**, 929.
18. SHARMA, O.P., TROWELL, J., COHEN, M., et al. (1967) Abnormal calcium metabolism in sarcoidosis. In *La Sarcoidose* (eds Turiaf, J. and Chabot, J.), p. 627. (Paris: Masson)
19. LEBACQ, E., VERHAEGEN, H. and DESMET, V. (1970) Renal involvement in sarcoidosis. *Postgrad. Med. J.*, **46**, 526.
20. MCCORT, J.J., WOOD, R.H., HAMILTON, J.B., et al. (1947) Sarcoidosis: A clinical and roentgenologic study of twenty-eight proved cases. *Arch. Intern. Med.*, **80**, 293.
21. CUMMINGS, M.M., Jr. (1959) Epidemiologic and clinical observations in sarcoidosis. *Ann. Intern. Med.*, **50**, 879.
22. MAYOCK, R.L., BERTRAND, P., MORRISON, C.E., et al. (1963) Manifestations of sarcoidosis: Analysis of 145 patients with a review of nine series selected from the literature. *Am. J. Med.*, **35**, 67.
23. TAYLOR, R.L., LYNCH, H.J. and WYNSOR, W.G., Jr. (1963) Seasonal influence of sunlight on hypercalcaemia of sarcoidosis. *Am. J. Med.*, **34**, 221.
24. SCADDING, J.G. (1967) *Sarcoidosis*. (London: Eyre and Spottiswoode)
25. MATHER, G. (1957) Calcium metabolism and bone changes in sarcoidosis. *Br. Med. J.*, **i**, 248.
26. PUTKONEN, T., HANNUKSELA, N. and HALME, H. (1965) Calcium and phosphorus metabolism in sarcoidosis. *Acta Med. Scand.*, **177**, 327.
27. GOLDSTEIN, R.A., ISRAEL, H.L., BECKER, K.L., et al. (1971) The infrequency of hypercalcemia in sarcoidosis. *Am. J. Med.*, **51**, 21.
28. JAMES, D.G., NEVILLE, E., SILTZBACH, L.E., et al. (1976) A worldwide review of sarcoidosis. *Ann. N.Y. Acad. Sci.*, **278**, 321.
29. HENNEMAN, P.H., CAROLL, F.L. and DEMPSEY, F.F. (1954) The mechanism responsible for hypercalciuria in sarcoidosis. *J. Clin. Invest.*, **33**, 941.
30. STERN, P.H., DEOLAZABAL, J. and BELL, N.H. (1980) Evidence for abnormal regulation of circulating 1-25-dihydroxyvitamin D in patients with sarcoidosis and normal calcium metabolism. *J. Clin. Invest.*, **66**, 852.
31. DELUCA, H.F. (1979) Vitamin D metabolism and function. *Arch. Intern. Med.*, **90**, 324.
32. PAPAPOULOS, S.E., CLEMENS, T.L., FRAHER, L.J., et al. (1979) 1,25-dihydroxycholecalciferol in the pathogenesis of the hypercalcemia of sarcoidosis. *Lancet*, **i**, 627.

33. KOIDE, Y., KUGAI, N., KIMURA, S., et al. (1981) Increased 1,25-dihydroxycholecalciferol as a cause of abnormal calcium metabolism in sarcoidosis. *J. Clin. Endocrinol. Metab.*, **52**, 494.
34. CHESNEY, R.W., HAMSTRA, A.J., DELUCA, H.F., et al. (1981) Elevated serum 1,25-dihydroxyvitamin D concentrations in the hypercalcemia of sarcoidosis: Correction by glucocorticoid therapy. *J. Pediatr.*, **98**, 919.
35. BARBOUR, G.L., COBURN, J.W., NORMANS, A.W., et al. (1981) Nonrenal hypercalcemia in sarcoidosis. *N. Engl. J. Med.*, **305**, 440.
36. ADAMS, J., SHARMA, O.P. and SINGER, F. (1983) Metabolism of 25-hydroxyvitamin D_3 by alveolar macrophages in sarcoidosis. *Clin. Res.*, **31**, 499A.
37. ABBASI, A.A., CHEMPLAVIL, J.K., FARAH, S., et al. (1979) Hypercalcemia in active pulmonary tuberculosis. *Ann. Intern. Med.*, **90**, 324.
38. RUDBERG-ROOS, I. (1962) Course and prognosis of sarcoidosis as observed in 296 cases. *Acta Tuberc. Scand.*, **41** (Suppl. 52), 1.
39. CUSHARD, W.G., SIMON, A.B. and CANTERBURY, J.M. (1972) Parathyroid function in sarcoidosis. *N. Engl. J. Med.*, **286**, 395.
40. LEBACQ, E.G., HENRION, I., MAYEUR, S., et al. (1980) Hypercalciuria in sarcoidosis with normocalcemia: pathogenesis and treatment. In *Proceedings of the Eighth International Conference on Sarcoidosis* (eds Williams, W.J. and Davies, B.H.), p. 215. (Cardiff: Alpha Omega)
41. SELROOS, O. (1969) The frequency, clinical picture and prognosis of pulmonary sarcoidosis in Finland. *Acta Med. Scand.*, **186** (Suppl. 503), 1.
42. HINMAN, L.M., STEVENS, C., MATTHAY, R. and GEE, J.B.L. (1979) Angiotensin convertase activities in human alveolar macrophages: effects of cigarette smoking and sarcoidosis. *Science*, **205**, 202.
43. LIEBERMAN, J. (1975) Elevation of serum angiotensin converting enzyme level in sarcoidosis. *Am. J. Med.*, **59**, 356.
44. FANBURG, B.L., SCHOENBERGER, M.D., BACHUS, B., et al. (1976) Elevated serum angiotensin-1 converting enzyme in sarcoidosis. *Am. Rev. Resp. Dis.*, **114**, 524.
45. ABBOY, R., KANADA, D. and SHARMA, O.P. (1980) Serum angiotensin converting enzyme in sarcoidosis. In *Sarcoidosis and Other Granulomatous Diseases* (eds Williams, W.J. and Davies, B.H.), p. 273. (Cardiff: Alpha Omega Publications)
46. SILVERSTEIN, E., FRIEDLAND, J. and LYONS, H.A. (1976) Elevation of angiotensin converting enzyme in granulomatous lymph nodes and serum in sarcoidosis: Clinical and possible pathogenic significance. *Ann. N.Y. Acad. Sci.*, **278**, 498.
47. GRONHAGEN-RISKA, C. (1979) Angiotensin converting enzyme. *Scand. J. Resp. Dis.*, **60**, 83.
48. KHOURY, F., TEASDALE, P.R., SMITH, L., et al. (1979) Angiotensin converting enzyme in sarcoidosis: A British study. *Br. J. Dis. Chest*, **73**, 382.
49. SCHALTZ, T., MILLER, W.C. and BEDROSSIAN, C.W.M. (1979) Clinical application of measurement of angiotensin converting enzyme level. *J. Am. Med. Assoc.*, **242**, 439.
50. LIEBERMAN, J., NOSSAL, A. and SCLESSNER, L.A. (1979) Serum angiotensin converting enzyme for diagnosis and therapeutic evaluation of sarcoidosis. *Am. Rev. Resp. Dis.*, **120**, 329.
51. STUDDY, P.R. and JAMES, D.G. (1981) The specificity and sensitivity of serum angiotensin converting enzyme in sarcoidosis and other diseases: Experience in twelve centres in six different countries. In *Sarcoidosis* (eds Chretien, J., Marsac, J. and Saltiei, J.C.), p. 32. (New York: Pergamon Press)
52. DEREMEE, R.A. and ROHRBACH, M.S. (1980) Serum angiotensin converting enzyme activity in evaluating the clinical course of sarcoidosis. *Ann. Intern. Med.*, **92**, 361.
53. SILVERSTEIN, E., FRIEDLAND, J. and STANEK, A.E., Jr (1981) Pathogenesis of sarcoidosis. Mechanism of angiotensin converting enzyme elevation: T-lymphocyte modulation of enzyme induction in mononuclear phagocytes: Enzyme properties. In *Sarcoidosis* (eds Chretien, J., Marsac, J. and Saltiel, J.C.), p. 319. (New York: Pergamon Press)
54. GRONHAGEN-RISKA, C., SELROOS, O., FROSETH, B., et al. (1980) Increased serum angiotensin converting enzyme (ACE) in sarcoidosis, silicosis and asbestosis. In *Sarcoidosis and Other Granulomatous Diseases* (eds Williams, W.J. and Davies, B.H.), p. 266. (Cardiff: Alpha Omega Publications)
55. SPRINCE, N.L., KAZEMI, H. and FANBURG, B.L. (1980) Serum angiotensin-1 converting enzyme in chronic beryllium disease. In *Sarcoidosis and Other Granulomatous Diseases* (eds Williams, W.J. and Davies, B.H.), p. 287. (Cardiff: Alpha Omega Publications)
56. STUDDY, P., BIRD, R., JAMES, D.G., et al. (1978) Serum angiotensin converting enzyme (ACE) in sarcoidosis and other granulomatous disorder. *Lancet*, **ii**, 1332.
57. HARA, A., SAWADA, H. FUKUYAMA, K., et al. (1981) Tissue angiotensin converting enzyme (ACE) in sarcoid and hypersensitivity granulomas. In *Sarcoidosis* (eds Chretien, J., Marsac, J. and Saltiel, J.C.), p. 351. (New York: Pergamon Press)
58. THOMAS, A.V., ANSARI, A., KHURANA, M., et al. (1979) Elevated serum angiotensin converting enzyme in miliary tuberculosis (Abstract). *Am. Rev. Respir. Dis.*, **119**, 86.

59. LIEBERMAN, J. and REA, T. (1977) Serum angiotensin converting enzyme in leprosy and coccidioidomycosis. *Ann. Intern. Med.*, **87**, 422.
60. LIEBERMAN, J. and BEUTLER, E. (1976) Elevation of serum angiotensin converting enzyme in Gaucher's disease. *N. Engl. J. Med.*, **294**, 442.
61. LIEBERMAN, J. and SASTRE, A. (1980) Serum angiotensin converting enzyme: Elevations in diabetes mellitus. *Ann. Intern. Med.*, **93**, 825.
62. MATTIOLLI, A., ZAKHEIM, R.M., MULLIS, K., *et al.* (1975) Angiotensin-1 converting enzyme activity in idiopathic respiratory distress syndrome of the newborn infant and in experimental alveolar hypoxia in mice. *J. Pediatr.*, **87**, 97.
63. SCHWEISFURTH, H. and WERNZE, H. (1979) Changes of serum angiotensin-1 converting enzyme in patients with viral hepatitis and liver cirrhosis. *Acta Hepato-gastroenterol.* **26**, 207.
64. JAMES, D.G. (1981) Conclusion: Angiotensin converting enzyme. In *Sarcoidosis* (eds Chretien, J., Marsac, J. and Saltiel, J.C.), p. 362. (Paris: Pergamon Press)
65. UEDA, E., KAWABE, T., TACHIBANA, T., *et al.* (1980) Serum angiotensin converting enzyme activity as an indicator of prognosis in sarcoidosis. *Am. Rev. Resp. Dis.*, **121**, 667.
66. SILTZBACH, L.E., KRAKOFF, L., DORPH, D., *et al.* (1980) Elevated levels of serum angiotensin converting enzyme and lysozyme levels in sarcoidosis. In *Sarcoidosis and Other Granulomatous Diseases* (eds Williams, W.J. and Davies, B.H.), p. 298. (Cardiff: Alpha Omega Publishing)
67. SELROOS, O. and KLOCKARS, M. (1977) Serum lysozyme in sarcoidosis: Evaluation of its usefulness in determination of disease activity. *Scand. J. Resp. Dis.*, **58**, 110.
68. CUMMISKEY, J.M., MELINN, M. and MCLAUGHLIN, H. (1978) Lysozyme levels in sarcoidosis. *Irish J. Med. Sci.*, **147**, 108.
69. PERILLE, P.E., KHAN, K. and FINCH, S.C. (1973) Serum lysozyme in pulmonary tuberculosis. *Am. J. Med. Sci.*, **265**, 297.
70. PASCUAL, R.S., GEE, J.B.L. and FINCH, S.C. (1973) Usefulness of serum lysozyme measurement in diagnosis and evaluation of sarcoidosis. *N. Engl. J. Med.*, **289**, 1074.
71. GILBERT, H.S. and SILTZBACH, L.E. (1980) Increased levels of circulating transcobalamin II in sarcoidosis. In *Sarcoidosis and Other Granulomatous Diseases* (eds Williams, W.J. and Davies, B.H.), p. 485. (Cardiff: Alpha Omega Publications)

Chapter 23

Gallium-67 scanning in sarcoidosis

Gallium-67 citrate

Gallium-67 is a cyclotron-produced radionuclide with a half-life of 78 hours. After an intravenous injection most of the isotope is bound to serum proteins except the remaining 10–20% which is excreted unchanged by the kidneys and gastrointestinal tract.

The technique

Gallium-67 scans are performed with crystal rectilinear scanners 47–72 hours after an injection of 50 mCi. kg^{-1}[^{67}Ga] citrate. In normal individuals rectilinear scans show some ^{67}Ga activity in the liver, spleen, spine, ribs and pelvis[1]. The lung scans may be classified as negative when the pulmonary concentration does not exceed the specific body background (*see Figure 23.1*). However, many observers use an index called the ^{67}Ga index to provide a semi-quantitative estimate of the degree of ^{67}Ga concentration in the lung. It is calculated by multiplying the estimated uptake area of the lung by the uptake intensity (graded 0–4) of that area, and by adding these products to obtain the total index value[2]. The highest possible ^{67}Ga index is 400 units; normal individuals show indices of 50 units or less. If the lung parenchyma has a ^{67}Ga index of more than 50 units, it is considered positive.

Gallium-67 uptake in various lung diseases

The high affinity of ^{67}Ga for carcinoma and metabolically active lesions is well recognized. The inflammatory lesions with cellular proliferation and increased protein synthesis show high concentration of ^{67}Ga. In contrast, ^{67}Ga lung scans on patients with chronic interstitial fibrosis and healed fibrotic tuberculosis show no uptake of gallium. This accumulation of gallium is non-specific for it is observed in a variety of clinical disorders[3,4]:

1. *Infections*—Bacterial pneumonias, lung abscess, tuberculosis, aspergillosis, blastomycosis, *Pneumocystis carinii*, cytomegalovirus, filariasis.

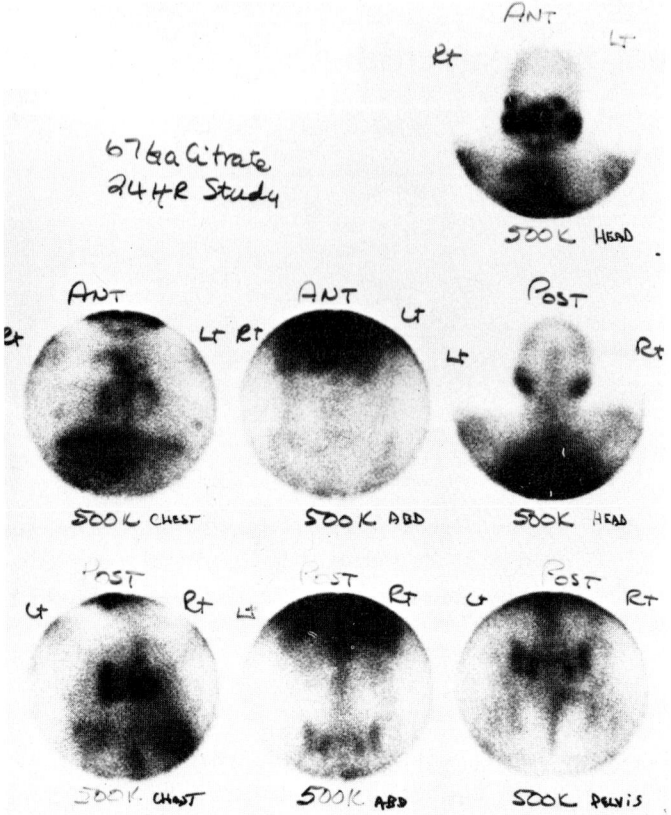

Figure 23.1 Gallium-67 body scan in a patient with acute sarcoidosis. Increased activity is noted in hilar areas and parotid and lacrimal glands. Normal intake is present in the liver and vertebral column. Gallium uptake by the lung parenchyma is negligible.

2. *Pneumoconiosis*—Asbestosis, coal worker's pneumoconiosis, silicosis.
3. *Immunological disorders*—Systemic lupus erythematosus, Wegener's granulomatosis, extrinsic allergic alveolitis, lymphocytic interstitial pneumonitis.
4. *Drug reactions*—Bleomycin toxicity, cyclophosphamide toxicity, radiation pneumonitis.
5. *Unknown aetiology*—Idiopathic pulmonary fibrosis, histiocytosis-X, sarcoidosis.
6. *Neoplasms*—Lung cancer (primary, secondary), lymphoma.

The test is of little value in establishing the specific diagnosis of a focal or generalized lung disease.

Gallium-67 uptake in sarcoidosis

Current views of the immunopathogenesis of pulmonary sarcoidosis suggest that the granuloma formation is preceded by a mononuclear cell alveolitis consisting of mononuclear phagocytes and T lymphocytes[5]. In order to study whether ^{67}Ga would be useful in staging the alveolitis of sarcoidosis, Line et al.[4] studied 41 patients with sarcoidosis. Two-thirds of the patients demonstrated significant pulmonary uptake (750 ^{67}Ga index units); 45% of patients showed index values of 100 units or more; 13% showed values of 200 units or more (see Figure 23.2). The authors also reported a strong correlation of ^{67}Ga index and the number of lymphocytes and T lymphocytes recovered from the lungs by bronchoalveolar lavage[2]. The data suggest that ^{67}Ga

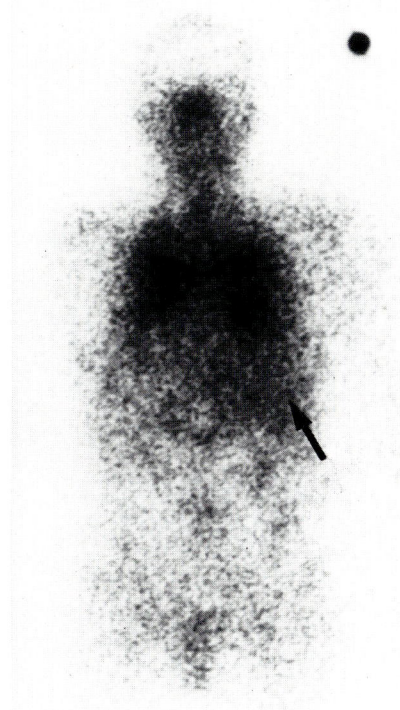

Figure 23.2 Gallium-67 scan showing high-intensity activity (alveolitis) in a patient with stage III disease (posterior view). Arrow indicates normal background activity in the liver.

accumulates in the immune effector cells, T lymphocytes and the mononuclear phagocytes and that the uptake reflects the intensity of sarcoid alveolitis. In addition to the ^{67}Ga accumulation in the lung, more than two-thirds of the patients with sarcoidosis show abnormal uptake by extrapulmonary tissues, including the parotid glands, lacrimal glands, spleen, peripheral lymph nodes, and the bone marrow[6].

Indications of gallium-67 scans in sarcoidosis

To establish the diagnosis of sarcoidosis

Gallium-67 uptake is not specific for sarcoidosis and does *not* establish the diagnosis of sarcoidosis. Nosal et al. suggested that the diagnostic sensitivity of gallium-67 scanning can be improved if it is combined with an elevated serum angiotensin converting enzyme activity. This is not so. We now know that serum angiotensin converting enzyme, like gallium-67 scanning, can be high in many clinical disorders unrelated to sarcoidosis (*see Table 22.1*). Two non-specific tests do not make one specific diagnosis!

To determine the degree of activity of sarcoid alveolitis

Based on ^{67}Ga scans and bronchoalveolar lavage studies, sarcoid alveolitis can be divided into 'high-intensity alveolitis' and 'low-intensity alveolitis'. In high-intensity alveolitis, the ^{67}Ga index is greater than 50 units, whereas in low-intensity alveolitis the index is either normal or less than 50 units[8].

To make therapy decisions, monitor treatment response and guide treatment dosage and duration

Untreated patients with 'high-intensity alveolitis' tend to show deterioration in about two-thirds of the patients; whereas 'low-intensity alveolitis' patients tend to remain stable. It is now apparent that the traditional monitors of the disease activity, e.g. symptoms, chest radiographs and lung function tests are not sensitive to activity of the disease and its response to corticosteroids[8, 9]. In such cases, ^{67}Ga scans are very useful in initiating and monitoring the response of corticosteroid therapy.

To assess the extent of pulmonary as well as extrapulmonary sarcoidosis

Not only is the ^{67}Ga scanning a more sensitive indicator of sarcoid alveolitis but it also increases our diagnostic sensitivity for such extrapulmonary lesions as parotid glands, inguinal and mesenteric adenitis and bone-marrow involvement[1, 6].

References

1. SIEMSEN, J.K., GREBE, S.F., SARGENT, E.N., *et al.* (1976) Gallium-67 scintigraphy of pulmonary diseases as a complement to radiography. *Radiology*, **118**, 371.
2. LINE, B.R., KEOGH, G.W., JONES, A.E., *et al.* (1981) Gallium-67 scanning to stage the alveolitis of sarcoidosis: Correlation with clinical studies, pulmonary function studies, and bronchoalveolar lavage. *Am. Rev. Resp. Dis.*, **123**, 440.
3. CRYSTAL, R.G., GADEK, J.K., FERRANS, V.J., *et al.* (1981) Interstitial lung disease: Current concepts of pathogenesis, staging and therapy. *Am. J. Med.*, **70**, 542.
4. LINE, B.R., HUNNINGHAKE, G.W., KEOGH, B.A., *et al.* (1983) Gallium-67 scanning as an indicator of the activity of sarcoidosis. In *Sarcoidosis and Other Granulomatous Diseases of the Lung* (ed. Fanburg, B.L.), p. 287. (New York: Marcel Dekker)
5. CRYSTAL, R., ROBERTS, W.C., HUNNINGHAKE, G.W., *et al.* (1980) Pulmonary sarcoidosis: A disease characterized and perpetuated by activated lung T lymphocytes. *Ann. Intern. Med.*, **94**, 73.
6. MISHKIN, F.S., TAKANA, T.T. and NIDEN, N.H. (1978) Abnormal gallium scan patterns of the salivary gland in pulmonary sarcoidosis. *Ann. Intern. Med.*, **89**, 933.
7. NOSAL, A., SCHLEISSNER, L.A., MISHKIN, F.S., *et al.* (1979) Angiotensin-I converting enzyme and gallium scan in noninvasive evaluation of sarcoidosis. *Ann. Intern. Med.* **90**, 328.
8. KEOGH, B.A., HUNNINGHAKE, G., LINE, B.R., *et al.* (1981) Alveolitis parameters as predicators of the natural history of pulmonary sarcoidosis. *Clin. Res.*, **49**, 447A.
9. KEOGH, B.A. and CRYSTAL, R.G. (1980) Pulmonary function testing in interstitial pulmonary disease: What does it tell us? *Chest*, **78**, 856.

Chapter 24
Diagnosis and biopsy procedures

Criteria for diagnosis

The criteria for establishing the diagnosis of sarcoidosis include: (1) a compatible clinical or radiological picture; (2) histological evidence of non-caseating granulomas; and (3) negative bacterial and fungal studies of biopsied tissue, sputum and other appropriate body fluids. If all three steps are not carried out the diagnosis of sarcoidosis remains in doubt since clinical or radiological features present too wide a differential diagnosis and histological evidence of non-caseating granulomas may be produced by many bacteria, viruses, fungi, chemicals and organic dust particles[1].

Strict adherence, however, to this three-step diagnostic work-up presents two major practical problems. First, the patient, particularly when asymptomatic, may not be willing to have any invasive procedure carried out. Secondly, biopsy procedures, depending on the site and technique used, carry definite, albeit small, risks of morbidity and even mortality. For many years, in such situations, chest physicians have looked on the Kveim-Siltzbach test as a specific and reliable diagnositic test. However, since the Kveim-Siltzbach antigen is not available commercially, the test, unfortunately, is of no use to practising physicians (see Chapter 21).

Although recently developed tests—including serum angiotensin converting enzyme, lysozyme and transcobalamin-II levels, gallium-67 lung scans and bronchoalveolar lavage lymphocyte count—have provided us with a better understanding of biochemical and immunological activity of sarcoidosis, they are of little help in establishing the specific diagnosis of sarcoidosis. These tests provide diagnostic help in those cases of sarcoidosis where there is a clear epidemiological, clinical and radiological evidence of the disease. Further studies are needed to confirm the usefulness and limits of these procedures in securing the diagnosis of the disease. Meanwhile, the definitive diagnosis of sarcoidosis still requires the demonstration of non-caseating granulomas in the involved tissue or tissues.

Biopsy procedures

Lung biopsy

For many years scalene-node biopsy, mediastinoscopy and thoractomy were the procedures commonly used to establish the diagnosis of pulmonary sarcoidosis.

However, the invention of the fibreoptic bronchoscope has relegated these techniques to the back seat[2]. Now, the transbronchial biopsy through a fibreoptic bronchoscope is the procedure of choice for obtaining tissue diagnosis in patients suspected of having pulmonary sarcoidosis regardless of the stage of the disease.

Table 24.1 combines the data reviewed by Whitcomb *et al.*, Teirstein from the Mount Sinai Hospital in New York, and our own data obtained at the Los Angeles County General Hospital in Los Angeles[3, 4]. About two-thirds to three-quarters of the patient with stage I disease had a positive transbronchial lung biopsy result. This is not surprising because parenchymal disease is present in almost all patients with sarcoidosis, particularly in stage I disease as demonstrated by Rosen and his col-

TABLE 24.1. Results of transbronchial lung biopsy in sarcoidosis

Chest X-ray stage*	Whitcomb et al.[3]			Teirstein[4]			Sharma†		
	Total	No. (%) biopsy	positive	Total	No. (%) biopsy	positive	Total	No. (%) biopsy	positive
0	2	2	(100)	—	—	—	2	1	(50)
I	39	27	(69)	21	13	(62)	19	14	(75)
II	40	32	(80)	36	31	(86)	37	34	(88)
III	29	24	(83)	54	48	(82)	21	17	(80)
IV	—	—	—	—	—	—	4	2	(50)
Total	110	85	(77)	114	91	(81)	83	68	(82)

* Chest X-ray stages: 0, normal; I, bilateral hilar lymphadenopathy; II, bilateral hilar lymphadenopathy and pulmonary infiltration; III, pulmonary infiltration and fibrosis; IV, advanced fibrosis and bullae formation.
† Unpublished observations from The Los Angeles County/University of Southern California Medical Center, Los Angeles, July 1975 to July 1982.

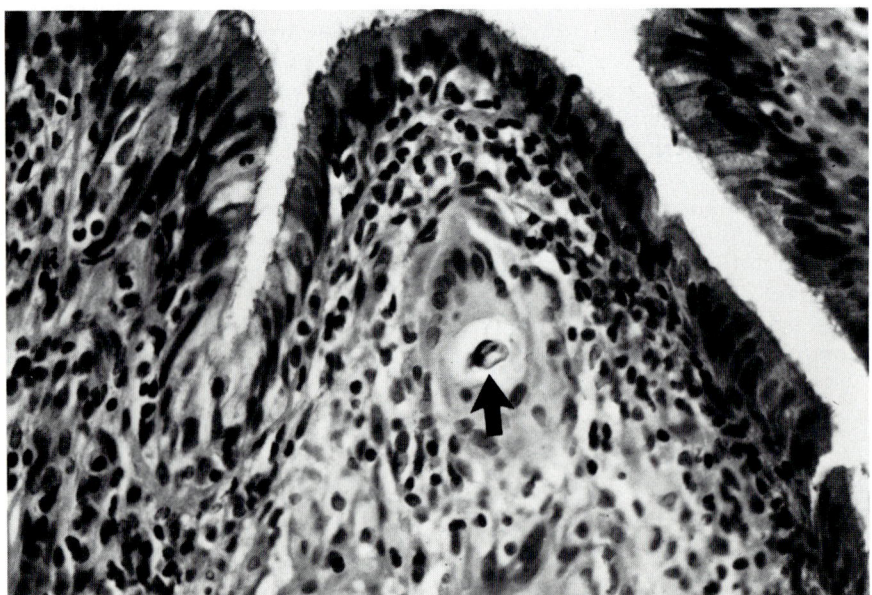

Figure 24.1 A biopsy specimen of the bronchial mucosa, obtained through a fibreoptic bronchoscope, showing a non-caseating granuloma with an asteroid body (arrow). (Haematoxylin and eosin. × 300.)

leagues[5]. They performed consecutive open lung biopsies in 21 patients with stage I sarcoidosis; non-caseating granulomas were found in all 21 (100%) patients. In patients with hilar and paratracheal adenopathy, we first perform a transbronchial biopsy and if a satisfactory diagnosis cannot be established then the patient is referred to a thoracic surgeon for a mediastinoscopy (see Figure 24.1).

In patients with stage II and III disease the incidence of positivity is much higher and depends on the number of biopsies and the expertise of the bronchoscopist. We generally obtain 4–6 transbronchial lung specimens. Gilman and Wang have demonstrated that a diagnostic yield of 90% can be secured with four transbronchial biopsy specimens[6]. Although Roethe et al. have increased their diagnostic accuracy to 95% by performing 10 biopsies[7], I do not feel that the increased cost (personnel time, burden on the laboratory, wear and tear of the instruments, increased fluoroscopy time, etc.) and the likelihood of more complications are justified in order to achieve the minimal gain in the diagnostic yields.

In experienced hands fibreoptic bronchoscopy is safe, relatively simple and inexpensive (compared with mediastinoscopy and an open lung biopsy). It is an efficient procedure with a high diagnostic yield[8,9]. However, certain routine precautions should be taken to avoid pneumothorax, bleeding, cardiac arrhythmias and vasovagal reactions[10,11].

Extrapulmonary biopsy sites

Sarcoidosis affects almost all the tissue systems in the body. Depending on the extent of the disease a number of biopsy sites may be available for the histological confirmation of the diagnosis. Before the advent of fibreoptic bronchoscopy, lymph-node (scalene, mediastinal, peripheral) biopsies were performed on as many as one-half of all the patients suspected of having sarcoidosis.[12] In the acute stage of sarcoidosis other fruitful sources of tissue biopsy include liver,[13] skeletal muscle[14] and lacrimal gland[15]. However, it should be remembered that in an asymptomatic person, particularly in a patient with erythema nodosum, presence of bilateral hilar adenopathy with or without paratracheal adenopathy is highly suggestive of sarcoidosis and may not require a biopsy confirmation especially if the serum angiotensin converting enzyme activity is significantly elevated. Later in the subacute stage, a nasal mucosa[16],

TABLE 24.2. Biopsy sites in sarcoidosis: Advantages and disadvantages

Biopsy procedure	Sensitivity*	Selectivity†	Hospitalization	Cost	Morbidity	Mortality
Transbronchial	High	High	No	Moderate	Low	None
Open lung	High	High	Yes	High	Moderate	Low
Mediastinoscopy	High	High	Yes	High	Moderate	Low
Scalene node	High	Moderate	Yes	High	Moderate	None
Liver	High	Low	No	Low	Very Low	None
Skin	Moderate	Moderate	No	Low	None	None
Muscle	Moderate	Moderate	No	Low	None	None
Conjunctiva‡	Moderate	Moderate	No	Low	None	None
Lacrimal	High	High	No	Low	None	None
Minor salivary glands‡	Moderate	Moderate	No	Low	None	None
Spleen‡	Moderate	Moderate	No	Low	Low	None

* Frequency of true positives.
† Low frequency of false-positive biopsies.
‡ Limited experience.

minor salivary gland[17], spleen[18], and conjunctiva[15] may provide a reliable source of epithelioid tubercles. Chronic skin lesions may provide histological evidence in some patients with advanced multisystem disease.

These techniques vary in sensitivity (frequency of true-positive biopsies), selectivity (frequency of false-positive biopsies), cost, morbidity, mortality and the need for hospitalization (see Table 24.2). The choice of the site depends on the interest of the physician and availability of various facilities.

Differential diagnosis

Many conditions can give rise to dyspnoea and diffuse pulmonary infiltration on the chest radiograph and thus may be confused with sarcoidosis. Some of the common pulmonary conditions encountered in the differential diagnosis of sarcoidosis are described below.

Extrinsic allergic alveolitis (hypersensitivity pneumonitis)

Frequent inhalation of the dust of mouldy hay or other vegetable allergens may produce diffuse non-caseating interstitial granulomatous pneumonitis, indistinguishable histologically from sarcoidosis. The history of exposure and immunological studies—positive skin tests and presence of precipitin antibodies against the offending antigen—are helpful in making the diagnosis (see Table 24.3).

TABLE 24.3 Differences between sarcoidosis and extrinsic allergic alveolitis

Features	Sarcoidosis	Extrinsic allergic alveolitis
Age (years)	20–50	Any
Symptoms	Asymptomatic, dyspnoea, fever and weight loss	Dyspnoea, malaise, weight loss
Multisystem involvement	Common: Eyes, skin, liver, spleen	None
Chest radiograph	Bilateral hilar adenopathy with or without pulmonary infiltration	No adenopathy. Basal or widespread infiltration
Delayed hypersensitivity	Depressed	Normal
Precipitin antibodies	Absent	Present
Bronchoalveolar lavage	T-lymphocyte predominance	T-lymphocyte predominance
Inhalational challenge	Not applicable	Positive
Treatment	Corticosteroids	Prevention, corticosteroids

Fibrosing alveolitis (idiopathic pulmonary fibrosis)

Fibrosing alveolitis is characterized by diffuse thickening of alveolar walls without any evidence of any occupational exposure or any other causative factors. Dyspnoea is the most common symptom; characteristic signs include superficial crepitations and clubbing of the fingers. The chest radiograph usually shows diffuse pulmonary infiltration and, in later stages, honeycombing. Antinuclear factor is found in 10% of patients and rheumatoid factor in 30%. Usually, an open lung biopsy is needed to establish the diagnosis.

Connective-tissue disease

Rheumatoid arthritis, progressive systemic sclerosis and systemic lupus erythematosus can all produce interstitial infiltration and fibrosis. However, clinical, immunological and histological differences between sarcoidosis and connective-tissue disorders are many and leave no room for any confusion between the two groups (*see Chapter 30*).

Pneumoconiosis

The radiographic and lung function abnormalities similar to those of sarcoidosis may occur in patients with asbestosis, silicosis and berylliosis. Berylliosis can also produce biochemical and immunological features similar to those seen in sarcoidosis (*see Table 24.4*).

TABLE 24.4. Sarcoidosis and berylliosis: A comparison

Features	*Sarcoidosis*	*Berylliosis*
Occupational history	Absent	Present
Dyspnoea	May be present	Usually present
Erythema nodosum	Present in acute form	Absent
Uveitis	Present (25%)	Absent
Lymphadenopathy	Common	Uncommon
Parotid/lacrimal enlargement	Present	Absent
Bone cysts	Present	Absent
Bilateral hilar lymphadenopathy	Common	Uncommon
Pulmonary infiltration	Common	Common
Depression of delayed-type hypersensitivity	Present	Present
Beryllium patch test	Negative	Positive
Histology	Granuloma	Granuloma
Bronchoalveolar lavage	Lymphocyte predominance	Lymphocyte predominance
Lymphocyte transformation in response to beryllium	Absent	Present
Treatment	Corticosteroids	Corticosteroids
Mortality (%)	5	27

Drugs

There are many drugs—including nitrofurantoin, hexamethonium, busulphan, cyclophosphamide, bleomycin and oxygen—that produce radiographic changes similar to that observed in sarcoidosis. However, there are at least five drugs that not only produce chest X-ray changes but also induce granulomatous reaction. These drugs are (1) talc (magnesium trisilicate); (2) methotrexate; (3) mineral oil; (4) BCG (bacille Calmette-Guérin); and (5) cromolyn sodium (Intal).

Miscellaneous

Miliary tuberculosis, histoplasmosis, coccidioidomycosis, lymphangitic carcinomatosis, diffuse amyloidosis, lymphoma and leukaemias and *Pneumocystis carinii* may all produce a chest X-ray appearance similar to sarcoidosis.

References

1. SHARMA, O.P. (1983) Diagnosis of sarcoidosis *Arch. Intern. Med.*, **43**, 1418.
2. IKEDA, S. (1970) Flexible bronchofiberscope. *Ann. Otol. Phenol. Laryngol.*, **79**, 916.
3. WHITCOMB, M.E., DOMBY, R.W., HAWLEY, P.C., *et al.* (1980) The role of fiberoptic bronchoscopy in the diagnosis of sarcoidosis. *Chest*, **74**, 205.
4. TEIRSTEIN, A.S. (1983) Fibre-optic bronchoscopy in the diagnosis of sarcoidosis. In *Sarcoidosis and Other Granulomatous Diseases of the Lung* (ed. Fanburg, B.L.), p. 323. (New York: Marcel Dekker.) (A very good overview of the subject.)
5. ROSEN, Y., AMOROSA, J.K., MOON, S., *et al.* (1977) Occurrence of lung granulomas in patients with stage I sarcoidosis. *Ann. J. Roentgenol.*, **129**, 1083.
6. GILMAN, M.J. and WANG, K.P. (1980) Transbronchial lung biopsy in sarcoidosis. An approach to determine optimal number of biopsies. *Am. Rev. Resp. Dis.*, **122**, 721.
7. ROETHE, R.A., FULLER, P.B., BYRD, R.B., *et al.* (1980) Transbronchial lung biopsy in sarcoidosis. *Chest*, **77**, 400.
8. SACKNER, M.A. (1974) Bronchofiberscopy: State of the Art. *Am. Rev. Resp. Dis.*, **109**, 63.
9. ZAVALA, D.C. (1978) Complications following fiberoptic bronchoscopy. The 'Good News' and the 'Bad News'. *Chest*, **73**, 783.
10. PEREIRA, W., Jr., KOVNAT, D.M. and SNIDER, G.L. (1978) A prospective cooperative study of complications following flexible fiberoptic bronchoscopy. *Chest*, **73**, 813.
11. SHRADER, D.L. and LAKSHMINARAYAN, S. (1978) The effect of fiberoptic bronchoscopy on cardiac rhythm. *Chest*, **73**, 821.
12. JAMES, D.G., NEVILLE, E., SILTZBACH, L.E., *et al.* (1976) A worldwide review of sarcoidosis. *Ann. N.Y. Acad. Sci.*, **278**, 321.
13. NEVILLE, E., PIYASENA, K.H.G. and JAMES, D.G. (1975) Granulomas of the liver. *Postgrad. Med. J.*, **51**, 361.
14. SCADDING, J.G. (1967) *Sarcoidosis.* (London: Eyre and Spottiswoode)
15. KARMA, A. (1979) Ophthalmic changes in sarcoidosis. *Acta Ophthalmol. (Suppl.)*, **141**.
16. NEVILLE, E., MILLS, R.G.S. and JAMES, D.G. (1976) Sarcoidosis of the upper respiratory tract and its relation to lupus pernio. *Ann. N.Y. Acad. Sci.*, **278**, 416.
17. NESSAN, V.J. and JACOWAY, J.R. (1979) Biopsy of minor salivary glands in the diagnosis of sarcoidosis. *N. Engl. J. Med.*, **301**, 922.
18. SELROOS, O. (1976) Fine needle aspiration biopsy of the spleen in diagnosis of sarcoidosis. *Ann. N.Y. Acad. Sci.*, **278**, 517.

Chapter 25
Treatment

Indications

Pulmonary sarcoidosis

Although corticosteroids are generally considered to be beneficial in treating pulmonary sarcoidosis, there is no single opinion regarding the indications for such treatment, the maximum effective dose, the duration, and the effect of therapy on the course of the granulomatous process. There are some who believe that corticosteroids do not alter the course of pulmonary sarcoidosis and that the treatment should be reserved to alleviate symptoms. Others believe that corticosteroids should be given, with the aim of preventing irreversible pulmonary fibrosis, to patients with pulmonary infiltration and active disease regardless of the presence or absence of symptoms[1].

Why is there such a difference of opinion? Partly because a large number of patients with sarcoidosis either undergo remission or follow a benign course, making controlled clinical studies well nigh difficult if not impossible; and partly because the cause of the disease is not known. However, most of the confusion has been created by unreliability of the clinical, radiological, physiological and biochemical data in predicting the activity, the extent and the course of the granulomatous process. Many of us treat our patients on the basis of lung function rather than on radiological findings; others recommend treating all patients with stage II or III disease; and others use symptoms as their guidelines for starting corticosteroids.

New tests for assessing activity of pulmonary sarcoidosis

Until recently we had no accurate measurement of granulomatous activity. Since the aim of the therapy is to prevent fibrosis, it is important to establish the activity and reversibility of the granulomatous process. There is now enough evidence that serum angiotensin converting enzyme (ACE), bronchoalveolar lavage (BAL) and ^{67}Ga lung scans reflect the index of sarcoid activity; however, some uncertainty remains about how the three methods correlate with each other[2]. It seems that serum ACE does not accurately reflect activity of the disease as assessed by the BAL lymphocyte count[3, 4]. There is a rough correlation between gallium scanning and serum ACE activity but not between gallium lung scans and BAL lymphocyte counts[5]. Much has yet to be learned about the usefulness of these tests in assessing the activity of sarcoidosis[6, 7].

In the meantime, combinations of the three tests should be used to assess the activity and extents of pulmonary involvement.

Role of corticosteroids

James et al.[8] studied 84 patients who were randomly allocated to 6 months of treatment with prednisone, oxyphenbutazone or placebo. Fifty-seven per cent of the patients improved with either prednisone or oxyphenbutazone treatment as opposed to only 17% observed with placebo. Although this study established short-term beneficial effects of corticosteroids, long-term data were not available to advocate lasting prolonged therapy. Yamamoto et al.[9] have followed the clinical course of 37 corticosteroid-treated patients and 37 untreated controls. The radiographic improvement at 3 months was higher in corticosteroid treatment. However, there was no difference in clinical or radiographic changes when the patients were followed up for more than 1 year.

Eule, Roth and Weide[10] divided sarcoid patients with stages I or II disease into two groups. The first group was treated with prednisone 40 mg daily which was reduced to 10–15 mg daily for 6 months. The second group was treated with a similar dose for 12 months. At 6 months, both groups showed greater improvement than the control group. At 12 months, the group receiving the treatment showed more improvement than the control group and the group in which treatment had been stopped. Johns et al.[11] treated approximately 250 patients over a 15-year period. They observed that long-term corticosteroid treatment is required for patients with symptomatic pulmonary sarcoidosis, and with maintenance doses of 10–15 mg daily clinical benefits far outweigh the infrequent problems associated with corticosteroids. Romer[12] followed up 243 patients for up to 10 years and in 87% the chest radiographic abnormalities improved within 2 years. The patients with hilar adenopathy had the best prognosis; 58% improved within 12 months, only 9% progressing to the infiltrative phase. In the patient with stage II disease, radiographic clearing occurred only in a quarter; 29% showed improvement and 10% disease progression. Of 11 patients with stage III disease only one improved spontaneously.

Who should be treated with corticosteroids?

The following points should be remembered:

1. Patients with bilateral hilar adenopathy (stage I) without symptoms and extrapulmonary involvement should be left untreated. A chest radiograph should be repeated after 6 months.
2. Patients with bilateral hilar adenopathy and infiltration (stage II) and symptoms (dyspnoea, cough, chest pain, exercise intolerance) should be treated with corticosteroids. Vital capacity, diffusing capacity, a chest radiograph and serum ACE activity should be used to monitor the course of the disease.
3. Patients with stage II disease who are asymptomatic should undergo ^{67}Ga and BAL lymphocyte studies. If the tests show high-intensity disease, the patient should be given corticosteroids. If sarcoidosis is of low activity then no therapy is needed and the patient should be examined again after 6 months.
4. Stage III disease. All patients should undergo ^{67}Ga and BAL lymphocyte studies. The treatment is almost always needed if the disease is active.
5. Stage IV disease (fibrosis and bullae formation). In these patients the assessment of

Indications 167

disease activity would be of great value because it is not unusual to find some activity by ^{67}Ga scans and bronchoalveolar lavage in an occasional patient with advanced sarcoidosis.

Extrapulmonary sarcoidosis

Fortunately, indications for the treatment of extrapulmonary involvement are straightforward and are not controversial.

Ocular sarcoidosis—All patients with sarcoidosis should have an adequate ophthalmic evaluation, including a slit-lamp examination. The response to therapy is particularly favourable in acute iridocyclitis or uveitis. Treatment at the early stage usually prevents further damage to the eye. Topical corticosteroids (prednisone acetate 1%) in the form of eye drops and ointments are effective for anterior uveitis. If there is no improvement within 2 weeks or if there is an evidence of posterior uveitis, concurrent use of systemic corticosteroids is strongly indicated.

Hypercalcaemia and hypercalciuria—Corticosteroids prevent urinary excretion of calcium and resultant nephrocalcinosis by blocking absorption from the gut. If calcium abnormality does not respond to corticosteroids, a trial with oral phosphates is indicated.

Myocardial involvement—Myocardial involvement may be indicated by heart block or cardiac arrhythmia and is an indication for corticoid therapy. Thallium-201 myocardial perfusion studies may demonstrate areas of myocardial involvement. An artificial pacemaker should be considered in the management of complete heart block (*see Figures 25.1 and 25.2*). In a Japanese study of cardiac pacemaker implantation in 33 cases (23 with endocardial and 10 with myocardial lesions), Sekiguchi *et al.*[13] observed that corticosteroids were effective in suppressing A-V block, atrial or ventricular arrhythmias and conduction disturbances in 16 (64%) out of 25 patients. After

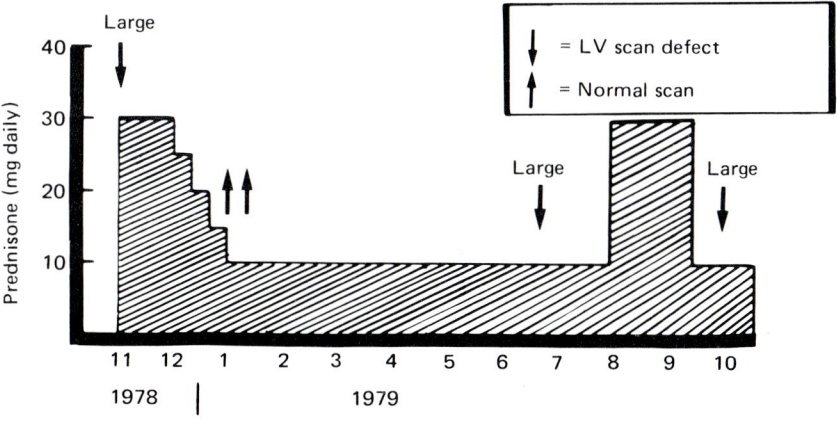

Figure 25.1 Graphic representation of scan defects' response to steroid therapy in a patient diagnosed as having multisystem sarcoidosis. The patient was on high doses of steroids initially; these were tapered off and discontinued 3 months after diagnosis, at which time palpitations were noted. Note how the large posterior-lateral wall defect ('Large' arrow) resolved after high doses of steroid ('Normal') and shows as such on a repeat scan ('Normal'). After some months on maintenance-level steroid doses the large defect returned and has remained. (Reproduced from *J. Natl. Med. Assoc.* (1982) **74**, 963, by courtesy of publishers.)

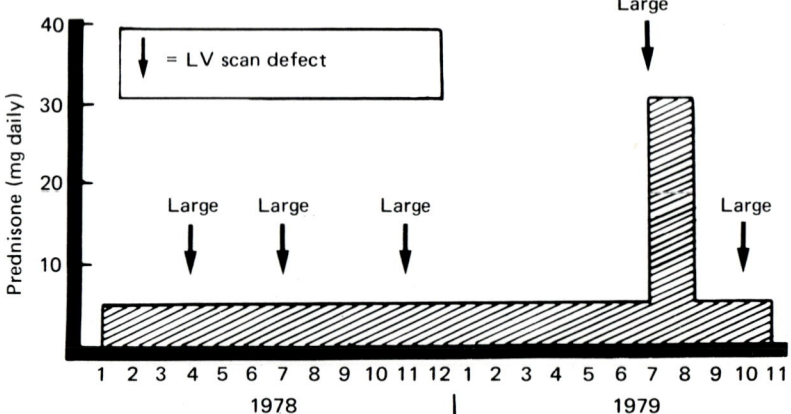

Figure 25.2 A patient with a large focal myocardial defect which remained as such in spite of a 6-week course of high doses of steroids ('Large' arrow at far right). (Reproduced from *J. Natl. Med. Assoc.* (1982) **74**, 963, by courtesy of publishers.)

the discontinuation of the steroid therapy one patient died suddenly and two other patients developed Stokes-Adams episodes. Nine of the 12 patients who died suddenly had not received corticosteroid therapy.

Neurological lesions—Diabetes insipidus, papilloedema and epilepsy caused by sarcoidosis respond well to corticosteroids.

Splenic involvement—Hypersplenism may cause anaemia, leucopenia and thrombocytopenia. The latter, if severe, may result in uncontrollable haemorrhage. Corticosteroids are very effective but splenectomy should be performed if bleeding is not controlled by medical therapy.

Liver involvement—Maddrey *et al.* recommended using corticosteroids when significant liver function abnormalities are found in association with inflammatory changes in liver biopsy[14]. Progressive liver disease is an indication for corticosteroid administration; however, portacaval surgery should be considered in patients with portal hypertension and bleeding oesophageal varices.

Glandular involvement—This is important if there is disordered function, e.g., dry eye due to lacrimal gland involvement and dry mouth due to parotid involvement.

Cutaneous lesions—Oral or local corticosteroids may cause regression of ugly skin rash, lupus pernio, scaly plaques and other chronic skin lesions. Corticosteroids and methotrexate are effective treatments of lupus pernio.

Sarcoidosis of the upper respiratory tract (SURT)—This indicates chronic persistent disease and almost always needs corticosteroids[15].

Arthritis, muscle and bone involvement—may occasionally require corticosteroid therapy. Colchicine is effective for the relief of acute bouts of joint inflammation.

Methods

Corticosteroids

We usually administer 20–40 mg prednisone daily in a single dose, gradually reducing this dosage to a maintenance level of about 5–10 mg daily for most of the indications given above. Alternate-day regimen can be used effectively with considerable reduction of side-effects associated with prolonged daily usage[16].

Acute uveitis, myocardial involvement, papilloedema and severe hypercalcaemia require somewhat higher dosages—60–80 mg prednisone. Local corticosteroids, as mentioned, are often effective for controlling low-grade uvetis and may be administered in the form of eye drops alone or reinforced by one subconjunctival injection.

An attempt should be made to treat cutaneous lesions by local corticosteroids alone. Intralesional injections of triamcinolone acetonide diluted with 1% procaine to a final concentration of 2–5 mg.ml^{-1} may be repeated at weekly intervals.

Chloroquine

Chloroquine has been found useful in the management of lupus pernio and pulmonary fibrosis, starting with 250 mg twice daily for 6 months[17, 18]. It may also be used concurrently with corticosteroids to reduce their dosage. Chloroquine administration may lead to irreversible retinopathy and blindness. Frequent and careful eye examination are mandatory.

Immunosuppressive drugs

Methotrexate[19], chlorambucil[20] and azathioprine[21] have been used with good results in a few patients who have not responded to corticosteroid therapy.

Oxyphenbutazone

In a British trial, oxyphenbutazone was found quite similar to corticosteroids in its effect on the radiological pulmonary findings and in the prevention of the evolution of the Kveim test. The drug is given in a dose of 100 mg four times daily for 3 months[8].

Colchicine

This has been found useful in the management of arthritis caused by sarcoidosis[22]. We prescribe 0.5 mg two or three times a day.

Levamisole

The drug augments delayed hypersensitivity both *in vitro* and *in vivo* in a variety of diseases including sarcoidosis and tuberculosis. Daddi *et al.* have treated 200 patients of sarcoidosis with levamisole. They contend that levamisole prevented relapses in those patients who were unsuccessfully treated with corticosteroids. More information is needed to justify the routine use of the drug in sarcoidosis[23].

Antituberculosis therapy

Prophylactic isoniazid in a dose of 300 mg once daily is given to those patients receiving corticosteroids who have a positive tuberculin test. Otherwise, antituberculosis drugs are not routinely indicated in sarcoidosis.

References

1. DEREMEE, R.A. (1977) The present status of treatment of pulmonary sarcoidosis: A house divided. *Chest*, **71**, 388.
2. CRYSTAL, R.G., ROBERTS, W., HUNNINGHAKE, G.W., *et al.* (1981) Pulmonary sarcoidosis: A disease characterized and perpetuated by activated T lymphocytes. *Ann. Intern. Med.*, **94**, 73.
3. SCHOENBERGER, C.I., LINE, B.R., KEOGH, B.A., *et al.* (1982) Lung inflammation in sarcoidosis: Comparison of serum angiotensin-converting levels with bronchoalveolar lavage and gallium-67 scanning assessment of the T-lymphocyte alveolitis. *Thorax*, **37**, 19.
4. ROSSMAN, M.D., DANKER, J.H., CARDILLO, M.E., *et al.* (1982) Pulmonary sarcoidosis: Correlation of serum angiotensin-converting enzyme with blood and bronchoalveolar lymphocytes. *Am. Rev. Resp. Dis.*, **125**, 366.
5. BEAUMONT, D., HERRY, J.Y., SAPENE, M., *et al.* (1982) Gallium-67 in the evaluation of sarcoidosis: Correlations with serum angiotensin-converting enzyme and bronchoalveolar lavage. *Thorax*, **37**, 11.
6. TURTON, C.W.G., GRUNDY, E., FIRTH, G., *et al.* (1979) Value of measuring serum angiotensin-converting enzyme and serum lysozyme in the management of sarcoidosis. *Thorax*, **34**, 57.
7. GREENING, A.P. (1982) Bronchoalveolar lavage. *Br. Med. J.*, **284**, 1896.
8. JAMES, D.G., CARSTAIRS, L.S. TROWELL, J. and SHARMA, O.P. (1967) Treatment of sarcoidosis: Report of a controlled therapeutic trial. *Lancet*, **ii**, 526.
9. YAMAMOTO, M., SAITO, N., TACHIBANA, T., *et al.* (1981) Effect of 18-month corticosteroid therapy to the Stage I and Stage II sarcoidosis patients. In *Proceedings of the IXth International Congress on Sarcoidosis* (eds Chretien, J., Marsac, J. and Saltiel, J.), p. 470. (Paris: Pergamon Press)
10. EULE, H., ROTH, I. and WEIDE, W. (1980) Clinical and functional results of a controlled trial of the value of prednisone therapy. In *Sarcoidosis and Other Granulomatous Diseases* (eds Jones Williams, W. and Davies, B.H.), p. 624. (Cardiff: Alpha Omega Publishers)
11. JOHNS, C.J., MACGREGOR, I., ZACHARY, J.B., *et al.* (1976) Extended experience in the long-term corticosteroid treatment of sarcoidosis. In *Proceedings of the Seventh International Conference on Sarcoidosis and Other Granulomatous Disorders* (ed. Siltzbach, L.E.). *Ann. N.Y. Acad. Sci.*, **278**, 722.
12. ROMER, F.K. (1982) Presentation of sarcoidosis and outcome of pulmonary changes. *Dan. Med. Bull.*, **29**, 27.
13. SEKIGUCHI, M., SUDA, T., FURNIE, T., *et al.* (1981) Long-term prognosis of cardiac sarcoidosis patients with permanent pacemaker implantation. In *Proceedings of the IXth International Congress on Sarcoidosis* (eds Chretien, J., Marsac, J. and Saltiel, J.), p. 658. (Paris: Pergamon Press)
14. MADDREY, W.C., JOHNS, J.C., BOITNOTT, J.K., *et al.* (1970) Sarcoidosis and chronic hepatic disease: A clinical and pathological study of 20 cases. *Medicine*, **49**, 375.
15. SHARMA, O.P. (1978) Sarcoidosis of the upper respiratory tract. *Arch. Intern. Med.*, **138**, 689.
16. BLOCK, A.J. and LIGHT, R.W. (1973) Alternate steroid therapy in diffuse pulmonary sarcoidosis. *Chest*, **63**, 495.
17. SILTZBACH, L.E. and TEIRSTEIN, A.S. (1964) Chloroquine therapy in 43 patients with intrathoracic and cutaneous sarcoidosis. *Acta Med. Scand. (Suppl.)*, **425**, 320.
18. BRITISH TUBERCULOSIS ASSOCIATION (1967) Chloroquine in treatment of sarcoidosis. *Tubercle*, **47**, 257.
19. ISRAEL, H. (1971) Effects of chlorambucil and methotrexate in sarcoidosis. In *Proceedings of the Fifth International Conference on Sarcoidosis* (eds Lavinsky, L. and Macholda, F.), p. 635. (Prague: Charles University)
20. SHARMA, O.P., HUGHES, D.T.D. and JAMES, D.G. (1971) Immunosuppressive therapy with azathioprine in sarcoidosis. In *Proceedings of the Fifth International Conference on Sarcoidosis* (eds Lavinsky, L. and Macholda, F.), p. 635. (Prague: Charles University)
21. JAMES, D.G. (1981) Lupus pernio is a valuable experimental model. In *Sarcoidosis and Other Granulomatous Disorders*, (eds Chretien, J., Marsac, J. and Saltiel, J.), p. 465. (Paris: Pergamon Press)
22. KAPLAN, H. (1963) Further experience with colchicine in the treatment of sarcoid arthritis. *N. Engl. J. Med.*, **268**, 761.
23. DADDI, G., GIOBBI, A., LUCCHESI, M., *et al.* (1981) Levamisolone and sarcoidosis. In *Sarcoidosis and other Granulomatous Disorders* (eds Chretien, J., Marsac, J. and Saltiel, J.), p. 657. (Paris: Pergamon Press)

Chapter 26
Sarcoidosis in children

Review of the literature indicates that sarcoidosis is not rare among children. Siltzbach and Greenberg described 18 children with a biopsy-confirmed diagnosis; five out of 18 (28%) were between 9 and 12 years of age and the remaining 13 were 13-15 years old. All children 12 years and under showed symptoms; whereas only six of 13 (46%) between 13 and 15 years of age showed symptoms markedly. Seven children were asymptomatic.

The children with symptoms were younger, had extensive disease, and the prognosis was less favourable[1]. Merton, Kirks and Grossman[2] observed chest radiograph abnormalities in 24 (92%) of 26 children under 17 years in age. Bilateral hilar adenopathy was present in all 24 patients. Bilateral paratracheal adenopathy with hilar adenopathy occurred in 88% of the children as compared with the 31-37% incidence observed in adults. According to Hetherington, skin rashes, uveitis, and arthritis are more common in children under 4 years of age[3]. Kendig reviewed 104 cases in patients 15 years old or younger and found that the distribution of organs involved in children was similar to that in adults[4].

It is now accepted that sarcoidosis occurs frequently in children and the diagnosis should be entertained in a child of any age who presents with a skin rash, uveitis, lymphadenopathy and pulmonary involvement. The prognosis in children is more favourable than in adults.

References

1. SILTZBACH, L.E. and GREENBERG, G.M. (1968) Childhood sarcoidosis: A study of 18 patients. *N. Engl. J. Med.*, **279**, 1239.
2. MERTEN, D., KIRKS, D.R. and GROSSMAN, H. (1980) Pulmonary sarcoidosis in childhood. *Am. J. Radiol.*, **135**, 673.
3. HETHERINGTON, S. (1982) Sarcoidosis in young children. *Am. J. Dis. Child.*, **136**, 13.
4. KENDIG, E.L., Jr. (1974) The clinical picture of sarcoidosis in children. *Pediatrics*, **54**, 289.

Chapter 27
Sarcoidosis in the aged

Sarcoidosis is a disorder of low mortality. Many patients live with it through their later years, and a few patients do not develop their first manifestation of the disorder until then. In a study of 115 patients with sarcoidosis, 11 (9%) were 60 years of age or older at the time of presentation. The most common symptoms were related to respiratory system (dyspnoea, cough and chest pain), occurring in about two-thirds of all the patients[1]. Remission is less likely to be achieved in elderly patients, particularly in those with extensive skin and bone lesions. However, early diagnosis and the initiation of effective therapy averts the complications of the disease.

Case report—In 1972, an 80-year-old woman visited a physician for the treatment of skin lesions. She was in excellent health until 1950 when she developed an erythematous 'butterfly' eruption on the face and a swollen right fifth digit. Physical examination showed erythematous, ulcerated nodules and plaques over both malar areas with serous exudation and crusting. Involvement of the left upper and lower eyelids resulted in near complete closure of the left eye (*see Plate 3.1a*). Collapse of the nasal septum and the crusting of the nasal mucosa were noted. The entire right fifth digit and right fourth digit about the proximal interphalangeal joint demonstrated fusiform violaceous swelling (*see Plate 3.1c*). Intradermal skin testing with tuberculin, coccidioidin, histoplasmin, Candida and Trichophyton were negative. The chest radiograph showed parenchymal linear infiltrations in the right upper lung zone and both lower lung fields. Radiographs of the hands showed cystic changes of the small bones. Biopsy specimens from the forearm and the face showed non-caseating granulomas. Cultures of the biopsy samples did not grow fungi or acid-fast bacilli. Guinea-pig inoculations were negative. The patient received prednisone 15 mg and chloroquine phosphate 500 mg daily. She also received weekly intralesional triamcinolone acetonide ($5\,mg.ml^{-1}$) injections to the left upper eyelid. After 10 months of therapy the chloroquine was discontinued and the prednisone was tapered to 5 mg daily. All skin lesions and soft-tissue swelling resolved completely leaving residual atrophic scars (*see Plate 3.1b,d*). The patient is now 92 years old and her sarcoidosis is in remission.

Comment—In the management of the disease in the aged, it is important to remember that a malignant disease of the lung, stomach, intestine and even uterus may give rise to a granulomatous reaction in the draining lymph nodes. The local sarcoid reaction must be distinguished from the multisystem sarcoidosis. Where there is a granulomatous reaction in the elderly, doubt the diagnosis of sarcoidosis; 'think of neoplasia' is a helpful dictum to follow.

References
1. SHARMA, O.P. (1973) Sarcoidosis in aged. *Geriatrics*, January, 76.

Chapter 28
Sarcoidosis and pregnancy

Effect of pregnancy on sarcoidosis

The conventional teaching is that pregnancy has a beneficial effect on sarcoidosis but the effect is temporary and lost during the puerperium[1-3]. In a few patients, the disease worsens after parturition; therefore, a chest radiograph should be obtained within 6 months after delivery. The pregnancy-related favourable response is probably due to increased cortisol levels. During the puerperium cortisol level drops, resulting in exacerbation of sarcoidosis. This cortisol-related fluctuation of the disease activity occurs not only in sarcoidosis but is observed in asthma, hay fever, psoriasis and rheumatoid arthritis.

Effect of sarcoidosis on pregnancy

Sarcoidosis does not affect pregnancy adversely. Siltzbach found no evidence of either spontaneous abortion or other complications in his study of 33 pregnancies carried to term[4]. Although there are reports of miscarriage and congenital fetal anomalies, the incidence of such problems is not different from that found in mothers without sarcoidosis[5,6]. Fertility is not affected by sarcoidosis. The uncomplicated disease does not constitute an indication for sterilization or therapeutic abortion. One maternal antepartum death has been reported by Given and DiBenedetto in a patient with sarcoidosis who developed pre-eclampsia[7].

References

1. AGHA, F.P., VADE, A., AMENDOLA, M.A. and COOPER, F.R. (1982) Effects of pregnancy on sarcoidosis. *Surg. Gynecol. Obstet.*, **155**, 817.
2. O'LEARY, J.A. (1962) Ten year study of sarcoidosis and pregnancy. *Am. J. Obstet. Gynecol.*, **84**, 462.
3. DINES, D.E. and BANNER, E.A. (1967) Sarcoidosis during pregnancy—improvement in pulmonary function. *J. Am. Med. Assoc.*, **200**, 150.
4. SILTZBACH, L.E. (1965) Sarcoidosis. In *Medical, Surgical and Gynecologic Complications of Pregnancy* (eds Rovinsky, J.J. and Guttmacher, A.F.), 2nd edn, p. 150. (Baltimore: William and Wilkins)
5. MAYOCK, R.L., SULLIVAN, R.D., GEENING, R.R., et al. (1957) Sarcoidosis and pregnancy. *J. Am. Med. Assoc.*, **164**, 158.
6. REISFIELD, D.R. (1958) Boeck's sarcoid and pregnancy. *Am. J. Obstet. Gynecol.*, **75**, 795.
7. GIVEN, F.R. and DIBENEDETTO, R.L. (1963) Sarcoidosis and pregnancy. *Obstet. Gynecol.*, **22**, 355.

Chapter 29
Infections in sarcoidosis

The occurrence of bacterial, viral and invasive fungal infection in sarcoidosis is no greater than that in the general population. The incidence of tuberculosis complicating sarcoidosis is less than 1%[1]. Aspergilloma is the common infectious complication of sarcoidosis. Mycetomas or fungus ball arise from saprophytic colonization of pre-existing lung cavities or bullae resulting from the parenchymal fibrosis and destruction[2].

Medical therapy is of doubtful value: amphotericin-B, nystatin and flucytosine have been tried unsuccessfully. Spontaneous lysis of aspergillomas occur in about 10% of the patients. Resection of an aspergilloma is indicated in patients with recurrent haemoptysis. The development of an aspergilloma is not related to prednisone therapy, extent of the intrathoracic disease and depression of delayed hypersensitivity.

Invasive aspergillosis is rare in sarcoidosis. However, the possibility should be considered when rapidly progressive pulmonary infiltrates and clinical deterioration occur in patients with steroid-treated sarcoidosis[3].

References

1. WINTERBAUER, R.H. and KRAEMER, K.G. (1976) The infectious complications of sarcoidosis. *Arch. Intern. Med.*, **136**, 1356.
2. VARKEY, B. and ROSE, H.D. (1976) Pulmonary aspergilloma. *Am. J. Med.*, **61**, 626.
3. WALDHORN, R.E., TSOU, E. and KERWIN, D.M. (1983) Invasive pulmonary aspergillosis associated with aspergilloma in sarcoidosis. *S. Med. J.*, **76**, 251.

Chapter 30
Sarcoidosis and autoimmunity

The presence of hyperglobulinaemia, defect in suppressor T-cell function, loss of self-tolerance to self-antigens with the appearance of auto-antibodies, uveitis and a favourable response to corticosteroid therapy have, in the minds of a few, suggested that autoimmune mechanisms play an important role in the pathogenesis of sarcoidosis. On the surface the assumption does not sound too unreasonable because it draws support from sporadic case reports describing the coexistence of sarcoidosis and other autoimmune disorders including systemic lupus erythematosus, progressive systemic sclerosis, thyroiditis, Addison's disease, Sjögren's syndrome and primary biliary cirrhosis.

Connective-tissue diseases

Rheumatoid arthritis

A relationship between sarcoidosis and connective-tissue diseases is far from evident. Though the rheumatoid factor is present in 20–40% of patients with sarcoidosis, in one study on 94 patients with sarcoidosis, Putkonen, Virkkunen and Wagner[1] found only one definite and one probable case of rheumatoid arthritis. The authors felt that the occurrence of sarcoidosis and rheumatoid arthritis together was no greater than would be expected in a normal population.

Systemic lupus erythematosus (SLE)

Teilum[2] described two patients in their early twenties who presented with joint pains, skin rash, anaemia and albuminuria. These patients were diagnosed as having systemic lupus erythematosus, but at autopsy multiple non-caseating granulomas were found in the lungs, blood vessels and lymph nodes. Pollack[3] described similar granulomatous appearances in serous membranes and mediastinal and oesophageal connective tissues. Dubois[4] examined 18 spleens from SLE patients and found two with loosely arranged non-caseating granulomas. In seven patients in which palmar tendon sheaths were examined, a solitary granuloma was found only in one patient.

Progressive systemic sclerosis (PSS)

Granulomas have been described in tendon sheaths of patients with PSS by Shulman, Kurban and Harvey[5]. In an extensive review of the literature for evidence suggesting a relationship between sarcoidosis and connective-tissue diseases, Wiesenhutter and Sharma[6] described three cases of sarcoidosis coexisting with PSS. In all of these patients PSS became manifest with symptoms of Raynaud's phenomenon, sclerodermatous changes of the hands and visceral involvement. In two patients sarcoidosis preceded the insidious development of PSS; whereas in the third patient the diagnosis of sarcoidosis and PSS were made at approximately the same time.

Sjögren's syndrome

As many as 50% of the patients with Sjögren's syndrome have an associated connective-tissue disease. James[7] found four cases of Sjögren's syndrome in a series of 200 patients. However, using more sensitive tests, the Schirmer test and instillation of Bengal pink, Crick, Hoyle and Smellie[8] found evidence of keratoconjunctivitis sicca in 70% of their cases of sarcoidosis. Turiaf[9] believes that the oculosalivary involvement identical with that of Sjögren's syndrome can occur in association with true sarcoidosis lasting over a number of years. Alarcon-Segovia et al. reported that clinical or subclinical evidence of Sjögren's syndrome occurs in more than 90% of patients with SLE[10] and PSS[11]. Thus, sarcoidosis as well as other autoimmune diseases may have a common origin with Sjögren's syndrome.

Autoimmune thyroiditis

The association of thyroiditis and sarcoidosis has been largely ignored by sarcoidologists. Mayock et al[12] in their study of 145 sarcoidosis patients mentioned in passing that two (1.4%) had clinical evidence of thyroiditis. Karlish and MacGregor[13] described four (1.3%) patients with clinical features of thyroiditis amongst their 300 sarcoidosis patients. Hancock reported five patients with thyrotoxicosis and sarcoidosis in a thyroid clinic composed of 2100 patients and concluded that such an association could result from an autoimmune disturbance resulting from loss of T-cell control[14].

Thrombocytopenia

About one-quarter of all patients with SLE have thrombocytopenia. Thrombocytopenia is far less common in sarcoidosis. Dickerman, Holbrook and Zinkham[15] presented two cases and reviewed 37 more cases of sarcoidosis complicated by thrombocytopenia. The authors postulated that immunological factors might be responsible for the shortened platelet life span in some of the patients with sarcoidosis.

Haemolytic anaemia

Dacie[16] reviewed 11 cases of haemolytic anaemia and sarcoidosis and concluded that the two conditions were related. The haemolytic anaemia may precede, coexist or post-date sarcoidosis by years. The clinical response is better with corticosteroids than with splenectomy, suggesting that the anaemia is not likely to be on the basis of hypersplenism. Sarcoidosis has been reported to coexist with haemagglutinin disease[17].

Primary biliary cirrhosis

Primary biliary cirrhosis (PBC) or chronic non-suppurative destructive cholangitis, a disease of middle-aged women, is characterized by progressive cholestatic liver injury, pruritus and hyperpigmentation of the skin. Non-caseating granulomas are found on liver biopsy in about half of the patients with the disease. PBC may occur in association with many immune disorders, including Sjögren's syndrome, CRST syndrome and renal tubular acidosis. Stanley et al.[18] described two middle-aged women with pruritus, liver biopsy findings of PBC, serum antimitochondrial antibodies and lung infiltrates. Both patients died of liver disease. Autopsy studies showed granulomas in the lungs. Maddrey studied four patients with PBC and lung infiltration[19]. Fagan, Moore-Gillon and Turner-Warwick reported the overlap of sarcoidosis and PBC in four women patients who had strongly positive antimitochondrial antibodies, hepatic granulomas and clinical evidence of pulmonary involvement (dyspnoea, dry cough, chest pain)[20]. In three of the four patients pulmonary granulomas were also found. It is clear that the two disorders—primary biliary cirrhosis and sarcoidosis—have certain similarities; both involve more than one organ, both have depressed delayed-type hypersensitivity and both are characterized by granuloma formation. Finally, the causes of both diseases remain unknown. Whether the sporadic association of sarcoidosis and primary biliary cirrhosis is accidental or reflects the underlying common immune mechanism remains to be established.

TASS syndrome

This is a rare clinical autoimmune syndrome which combines the features of thyroiditis, Addison's disease, Sjögren's syndrome and sarcoidosis[21].

Comment—Immunological abnormalities in sarcoidosis are consistent with the assumption that there is a defect in the suppressor regulatory system. The apparent similarity of this immunological profile to the abnormalities found in animal models of autoimmunity and human SLE raises, once more, the possibility that some, yet undiscovered, relationship exists between sarcoidosis and autoimmune disorders. However, the inclusion of sarcoidosis into the group of autoimmune disorders cannot be accepted. It would be interesting to examine sarcoidosis by a battery of newly developed tests used for SLE and other related disorders. It is generally accepted that major histocompatibility complex genes confer susceptibility toward the development of autoimmune disorders. Sjögren's syndrome[22] and autoimmune thyroid disease[23] appear to be associated with HLA-B8 and HLA-DRW3: histocompatibility antigens. Neville et al.[24] have pointed out that sarcoidosis patients in London with HLA-B8 are likely to have arthritis, erythema nodosum, or both. However, not all patients with these manifestations have B8 antigen and not all with B8 antigen will develop these lesions[25]. Clearly, other factors are important. More genetic markers are needed to increase understanding of the mechanisms influencing the association of sarcoidosis and autoimmune disorders.

References

1. PUTKONEN, T., VIRKKUNEN, M. and WAGNER, O. (1965) Joint involvement in sarcoidosis with special reference to the existence of sarcoidosis and rheumatoid arthritis. *Acta Pneum. Scand.*, **11**, 53.
2. TEILUM, G. (1945) Miliary epithelioid-cell granulomas in lupus erythematosus disseminatus. *Acta Pathol. Microbiol. Scand.*, **22**, 73.
3. POLLACK, A.D. (1959) Some observations on the pathology of systemic lupus erythematosus. *J. Mt. Sinai Hosp.*, **26**, 224.
4. DUBOIS, E.L. (1974) *Lupus Erythematosus*, 2nd edn. (Los Angeles: University of Southern California Press)
5. SHULMAN, L.E., KURBAN, A.K. and HARVEY, A.M. (1961) Tendon friction rubs in progressive system sclerosis (scleroderma). *Trans. Assoc. Am. Phys.*, **74**, 378.
6. WIESENHUTTER, C.W. and SHARMA, O.P. (1979) Is sarcoidosis an autoimmune disease? Report of four cases and review of the literature. *Semin. Arthr. Rheum.*, **9**, 124.
7. JAMES, D.G. (1959) Ocular sarcoidosis. *Am. J. Med.*, **26**, 331.
8. CRICK, R.P., HOYLE, C. and SMELLIE, H. (1961) The eye in sarcoidosis. *Br. J. Ophthalmol.*, **45**, 461.
9. TURIAF, J. and BATTESI, J.P. (1976) Gougerot–Sjögren's syndrome in sarcoidosis. *Ann. N.Y. Acad. Sci.*, **278**, 401.
10. ALARCON-SEGOVIA, D., IBANEZ, G., VELAZQUEZ-FORERO, F., *et al.* (1974) Sjögren's syndrome in systemic lupus erythematosus. *Ann. Intern. Med.*, **81**, 577.
11. ALARCON-SEGOVIA, D., IBANEZ, G., VELAZQUEZ-FORERO, F., *et al.* (1974) Sjögren's syndrome in progressive systemic sclerosis (scleroderma). *Am. J. Med.*, **57**, 78.
12. MAYOCK, R.L., BERTRAND, P., MORRISON, C.E., *et al.* (1963) Manifestations of sarcoidosis. Analysis of 145 patients with a review of nine series selected from the literature. *Am. J. Med.*, **35**, 67.
13. KARLISH, A.J. and MACGREGOR, G.A. (1970) Sarcoidosis, thyroiditis and Addison's disease. *Lancet*, **ii**, 330.
14. HANCOCK, B.W. and MILLARD, L.G. (1976) Sarcoidosis and thyrotoxicosis: A study of five patients. *Br. J. Dis. Chest*, **70**, 129.
15. DICKERMAN, J.D., HOLBROOK, P.R. and ZINKHAM, W.H. (1972) Etiology and therapy of thrombocytopenia associated with sarcoidosis. *J. Pediatr.*, **81**, 758.
16. DACIE, J.V. (1967) *The Hemolytic Anaemias*, Vol. III, 2nd edn., p. 921. (London: Churchill Livingstone)
17. PALAZZO, E. OBERLING, F., NORTH, M.L., *et al.* (1972) Sarcoidosis and cold haemagglutinin disease. *Acta Haematol.*, **48**, 331.
18. STANLEY, N.N., FOX, R.A., WHIMSTER, W.F., *et al.* (1972) Primary biliary cirrhosis or sarcoidosis: or both. *N. Engl. J. Med.*, **287**, 1282.
19. MADDREY, W.C. (1983) Sarcoidosis and primary biliary cirrhosis: Associated disorders. *N. Engl. J. Med.*, **308**, 588.
20. FAGAN, E.A., MOORE-GILLON, J.C. and TURNER-WARWICK, M. (1983) Multiorgan granulomas and mitochondrial antibodies. *N. Engl. J. Med.*, **308**, 572.
21. SEINFELD, E.D. and SHARMA, O.P. (1983) The TASS syndrome. *Proc. R. Soc. Med.*, **76**, 883.
22. MOUTSOPOULOS, H.M., MANN, D.L., JOHNSON, A.H., *et al.* (1979) Genetic differences between primary and secondary sicca syndrome. *N. Engl. J. Med.*, **301**, 761.
23. NOENS, H. and FARID, N.R. (1978) Hashimoto's thyroiditis is associated with HLA-DRW3. *N. Engl. J. Med.*, **299**, 133.
24. NEVILLE, E., JAMES, D.G, BREWERTON, D.A. *et al.* (1980) *HLA antigens and clinical features of sarcoidosis*. In *Proceedings of the Eight International Conference on Sarcoidosis and Other Granulomatous Diseases* (eds Williams, J.W. and Davies, B.H.), p. 201. (Cardiff: Alpha Omega Publications)
25. EISENBERG, H., TERASAKI, P., SHARMA, O.P., *et al.* (1978) HLA associated studies in Black patients with sarcoidosis. *Tiss. Antigens*, **11**, 484.

Chapter 31
Sarcoidosis, lymphoma and malignancy

It is well known that 'sarcoid reaction' or 'sarcoid-like' granulomas may be found in regional lymph nodes draining a carcinoma or a lymphoma. Granulomas have also been found amongst the tumour cells at the site of the primary neoplasm[1]. This local reaction should not be confused with systemic sarcoidosis. Jefferson, Smith and Taylor[2] described two patients with sarcoidosis who developed bronchial carcinoma; one, a man aged 52 with bilateral hilar adenopathy and cutaneous lesions, who developed bronchial carcinoma and the other, a man aged 45 with extensive parenchymal fibrosis, who died of Oat-cell carcinoma. Sarkar described a 36-year-old housewife with diffuse pulmonary infiltration and a positive Kveim test who developed an anaplastic tumour[3].

Is there an increase in the incidence of lung cancer or lymphoma in patients with sarcoidosis? In a 10-year study of 2544 patients with pulmonary sarcoidosis, 48 patients developed a malignant tumour; whereas only 33.8 cases were expected if sarcoidosis patient had had the same rate as the general population ($0.02 > P > 0.01$). Malignant lymphomas occurred 11 times and lung cancer three times more frequently than expected[4]. In an early study, Brincker found five cases of true sarcoidosis amongst 1500 cases of malignant lymphoma[5]. These observations suggest that an association may exist between cancer and sarcoidosis and it may result from immunological deficiency in patients with sarcoidosis.

Occasionally, a neoplasm may produce bilateral hilar adenopathy and create a diagnostic problem. Welsh and Welsh have described a clear-cell carcinoma of the kidney which produced bilateral hilar adenopathy 2 years after the initial nephrectomy. The diagnosis of metastatic renal lesion was confirmed by a mediastinoscopy[6].

References

1. ELLMAN, P. and HANSON, A. (1958) The coexistence of bronchial carcinoma and sarcoidosis. *Br. J. Tuberc.*, **50**, 219.
2. JEFFERSON, J.M., SMITH, W.T. and TAYLOR, A.B. (1954) Sarcoidosis and bronchial carcinoma. *Thorax*, **1**, 291.
3. SARKAR, T.K. (1970) Anaplastic carcinoma of the lung in sarcoidosis. *Br. J. Clin. Pract.*, **24**, 297.
4. BRINCKER, H. and WILBEK, E. (1974) The incidence of malignant tumours in patients with sarcoidosis. *Br. J. Cancer*, **29**, 247.
5. BRINCKER, H. (1972) Sarcoid reactions and sarcoidosis in Hodgkin's disease and other malignant lymphomata. *Br. J. Cancer*, **26**, 120.
6. WELSH, L. and WELSH, J.L. (1977) Problems of diagnosis in the evaluation of mediastinal sarcoidosis. *Laryngoscope*, **87**, 1635.

Chapter 32
Miscellaneous

Sarcoidosis and amyloidosis

The development of secondary (reactive) amyloidosis following long-standing infections due to tuberculosis, syphilis, leprosy and osteomyelitis is well known. There are, at least, two case reports that describe the occurrence of amyloidosis in patients with chronic sarcoidosis[1,2]. It is worth remembering that pulmonary amyloidosis can produce hilar lymphadenopathy—unilateral or bilateral—and diffuse nodular infiltration[3].

Sarcoidosis and clubbing

Clubbing of the fingers has long been considered an uncommon manifestation of sarcoidosis[4]. Of 136 histologically proved sarcoidosis patients, only four were found to have clinically clubbed fingers[5]. However, using a micrometer to measure clubbing, Chusid was able to demonstrate some degree of finger clubbing in 64 (53.3%) out of 120 patients with sarcoidosis. The clubbing occurred more frequently in patients with stage II or stage III disease[6,7].

References

1. FRESKO, D. and LAZARUS, S.S. (1982) Reactive systemic amyloidosis complicating longstanding sarcoidosis. *N.Y. State J. Med.*, **82**, 232.
2. SWANTON, R.H., PETERS, D.K. and BURN, J.L. (1971) Sarcoidosis and amyloidosis. *Proc. R. Soc. Med.*, **64**, 1002.
3. KANADA, D.J. and SHARMA. P. (1979) Long-term survival with diffuse pulmonary amyloidosis. *Am. J. Med.*, **67**, 879.
4. YOUNG, R.C., TITUS-DILLON, P., SCHNEIDER, M.L., *et al.* (1970) Sarcoidosis in Washington, D.C. *Arch Intern. Med.*, **125**, 102.
5. YANCEY, J., LUXFORD, W. and SHARMA, O.P. (1972) Clubbing in sarcoidosis. *J. Am. Med. Assoc.*, **222**, 582.
6. CHUSID, E.L. (1980) Clubbing of the fingers in sarcoidosis: A critical assessment. In *Sarcoidosis and Other Granulomatous Diseases* (eds Williams, W.J. and Davies, B.H.), p. 543. (Cardiff: Alpha Omega Publishers)
7. WARING, W.W., WILKINSON, R.W., WIEKE, R.R., *et al.* (1971) Quantitation of digital clubbing in children. *Ann. Rev. Resp. Dis.*, **104**, 166.

Index

Abortion, spontaneous, 173
Acne scars, sarcoidosis, 71
Acute (subacute) sarcoidosis, 24, 28
Addisonian crisis, 116
Addison's disease, 116
Adenopathy, mediastinal, 31
Adrenals, sarcoid involvement, 116
Age, sarcoidosis distribution, 5
Aged, sarcoidosis, 172
Airway obstruction, pulmonary sarcoidosis, 61
Alcohol-induced pain, Hodgkin's disease, 80
Alkaline phosphatase, serum levels, 89, 90, 91
Alopecia, sarcoid, 75
Alveolar sarcoidosis, 34–5, 36
Alveolitis, 16
    allergic, extrinsic, 21, 162
    fibrosing, 162
Amyloidosis,
    diffuse, 163
    secondary, 180
Anaemia,
    haemolytic, 176–7
    sarcoidosis, 143
Anergy, cutaneous, 132–4
Angiolupoid lesions, 65
Angiotensin converting enzyme (ACE), 149–51, 161, 165
    corticosteroid effects, 78
    source in sarcoidosis, 150
Angiotensin II, hypothalamic overactivity, 115
Antibody formation, 136
Arthralgias, migrating, transient, 108–9
Arthritis,
    acute relapsing, 109
    monoarticular, 109–10
    sarcoid, 107–11
        differential diagnosis, 110
        HLA-B 7, 8
        treatment, 168, 169
Asbestosis, 163
Ascites, 123
Aspergilloma,
    pulmonary sarcoid, 16
    sarcoid-associated, 174
    spontaneous lysis, 174
Asteroid (stellate) bodies, sarcoid granuloma, 15
Auditory nerves, sarcoidosis, 103
Autoimmune disease, sarcoidosis-associated, 9, 137, 175–8
Autoimmune thyroiditis, 176
Autoimmunity, 9, 137, 175–8

B cells, 127, 132
Bacterial infections, sarcoid differences, 19–20
Band keratopathy, 78
BCG vaccination, sarcoidosis, test effects, 133–4
Beclomethasone diproprionate nasal spray, 125
Berylliosis,
    conchoidal bodies, 15
    differences from sarcoid, 183
Beryllium granulomatosis, 9, 10, 20
Biliary cirrhosis, primary (PBC), 177
Bilirubin, serum, sarcoidosis, 90
Biopsy procedures, 159–62
    sensitivity, 161
Blastomycosis, 20
Blood, laboratory investigations, 143–5
Boeck's sarcoid, 2
Bone cysts, 107, 108
    lupus pernio, 64, 66
    sarcoid granulomas, 19
Bone lesions, 107, 108, 109
Bone marrow, sarcoid involvement, 83, 85–7
Breasts, sarcoidosis, 131
Broncheoalveolar lavage (BAL), 138–9, 159, 165
    alveolitis intensity, 139
Bronchial carcinoma, 179
Brucellosis, sarcoid differences, 20
Bullae, pulmonary, 38–9, 41

Calcium balance studies, sarcoidosis, 148

Carcinoma,
  bronchial, 179
  lymph glands, 163
  oat-cell, 179
Cardiac arrhythmias, myocardial sarcoidosis, 98
Cardiac pacemakers, myocardial sarcoidosis, 167–8
Cat scratch disease, 20
Cataracts, 78
Cavitary sarcoidosis, 52–3, 55
  diagnosis, 53
Centrospheres, sarcoid granuloma, 15
Cerebrospinal fluid, neurosarcoidosis, 105
Chest radiographs, chronic sarcoidosis, 28
Children, sarcoidosis, 171
Chloroquine,
  dosages, 169
  lupus pernio, 64, 169
Chlorpromazine, prolactin response, 115
Choroidoretinitis, 77
Chronic sarcoidosis, symptoms, 28
Cirrhosis, biliary, primary (PBC), 177
Clay eating, 9
Clinical features, 22–8
Coccidioidomycosis, 20, 163
Colchicine, bone and joint sarcoid, 168, 169
Complement, serum, activity increase, 136
Computed tomography scans, cranial, 105
Concanavalin A, lymphocyte stimulation, 135
Conchoidal bodies, 13–15
Conduction disturbances, myocardial, 98
Congestive heart failure, myocardial sarcoidosis, 98–9
Conjunctiva, biopsy, 162
Conjunctival follicles, 77
Conjunctivitis, 77
Connective tissue diseases, 163, 175–6
Coomb's test, 143
Cor pulmonale, 16
Corticosteroids,
  dosages, 168–9
  1,25-hydroxyvitamin D inhibition, 149
  patient selection, 166–7
  pulmonary sarcoidosis, 166–8
  sarcoid splenomegaly, 82, 84
Cranial computed tomography scans, 105
Cranial nerves, sarcoidosis, 102–3
Crohn's disease, 123
CRST syndrome, 177
Cryptococcosis, 20
Crystalline inclusions, sarcoid granuloma, 15
Cutaneous anergy, 132–4
Cutaneous plaques, 65, 67, 68–9
Cutaneous sarcoidosis, iritis association, 3
Cytoplasmic vacuoles, sarcoid granuloma, 15

Darier-Roussy sarcoid, 69
  ulceration, 73–4, 75
Deafness, sarcoidosis, 103
Delayed-hypersensitivity cells, 132
  see also Hypersensitivity

Diabetes insipidus, 114–15
  corticosteroids, 168
Diagnosis,
  criteria, 159
  differential, 162–3
  gallium-67 scans, 157–8
  see also Biopsy procedures; Laboratory tests
1,25-Dihydroxyvitamin D, 148–9
  corticosteroid inhibition, 149
L-dopa, prolactin response, 115
Drug addicts, talc granulomatosis, 20
Drug reactions,
  granulomatous, 9, 156, 183
  pulmonary, 9
    gallium-67 uptake, 156
Dwarfism, 115

Eighth nerve involvement, 103
Elderly, sarcoidosis, 172
Electroencephalograms, neurosarcoidosis, 105
Endobronchial sarcoidosis, 40, 42
Endometrial sarcoidosis, 130
Endomyocardial biopsy, 100
Eosinophilia, 144
  peripheral infiltration (PIE syndrome), 56–7
Epididymitis, sarcoid, 129, 130
Epilepsy, corticosteroids, 168
Epithelioid cells, sarcoid granuloma, 11
Epstein-Barr virus, antibodies in sarcoid, 9
Erythema nodosum, 144–5
  bilateral hilar adenopathy, 161
  sarcoidosis, 71, 75
Erythrocyte sedimentation rate (ESR), 144–5
Exophthalmos, 78
Extrapulmonary sarcoidosis, treatment, 167–8

Facial nerve, sarcoidosis, 102–3
Fallopian tubes, sarcoidosis, 130
Familial sarcoidosis, 6–7
Feet, sarcoid involvement, 107
Fertility, sarcoidosis and, 173
Finger clubbing, sarcoid-associated, 180
Fröhlich's syndrome, 115

Gallium-67
  scanning, 155–8, 159
    indications, 157–8
    technique, 155
  uptake
    lung diseases, 155–6
    sarcoidosis, 156–7, 165
Gastric mucosa,
  granulomatous infiltration, 123
  symptomless granulomas, 122
Gastric sarcoidosis, 122–3
Gastric ulcers, granulomatous, 122
Gastrointestinal sarcoidosis, 122–4
Giant cells, sarcoid granuloma, 13

Glomerular disease, sarcoidosis, 94
Glossopharyngeal nerve, sarcoidosis, 103
Granulomas,
 muscle, asymptomatic, 111
 sarcoid,
  antigen immune response, 10
  components, 11–16
  differential diagnosis, 19–21
  electron microscopy, 15
  local, 21
  natural history, 15
  necrotizing, 21
  shape, 10
  stages, 11

Haemolytic anaemia, 176–7
Hair spray inhalation, 9
Hands, sarcoid involvement, 107, 108, 109, 180
Heart valves, sarcoidosis, 99
Heerfordt's syndrome, 3, 24, 76
Helper-inducer cells, 132
Herpes-like virus, antibodies in sarcoid, 9
Hilar calcification, 57–9
 causes, 59
Hilar lymphadenopathy,
 bilateral, 29–31
  bronchial carcinoma, 179
  causes, 30
  corticosteroids, 166–7
  erythema nodosum, 161
 parenchymal infiltration, 31–5
 unilateral, causes, 30
Histoplasmin antigen skin test, 134
Histoplasmosis, 20, 163
HLA typing, 7
HLA-B7 phenotypes, 7
Hodgkin's disease, alcohol-induced pain, 80
Homograft survival, 135
Humoral responses, sarcoidosis, 136–7
Hutchinson's lupus, 64
Hydatid cyst rupture, granulomatous reactions, 20
Hydrocephalus, neurosarcoidosis, 105
Hydroxyproline excretion, 145
Hypercalcaemia, 93, 95
 causes, 148–9
 frequency variations, 145–6
 incidence, 145–8
 parathyroid role, 149
 sarcoidosis, 145–9
 sun exposure effects, 147–8
 treatment, 167
Hypercalciuria, 93, 95, 145
 treatment, 167
Hypergammaglobulinaemia, 3, 9, 136
Hypersensitivity, delayed,
 cells, 132
 in vitro changes, 134–6
 suppression in sarcoidosis, 135–6
Hypersplenism,
 red cell destruction, 143

Hypersplenism (*cont.*)
 treatment, 168
Hypertension, pulmonary, pulmonary sarcoidosis, 61
Hyperthyroidism, 116
Hypogammaglobulinaemia, 136
Hypopituitarism, 115
Hypothalamus, sarcoid involvement, 103
Hypothyroidism, 115–16
Hypoxaemia, pulmonary sarcoidosis, 60

Ichthyosis, sarcoid, 75
Immune complexes, sarcoidosis, 137
Immunity,
 cell-mediated, 10
 humoral, 136–7
Immunoglobulins, abnormalities, 136
Immunological diseases, gallium-67 uptake, 156
Immunosuppressive drugs, 169
Infantilism, 115
Infections,
 pulmonary, gallium-67 uptake, 155–6
 sarcoidosis and, 174
Intestines, sarcoidosis, 123
Iridocyclitis, 76
Irish, sarcoidosis prevalence, 4
Isoniazid, prophylactic, 169

Joints, sarcoid involvement, 107–11

Keloids, sarcoidosis, 71
Keratic precipitates,
 eye anterior chamber, 77
 'mutton fat', 76
Keratoconjunctivitis sicca, 77, 78
Keratopathy, band, 78
Kidneys, sarcoidosis, 93–6
Kveim-Siltzbach test, 137–8, 159
 oxyphenbutazone effects, 169

Laboratory tests, 143–54
Lacrimal glands, 118–21
 biopsy, 161
 see also Keratoconjunctivitis sicca
Landry-Guillain-Barré syndrome, 104
Laryngeal sarcoidosis, 127–8
Leprosy, sarcoid differences, 20
Leukaemia, 163
Leukaemoid reaction, 143
Leukopenia, 143
Levamisole, sarcoid relapse prevention, 169
Leydig cell dysfunction, 129
Linitis plastica syndrome, 123
Liver,
 biopsy, 161
 failure, sarcoidosis, 90
 function tests, 90, 91

Liver (*cont.*)
  granulomas, 89–90
  sarcoidosis, 89–92
Löfgren's syndrome, 3, 29–31, 161, 166–7, 179
Lung biopsy, pulmonary sarcoidosis, 159–61
Lung functions, pulmonary sarcoidosis, 59–61
Lung volumes, pulmonary sarcoidosis, 59–61
Lupus pernio, 64–6
  bone lesions, 2–3, 64, 66
  chloroquine, 64, 169
  nasal mucosa, 125–6
  ulceration, 73–4, 75
Lymphadenopathy, 21
  peripheral, 80–82
  see also Hilar lymphadenopathy
Lymphocytes,
  sarcoid granuloma, 13
  transformation, 135
Lymphogranuloma benignum, 3
Lymphogranuloma inguinale, conchoidal bodies, 15
Lymphoma, 163, 179
Lymphopenia, 134
Lysozyme, serum, 151, 159

Macroglobulinaemia, 137
Maculopapular eruptions, 67–8, 70–1
Mediastinal sarcoidosis, salivary glands, 118
Mediastinoscopy, 159
Meningitis, 104
Mikulicz syndrome, 118
Monocytes, peripheral blood, function in sarcoidosis, 135
Monocytosis, 144
Mortimer's malady, 2
Mumps-influenza-Newcastle viruses, 9
Muscles,
  palpable sarcoid nodules, 112
  sarcoid involvement, 111–12
'Mutton fat' keratic precipitates, 76
Mycetoma, sarcoid-associated, 174
Mycobacteria, atypical, sarcoid aetiology, 8
Myocardial infarction-like disease, 99
Myocardial perfusion, thallium-201 studies, 100
Myocardial sarcoidosis, 97–100
  diagnosis, 98–100
  ECG abnormalities, 99–100
  rhythm changes, 98
  sudden death, 98
  treatment, 167–8
Myocardium, granulomas, 16, 19
Myopathy,
  chronic, sarcoid, 112
  isolated, sarcoid, 112

Nails, dystrophic, lupus pernio, 64, 66
Nasal mucosa,
  biopsy, 161
  lupus pernio, 125–6

Nasal septum, sarcoidosis, 125–6
Negroes,
  bone lesions, 107
  maculopapular eruptions, 68, 70–1
  psoriasiform sarcoid, 75
  sarcoidosis,
    prevalence, 4–5
    sex distribution, 5–6
Nephrocalcinosis, 93, 95
Nephrolithiasis, 93, 95
Neuroendocrine sarcoidosis, 114–15
Neurosarcoidosis, 102–6
  clinical diagnosis, 102
  EMG studies, 104
Nodular sarcoidosis, 37, 51–2, 54
Null cells, 132

Oat-cell carcinoma, 179
Ocular sarcoidosis, 76–9
  diagnosis, 78–9
  treatment, 167
Oesophagus,
  granulomas, 122
  varices, portacaval surgery, 168
Oidiomycin skin test, 134
Optic nerve, sarcoidosis, 103
Oxyphenbutazone therapy, 169

Palate, sarcoidosis, 128
Pancreas, sarcoidosis, 123
Papilloedema, 103
  corticosteroids, 168
Parasitic disease, granulomatous reactions, 20
Parathyroids,
  role in hypercalcaemia, 147–8
  sarcoid involvement, 116
Parenchymal infiltration, 35–8
  acinar (alveolar), 36, 40
  hilar lymphadenopathy, 31–5
  nodular, 37, 51–2, 54
  retronodular, 36–9
Parotid glands, 118–21
  enlargement, facial nerve palsy, 102
Pathogenesis, 16–19
Peanut dust inhalation, 9
Penis, sarcoidosis, 129
Pericardial effusion, myocardial sarcoidosis, 99
Peripheral neuropathy, 104
Periphlebitis retinae, 78
Peritoneum, sarcoidosis, 123
Pertussis antigen skin tests, 134
Phosphate, serum levels, 149
Phytohaemagglutinin (PHA), lymphocyte stimulation, 135
PIE syndrome, 56–7
Pine pollen allergy, 9
Pituitary, sarcoid involvement, 114
Pleural effusion,
  laboratory tests, 44
  pulmonary sarcoidosis, 42, 44, 47–50

Pneumoconiosis, differences from sarcoid, 163
Pneumocystis carinii infections, 163
Pneumonitis, hypersensitivity, 21, 162
Pneumothorax,
    pulmonary sarcoidosis, 45-6, 50, 52
    steroid therapy effects, 46
Polyarthritis,
    chronic persistent, 109-10
    migratory, 109
Polycythaemia, 143
Polymyositis, sarcoid, 112
Portal hypertension, 90
    treatment, 168
Prednisone,
    hypercalcaemia, 148
    topical, ocular sarcoidosis, 167
Pregnancy, sarcoidosis effects, 173
Progressive systemic sclerosis (PSS), 163, 176
Prolactin levels, disseminated sarcoidosis, 115
Proptosis, 78
Prostate gland, 129
Proteins, serum, abnormalities, 136
Proteinuria, 145
Psoriasiform sarcoid, negroes, 75
Psychiatric disorders, neurosarcoidosis, 104-5
Pulmonary fibrosis,
    chloroquine, 169
    idiopathic, 162
    irreversible, 38-9, 41
Pulmonary granulomata,
    drug-associated, 9, 156, 183
    pathogenesis, 16-19
Pulmonary granuloms,
    drug-associated, 9, 156, 183
    asymptomatic, 23
    lung biopsy, 159-61
    lung functions, 59-61
    stage 0, 29
    stage I, 29-31
    stage II, 31-5
        differential diagnosis, 34-5
    stage III, 35-8
        differential diagnosis, 37
    stage IV, 38-9, 41
    stages, 29-40
    treatment, 165-7

Renal arteritis, granulomatous, 94-5
Renal parenchyma, granulomas, 93-4
Renal tubular acidosis, 177
Reproductive system,
    female, sarcoidosis, 130-1
    male, sarcoidosis, 129-30
Residual bodies, sarcoid granuloma, 15
Respiratory symptoms, 23-4
Respiratory tract, upper, sarcoidosis, 168
Retina, haemorrhages, 78
Retinitis proliferans, 78
Rheumatoid arthritis, 163, 175
Rheumatoid factor (RF), 127

Sarcoid alveolitis, activity degree, gallium-67 scans, 158
'Sarcoid reaction', 79
Sarcoidosis,
    activity monitoring, ACE, 150
    brother-sister relationship, 6
    coexistent autoimmune diseases, 9, 137, 175-8
    descriptive definition, 1
    extent, gallium-67 scans, 158
    genetic predisposition, 9
    historical aspects, 2-3
    immunological aspects, 3, 9-10, 132-42
    multisystem involvement recognition, 2-3
    patient classification, 24
    pregnancy effects, 173
    presentation modes, 22-3
    prevalence,
        age distribution, 5
        geographic aspects, 4
    recessive inheritance, 6
    recovery, cutaneous anergy, 133
    sex distribution, 5-6
    tuberculosis superimposition, test effects, 133-4
    see also various organs, regions, types
Scalene node biopsy, 159
Scars, sarcoidosis, 71, 72
Schaumann bodies, 13-15
Scrotum, sarcoidosis, 129
Seizures, sarcoidosis, 104
Seminal vesicles, 129
Serum complement, activity increase, 136
Serum inhibitors, 135
Serum lysozyme, 151, 159
Serum phosphate levels, 149
Serum protein abnormalities, 136
Silica, granulomatosis, 21
Silicosis, 163
    hilar calcification, 57
Sjögren's syndrome, 118
Skeletal muscle, biopsy, 161
Skin plaques, 65, 67, 68-9
Space-occupying lesions, intracranial, 103-4
Spermatic cord, sarcoidosis, 129
Spinal cord, neurosarcoidosis, 105
Spleen, biopsy, 162
Splenomegaly, sarcoid, 82-3, 84, 85
Stomach, sarcoidosis, 122-3
Subcutaneous nodules (Darier-Roussy sarcoid), 69
    ulceration, 73-4, 75
Sun exposure, hypercalcaemia and, 147-8
Suppressor-cytotoxic cells, 132
Syphilis, granulomas, sarcoid differences, 20
Systemic lupus erythematosus (SLE), 163, 175
Systemic sclerosis, progressive (PSS), 163, 176

T cells, 132
    activated, 135
Talc (magnesium silicate) granulomas, 10, 20
TASS syndrome, 177
Testis, sarcoidosis, 129

Thallium-201, myocardial perfusion studies, 100
Thoracotomy, 159
Thrombocytopenia, 144, 176
Thyroid, sarcoid involvement, 115–116
Thyroiditis, autoimmune, 176
Thyrotropin releasing hormone (TRH), prolactin response, 115
Tongue, sarcoidosis, 128
Tonsils, sarcoidosis, 128
Trachea, sarcoidosis, 128
Transcobalamin II, 151, 159
Treatment,
  indications, 165–8
  methods, 168–9
  prior gallium-67 scans, 158
Tubercle bacillus, sarcoid aetiology, 8
Tubercular granulomas, sarcoid differences, 19
Tuberculin sensitivity,
  cortisone effects, 133
  regained, 133
Tuberculin test, 132–3
  BCG vaccination effects, 133–4
Tuberculosis,
  conchoidal bodies, 15
  miliary, 163
  sarcoid-associated, 174
    test effects, 133–4
Twins, sarcoidosis, 7

Urinary bladder, 129
Urine, laboratory tests, 145
Uropathy, obstructive, 93, 95
Uterus, sarcoidosis, 130
Uveal tract, fibrinosis, associated disorders, 16
Uveitis,
  chronic, 76–7
  granulomatous, 76–7
  posterior, 77
  subacute, 76
  see also Heerfordt's syndrome

Vaccination scars, sarcoidosis, 71
Vagus nerve, sarcoidosis, 103
Ventilation control, pulmonary sarcoidosis, 61
Ventilation perfusion relationship, 61
Ventricular aneurysm, myocardial sarcoidosis, 99
Viruses, sarcoid aetiology, 9
Visual defects, sarcoidosis, 103
Vitamin B_{12} binding capacity (VBBC), 151

West Indians, sarcoidosis prevalence, 4

Zirconium granulomatosis, 9, 21